Psychological Assessment, Psychiatric Diagnosis, & Treatment Planning

PSYCHOLOGICAL ASSESSMENT, PSYCHIATRIC DIAGNOSIS, & TREATMENT PLANNING

Stephen W. Hurt, Ph.D.

Marvin Reznikoff, Ph.D.

and

John F. Clarkin, Ph.D.

BRUNNER/MAZEL Publishers • New York

Library of Congress Cataloging-in-Publication Data
Hurt, Stephen W.
    Psychological assessment, psychiatric diagnosis & treatment
planning / by Stephen W. Hurt, Marvin Reznikoff, John F. Clarkin.
      p. cm.
    Includes bibliographical references and index.
    ISBN 0-87630-607-5
    1. Psychological tests. 2. Mental illness—Diagnosis. 3. Mental
illness—Treatment. I. Reznikoff, Marvin. II. Clarkin, John F.
III. Title.
    [DNLM: 1. Mental Disorders—diagnosis. 2. Patient Care Planning.
3. Psychological Tests. WM 141 H967p]
RC473.P79H87 1990
616.89'075—dc20
DNLM/DLC
for Library of Congress   90-15146
                                                               CIP

Published by
BRUNNER/MAZEL, INC.
19 Union Square
New York, New York 10003

Designed by Tere LoPrete

Manufactured in the United States of America

10 9 8 7 6 5 4 3 2 1

Contents

❖

Foreword

The critical role of psychological assessment in treatment planning has been increasingly recognized in recent years as social and economic factors have brought about significant changes in diagnostic approaches and psychotherapeutic intervention strategies. An adequate treatment plan is the necessary first step in helping clients and patients who seek assistance from mental health service providers to alleviate their suffering, and psychological assessment is basic to effective treatment planning. Traditionally, the major goal of psychological testing has been to describe the psychopathology and personality dynamics of the patient. Consequently, significant questions relating to optimal intervention procedures are often neglected.

This volume is unique in its dual focus on the role of psychological assessment in clarifying diagnostic issues and the contribution of assessment to treatment planning. In providing case examples of commonly encountered diagnostic questions, the authors draw upon a broad range of psychiatric patients who were referred for comprehensive psychological assessment. These case materials were available to the authors on the basis of their long-term association with a freestanding psychiatric hospital that admits more than a thousand patients a year.

The cases described were referred for extensive psychological assessment with traditional assessment instruments such as the WAIS, the MMPI, the Rorschach, the Thematic Apperception Test, the Bender Gestalt, and figure drawings. The inclusion of the raw data of assessment makes these cases especially useful for classroom instruction and in the supervision of clinical practicum work.

Prior to the presentation of the history, mental status and psychological assessment findings for individual cases, the diagnostic criteria for the DSM-III-R category for which each case is representative are reviewed by the authors. Both simple and complex cases representing the most important DSM-III-R diagnostic categories are evaluated and discussed in this volume.

The results of psychological testing are integrated with detailed case materials, including the patient's chief presenting complaint, a history of the present illness, and the results of the mental status examination. The tables that accompany the description of each case provide rich summaries of the clinical and psychological information that not only clarify the diagnostic decision but also serve to provide information on psychodynamic issues, personality functioning, cognitive abilities, and social and environmental pressures that impinge on the patient.

Since the information on which an initial diagnostic formulation is based is generally available to the psychologist prior to the assessment consultation, it provides the contextual framework for identifying the major diagnostic issues and significant factors that must be considered in treatment planning. While psychiatric diagnostic questions are typically the chief reason that most patients are referred for psychological testing, assessment data not only answer such questions, but may be even more important in the formulation of a comprehensive treatment plan.

The richness of the interpretations of the psychological test data reflects the extensive research and clinical experience of the authors in the field of psychological assessment, differential diagnosis and treatment planning, treatment in various clinical settings, and teaching of graduate students and interns.

Although this book will prove especially valuable for clinical psychologists and students of psychological assessment, it will also be highly useful for other mental health professionals who are involved in providing clinical services. Psychiatrists, social workers, nurses, and counselors will gain a beneficial understanding of how the data of psychological assessment contribute to the clarification of diagnostic issues and, especially, to the development of an optimal treatment plan.

CHARLES D. SPIELBERGER, Ph.D.
Graduate Research Professor of Psychology
University of South Florida, Tampa

❖

Preface

Our purpose in writing this book was to examine the relationship between the psychological assessments commonly carried out by clinical psychologists and the treatment planning situation faced by the provider of clinical services. We chose as our setting the psychiatric hospital. This is the principal setting in which psychological assessments are carried out and it is the principal setting in which many mental health professionals receive a significant portion of their training early in their careers. It is to these professionals, whether psychologists, psychiatrists, nurses, social workers, counsellors, or case managers, that we address this book.

The book is intended for both practicing professionals and for those in training. The practicing professional will derive considerable benefit, we believe, from reviewing the psychological assessment from the standpoint of treatment planning. Although recent changes in the official diagnostic nomenclature of the American Psychiatric Association have emphasized more behavioral and operational criteria for psychiatric diagnoses, practicing professionals often recognize that formal diagnostic procedures do not *per se* provide sufficient information for developing a treatment plan. The present climate of patient advocacy, informed consent, and choice of services would serve in themselves to make the treatment planning process a more collaborative effort. This book is intended to illustrate the many ways in which psychological testing can contribute to that effort for the benefit of both the patient and the treatment provider.

For the professional in training, the book also provides an introduction to the system of psychiatric diagnosis and case formulation. In providing many of the details of the case histories and the testing data, we hope the book will serve as a guide for those in training. In our formulation of the testing material, the student will find in our approach much that is traditionally taught in clinical psychology. There is also much that is relatively new. Our emphasis on the role of the psychological assessment in treatment planning and our organization and presentation of the testing material in light of the areas critical for this endeavor have novel elements.

In selecting the cases for the book, we chose cases where the treatment planning issues were addressed by the data from the psychological assessment. In order to preserve the vitality of the material, we made as few changes in the original test materials and the clinical situations of the cases as were compatible with preserving the confidentiality of the individuals. The cases are presented in the order in which the diagnostic groupings of DSM-III-R are presented, beginning with disorders usually first evident in infancy, childhood, or adolescence and ending with the Axis II personality disorders.

The cases represent a range of DSM-III-R categories. The categories are those most frequently encountered in the diagnostic situations of the psychiatric hospital. Each disorder is briefly introduced in terms of its current psychiatric definition. Each disorder is represented by two cases. One of these cases has been chosen because it represents a comparatively clear case in which virtually all of the DSM-III-R diagnostic criteria for the disorder are manifest. The second case has been chosen because although a sufficient number of diagnostic criteria are present to support the diagnosis, some elements of ambiguity remain. Each presentation gives the referral questions, as they arose in the context of the hospital treatment situation, the current status, historical material, test responses, formal scoring and tabulation of these responses where applicable, the psychological report and recommendations, as well as other information pertaining to treatment. Finally, a brief, comparative discussion of the two cases is used to explore differences and similarities in the diagnostic and treatment planning issues pertinent to the two cases.

In choosing the cases and preparing the final materials for the book, we received a tremendous amount of help from several individuals. Case materials which could not be found in our hospital files were contributed by our colleague, Dr. Mark Schwartz. We would like to thank him for his contribution of these materials. Ms. Lisa Gerstein helped to compile and select from among over 400 cases initially screened a set of 120 cases which were reviewed for possible inclusion. She devoted an entire summer and a good part of the fall to scoring and tabulating the material from these cases so that our selection of case material could be as representative of our hospital population as possible. Ms. Sharon Daly subsequently rescored the final case material chosen for the book and helped to insure that all relevant materials were prepared with equal care and attention to detail. These are time-consuming tasks and we are grateful to both Ms. Gerstein and Ms. Daly for their attention to these matters. Ms. Nina Huza and Ms. Jane Drenga prepared the initial typed drafts of much of the case material. Their many years of experience in deciphering the usually cryptic verbatim transcripts of the examiners made the final editing of the case materials almost a pleasant task.

The material presented here has also benefited from the contributions of several groups of trainees in the psychology internship program of The New York Hospital's Westchester Division. They reviewed previous drafts of these cases as the book was under preparation. They were helpful in pointing out areas that needed further clarification and helped us to gauge the level at which the material could be presented effectively. We would also like to thank several individuals for taking the time to read various sections of the manuscript. Mrs. Ruth Heim deserves particular mention for having read the manuscript in its entirety and providing many helpful editorial suggestions. Finally, we wish to thank our spouses and children. They rather graciously bore with us during the course of this enterprise and their forbearance is much appreciated.

In reviewing the clinical and psychological material from the cases, we have focused on six areas that are central to treatment planning: symptoms/diagnosis, personality factors, cognitive abilities, psychodynamics (including defenses and motivations), therapeutic enabling factors, and environmental demand and social adjustment. For each clinical case, we summarize the information for these six areas as obtained from the clinical workup and the psychological testing. By examining these tables across the patients presented here, one can come to some conclusions as to the nature and amount of information that is ordinarily obtained from the clinical workup and psychological assessment.

The process of writing this book was an in-depth exploration for the authors of examining, with actual cases, how the test findings overlapped the clinical data, either confirming or differing with it, as well as the complementary relationship between test and clinical data in arriving at a comprehensive clinical formulation. Having completed our work, we can make some generalizations.

1) Referrals for diagnostic consultations still constitute the chief reason for psychological testing referrals, despite the relatively clear and operational criteria of DSM-III and DSM-III-R. Among the more frequent questions are those concerning the presence or absence of thought disorder in patients who do not evidence pathological thinking in clinical interviews but who are suspected of being more disturbed. Questions also arise as to the presence of affective symptoms such as depression with patients who deny any direct experience of such an affect.

2) Cognitive and intellectual functioning is quite relevant for planning treatment interventions, especially with regard to verbal therapies that depend upon making abstractions about one's motivations and behaviors.

The clinical interview and the mental status examination, in particular, yield some critical information about this area of functioning. However, the use of structured tests with their sets of standardized stimuli, formal scoring procedures, and norms provide an accurate picture of the relative strengths and weaknesses of the patient's intellectual abilities.

3) The same surface behaviors and/or symptoms may be accompanied by quite different constellations of cognitions and motivations in different patients. This is an area in which tests are extremely helpful. Projective tests are particularly effective in circumventing a patient's conscious defensive operations and providing data on the possible underlying conflicts which motivate seemingly contradictory aspects of a patient's behavior.

4) The ability and motivation of the patient to establish a positive therapeutic alliance can be effectively evaluated in the testing situation. The tests, particularly the TAT, are extremely useful in assessing the patient's attitudes, self-concept and interpersonal relationship style. This information can play a crucial role in developing a treatment plan in situations in which a choice of several equally successful treatment strategies is possible.

5) The role of the psychological examination and the manner in which information gathered during the examination is explained to the referring source and to the patient provide an excellent opportunity to help prepare the way for a successful treatment intervention. Treatment planning is, at its best, a collaborative effort. The information gathered during the course of a psychological assessment can provide an opportunity to effect this collaboration by helping to place the referring questions in a treatment context and by providing a common frame of reference for both the referring source and the patient.

In making these generalizations, we wish to emphasize the value of psychological testing to the treatment planning process. Although we have come away from this enterprise firmly convinced that psychological assessment indeed can serve to enhance the collaborative efforts required for successful treatment interventions, we must finally leave it to the reader to judge the success of our efforts.

Psychological Assessment, Psychiatric Diagnosis, & Treatment Planning

CHAPTER 1

Psychological Testing and Psychiatric Diagnosis

In the broader sense, the purpose of psychological testing is to assess individual differences on one or more psychological variables. Clinical psychological testing as discussed in this book constitutes a specialized area of psychological testing that focuses on differentiating individuals in clinical inpatient and outpatient populations on the basis of the nature and degree of psychopathology. There are, of course, many other types of diagnostic testing, especially in the fields of medicine and education.

The meaningfulness of psychodiagnostic testing is obviously based upon the premise that there exists a taxonomy for classifying psychopathology into reliable diagnostic categories. Devising such a diagnostic classification system or nosology, however, has proven a very formidable task. Over a period of 35 years, the American Psychiatric Association has published four *Diagnostic and Statistical Manuals* (DSMs) (1952, 1968, 1980, 1987) with an additional version now in preparation. Each successive manual has offered more explicit and comprehensive diagnostic criteria in not always fruitful efforts to make the process of differential diagnosis more reliable.

In this introductory chapter, a selective history of psychological testing will be given, including an evaluation of its current status. *Psychological Testing* (1988) by Anne Anastasi has been an invaluable source of guidance and information for the preparation of the first section of this chapter and is highly recommended as an exhaustive treatment of the subject. Within the framework of the various DSM editions, an overview of past efforts to develop reliable and readily applicable diagnostic schema will also be presented.

HISTORY OF PSYCHOLOGICAL TESTING AND ASSESSMENT

Early Testing Efforts

Anastasi (1988) defines the traditional function of psychological tests as having been "to measure differences between individuals or between the reactions of the same individuals on different occasions." Another leading authority on psychological testing, Cronbach (1949) states that what a test entails is a "systematic procedure for comparing the behavior of two or more persons."

Contemporary psychological testing, perceived as the utilization of standardized instruments to measure various psychological functions, has its major roots in the nineteenth century. However, it is of interest to note that a comparatively well-developed program of oral civil service examinations seems to have existed in China more than 4,000 years ago (Wiggins, 1973). By the fourteenth century, the Chinese civil service selection program boasted a network of local testing centers across the nation which administered written examinations of an essay type in specially constructed testing booths. The Greeks some 3,000 years ago also employed testing procedures incorporating them in their educational system (Anastasi, 1988).

The impetus for the development of psychological tests in the nineteenth century can be traced to the growing concern with humane treatment of the mentally deficient and the insane. This, in turn, gave rise to a need to identify, differentiate between, and classify mentally impaired individuals in some sort of systematic fashion. In France, Esquirol, for example, endeavored to distinguish varying degrees of mental retardation by assessing language skills. Seguin, another French physician who subsequently came to America, experimented with methods of training the mentally deficient and developed a form board akin to a jigsaw puzzle which is still a part of performance intelligence scales.

The focuses of the experimental psychologists of the nineteenth century were largely on measuring sensory phenomena and developing generalized principles of behavior. This approach is typified by Wundt, who established a laboratory in Leipzig in 1879 where a number of the early experimental psychologists studied. When individual differences were observed under standardized conditions, they were ordinarily ascribed to a form of human error. By contrast, in the 1880s, Sir Francis Galton, the English biologist, grasped the importance of accurately assessing individual differences and similarities in connection with his research on heredity and, in effect, fathered contemporary psychological testing.

Rather than studying mental processes exhaustively in a few people, Galton was more interested in less intensive investigations of large numbers of individuals. Furthermore, he did not confine his studies to simple sensorimotor functions, but broadened his investigative approaches to include questionnaires and rating scales and devised statistical methods for analyzing his findings on individual differences.

Galton believed that sensory discrimination and reaction time tests could evaluate intellectual ability, a point of view shared by the American psychologist Cattell. Cattell, stimulated by contact with Galton, developed his own series of simple measures for assessing individual differences in intelligence, also emphasizing in his battery sensory tasks and speed of response which lent themselves to precise measurement. For the first time in the psychological literature, Cattell employed the term "mental tests" in an article written in 1890 describing a series of tests administered to college students to appraise intellectual functioning.

In approximately the same period, the German psychiatrist Kraepelin, who was a prime mover in the classification of mental illness, devised a battery of tests, tapping, among other factors, memory and fatigue susceptibility. Kraepelin was interested principally in using his tests with clinical populations. Ferrari, an Italian psychologist, was also concerned with evaluating psychopathology through a diverse series of tests encompassing motor skills, physiological measures, and even interpretation of pictures.

It remained for Binet, however, to add new scope and direction to testing. In an article appearing in 1895, Binet and Henri criticized the intelligence tests of the time as too simplistic, narrowly focused, and based on the dubious assumption that intelligence was fundamentally reducible to motor speed and sensation. They asserted, additionally, that more meaningful complex functions would not pose major measurement difficulties in that there was far greater individual variability in such functions.

Mental Tests During the First Part of the Twentieth Century

Binet, working collaboratively with Simon, constructed an intelligence scale in 1905 which advanced the assessment of intelligence from measuring very delimited, specialized abilities to covering such functions as reasoning, judgment, and comprehension. This first far broader intelligence scale, however, still included some perceptual and sensory problems among its 30 tasks arranged in order of increasing difficulty. As a part of a 1908 modification of this scale, the tasks were grouped according to age levels based on a normal sample of children between three and 13 years. This gave rise to the concept of mental age. There were a number of other revisions of the test—the best known of which was the 1916 Stanford-Binet developed by Terman at Stanford University. This version was the first to utilize a ratio between mental age and chronological age to yield an intelligence quotient or IQ.

The advent of World War I was accompanied by a practical need to evaluate the intellectual level of large numbers of recruits. The Binet scale, requiring individual administration and a trained examiner, was clearly not a suitable instrument for this mass testing operation. As a consequence, considerable effort was directed toward developing procedures which could be administered easily and rapidly to large groups of individuals.

The Army Alpha and Beta ultimately produced by Army psychologists for large-scale testing relied to a considerable degree upon Otis's unpublished group intelligence test which utilized multiple-choice items for the first time. The Army Beta was a non-language scale specifically devised for illiterates and those with very limited knowledge of English. These Army group intelligence tests were adopted subsequently for a variety of civilian populations but, unfortunately, were applied indiscriminately without adequate recognition of their technical crudeness and limitations.

Also developed during World War I to address another dimension of the process of screening recruits for military service was Woodworth's Personal Data Sheet. This inventory was designed to identify men who would not be suitable for the military by tallying the number of psychological symptoms they reported about themselves in response to written questions. Although the Personal Data Sheet was not in sufficiently finished form to be actually utilized during World War I, it was revised for civilian use and served as the prototype for subsequent personality inventories.

The Projective Tests

While the test boon of the 1920s, which also included the development of tests of special aptitudes, highlighted the attempts of psychologists to construct more sophisticated and diverse instruments, psychiatrists and psychoanalysts were employing different methodologies. Using clinical interviews and observational techniques, clinicians such as Freud explored the intricacies of personality in terms of conscious thoughts and emotions as well as in areas less subject to rational controls and not within the individual's full awareness. These approaches, which raised important diagnostic, therapeutic, and prognostic questions and issues, also provided an impetus for a new kind of test, namely, the projective technique. This procedure was developed to tap basic personality structure and underlying dynamics, essentially by analyzing an individual's interpretations of ambiguous or unstructured stimuli.

One of the earliest projective devices was a word association test developed by Jung (1910), among others. Through this approach, a subject's reactions and associations to an emotionally-toned series of words were examined from the standpoints of speed and content of response, as well as for other behavioral concomitants. However, the test having the greatest impact on the future course of clinical psychology was doubtlessly the Rorschach.

Psychology is indebted to Kerner for first recognizing the potential present in inkblots for studying personality. In a book entitled, *Kleksographien*, published in Germany in 1857, Kerner observed that inkblots appeared to impose their own meaning upon the interpreter (Klopfer & Kelly, 1942). He did not fully realize, however, that significant individual differences in inkblot interpretation existed and could form the basis for personality assessment.

Hermann Rorschach, a Swiss psychiatrist, had a long-standing investment in developing the diagnostic possibilities of inkblots. For a 10-year period, he experimented with thousands of inkblots, administering them to different groups of psychiatric patients and also to nonpsychiatric populations for purposes of comparison. His goals were to select a set of blots and develop a scoring procedure which could differentially identify various forms of psychopathology.

The results of Rorschach's formidable labors were published in his monograph *Psychodiagnostik* in 1921 which was later translated and reprinted in English (Rorschach, 1942). This monograph reproduced the five achromatic and five chromatic blots, still currently in use, and also presented the basic Rorschach scoring system which notably placed its emphasis on the formal characteristic of the subject's percepts rather than on the content of the responses.

After Rorschach's unfortunate death shortly after the publication of his monograph, his close associate, Oberholzer, continued his work. David Levy, an American psychiatrist, studied under Oberholzer in 1923–1924 and introduced the Rorschach to the United States. Influenced by Levy, Beck, then a doctoral student at Columbia, also sought to train with Oberholzer and wrote the first American dissertation on the Rorschach method.

Klopfer, Piotrowski and Rapaport are numbered among the many psychologists in the United States who subsequently made major Rorschach contributions. More recently, Holtzman (1968) developed a new series of inkblots which can be administered and evaluated under more controlled conditions. Also gaining prominence has been Exner's (1974) comprehensive system which endeavors to enhance the scoring and interpretive precision and reliability of the Rorschach technique. Rorschach content interpretation has also been examined more critically (Aronow & Reznikoff, 1976; Schafer, 1954)

Stimulated by the enthusiasm that initially greeted the appearance of the Rorschach, other instruments emerged on the projective landscape and rather quickly gained a substantial following. Noteworthy among these was the Thematic Apperception Test (TAT) which was developed by Murray and his collaborators at the Harvard Psychological Clinic.

Although an earlier report on the TAT was published by Morgan and Murray (1935), it was not until three years later when Murray's seminal book, *Explorations in Personality* (1938), appeared and integrated the TAT with a broad theory of personality, that it achieved prominence. Compared with the Rorschach, the TAT presents pictures which are clearly more structured than the Rorschach inkblots but, nevertheless, are sufficiently ambiguous to be perceived (apperceived) by the individual from the standpoint of prior experience. The examinee is requested to make up stories to various cards in the set of 30 black and white pictures depicting sundry situations, plus one blank card. The stories are to cover what is transpiring in the picture, the events leading up to it, the outcome, and the feelings and thoughts of the characters. These stories are analyzed primarily in terms of such content variables as main theme, conflicts and defenses. Particularly useful normative data on TAT themes have been published by Eron (1950, 1953).

Murray's TAT in its original form is still clearly the test of choice for a variety of populations covering a wide age range. However, over a period of time, there have been various modifications and extensions of the TAT proposed for special groups, including an animal form, the Children's Apperception Test (CAT) for young children, and an adaptation of the CAT designated as the CAT-H, for older children which depicts the same situations as the animal version but uses humans rather than animals in the pictures (Bellak, 1975). There are, additionally, several versions devised specifically for the elderly, with sets of pictures reflecting typical problems of older people. The Gerontological Apperception Test (Wolk & Wolk, 1971) and the Senior Apperception Technique known as the SAT (Bellak & Bellak, 1973) are two such thematic tests.

Another major and enduring projective instrument of a very different type which has retained a prominent place in the history of testing is the Bender-Gestalt Test (Bender Visual Motor Gestalt Test). This test, constructed by Bender, was first described in a research monograph (Bender, 1938) and is essentially based on the manner in which the examinee copies nine simple, geometric designs, taken one at a time. Frequently, a second recall phase of the test is administered after the copy portion is completed. Bender selected her designs from those used by the Gestaltist Wertheimer in his research on visual perception. In her original analyses of the test,

Bender emphasized gestalt configurational principles and visual-motor maturation. There has, however, been a steady and impressive flow of studies on the Bender-Gestalt Test since its publication, ordinarily employing the same nine designs but modifying and expanding administrative and interpretative approaches to embrace the detection of organic disorders and to provide a projective test for the diagnosis of emotional difficulties.

While most clinicians interpret organizational features of the Bender test performance and distortions of the reproductions of the designs in an intuitive fashion, several objective scoring systems have been devised. For adults, the Pascal-Suttell scoring scheme (1951) is probably the best standardized and most widely known. It has proven useful in the differential diagnosis of groups with organic pathology from both normals and groups of psychotic patients. Koppitz (1964, 1975) focused on establishing norms for children. In extensive standardization studies of the Bender-Gestalt as a nonverbal developmental scale for ages 5 to 10, Koppitz found moderate to high correlations with standard intelligence tests up until age 10. Additionally, significant differences occurred between the scores of normals and brain-damaged children on her developmental scale. Apart from her Bender-Gestalt developmental scoring procedures, Koppitz lists 10 indicators for the detection of emotional problems in children when the projective aspects of the tests are utilized.

In contrast to the ostensible simplicity of the copy task of the Bender-Gestalt Test, drawing of human figures, another clinical tool of long-standing importance, provides the opportunity for far more creativity. The least structured of all of the projective techniques, human figure drawing was initially used solely as a nonverbal measure of intellectual level in the form of the Goodenough Draw-A-Man Test (1926). This test, tapping observational accuracy and conceptual thinking rather than artistic ability in depicting the human figure, remained unrevised as an intelligence scale until 1963 when it was modified, extended and restandardized by Harris (1963).

Although Goodenough appeared to recognize the potential of her figure drawing test for personality as well as intellectual evaluation, it was Machover (1949) who first gave the technique projective test status. Departing from the observation that children receiving the same IQ on the Goodenough scale were producing very different drawings, Machover devoted herself to studying the instrument from the vantage point of its ability to reveal aspects of self concept, attitudes toward people, and other personality variables.

The Draw-A-Person Test (DAP), as it is commonly known, generally requires the examinee to draw a human figure and then an individual of the opposite sex. Associations are typically obtained to the drawings. Currently, there is no generally accepted systematic scoring procedure or interpretive approach for drawings. Among the drawing characteristics which are often interpreted are comparative size and detailing of the figures and their respective body parts, location on the page, and line quality and shading.

Over the years, a number of variations of the DAP test have been proposed, including tree and animal drawings (Hammer, 1958) and family drawings (Hulse, 1952). None has achieved the popularity of the DAP. Figure drawings share with the Bender-Gestalt Test special usefulness in the personality assessment of illiterate or foreign individuals and for the evaluation of spatial difficulties associated with brain damage.

The sentence completion method perhaps can be most accurately regarded as falling between a projective technique and a questionnaire. It can appropriately be considered an extension of the Word Association Test. Rather than responding to a single stimulus word as in the Word Association Test, the examinee completes a fragmentary sentence. It has largely been a "custom" test in that a set of sentence stems are often designed specifically to explore a particular personality variable. Thus, there are many sentence completion forms. Among the earlier forms was one published by Tendler (1930) who perceived his test as probing emotional insight. In studying language and thought processes, Cameron (1938a, 1938b) contrasted schizophrenics and senile patients with normal groups utilizing sentence completion tests. Rohde (1946) developed a sentence completion form with a format for scoring based on Murray's personality theory.

A different scoring approach is employed in conjunction with the widely used Rotter Incomplete Sentence Completion Blank. This particular Sentence Completion Test consists of 40 stems which can be assessed on a 7-point scale for adjustment-maladjustment according to a manual (Rotter & Rafferty, 1950) which provides illustrative examples for each scoring category. The sentence completion, however, often tends to be dealt with less formally in actual clinical practice. Typically, the clinician looks for such factors as conflicted, avoidant, and inconsistent completions, overly lengthy and excessively precise responses, and unusual language as well as behavioral indicators of tension or discomfort accompanying certain answers.

The Minnesota Multiphasic Personality Inventory

While projective tests were enjoying an extraordinary growth spurt, the self-report personality questionnaire was far from moribund. Some clinicians remained convinced that inventories of this type could provide diagnostic information more efficiently and less expensively than projectives. In the late 1930s, Hathaway and McKinley developed the Minnesota Multiphasic Personality Inventory (MMPI) and a version of it then designated as the Multiphasic Personality Schedule was published in an article on assessing depression (Hathaway & McKinley, 1942). No test has been more influential than the MMPI. At this point in time, well over 5,000 references have been published about this instrument and it has had a significant impact on the growth of the field of clinical psychology beginning with World War II.

The 550 statements on the MMPI to which the examinee can respond "true," "false," or "cannot say" cover 26 different content areas, including religious and political attitudes, psychosomatic conditions, obsessive states, and family and marital affairs. The original test provided scores on nine scales used in traditional psychiatric diagnosis based on Kraepelin's classification scheme. These "clinical scales" were developed empirically and are composed of items which differentiated between specific clinical groups, most of which were about 50 patients in size, and a normal control group of about 700 individuals. The latter represented a cross section of the Minnesota population and were recruited when they visited the University of Minnesota hospitals.

A special aspect of the MMPI is the inclusion of three "validity" scales to check on carelessness, confusion, malingering, and the presence of a response set as well as attitudes toward taking the test. Since the initial publication of the MMPI, the 550 statements have comprised an item pool for the development of approximately 300 new scales. One of these, the Social Introversion Scale (Si), is now regularly included in the MMPI. These new scales vary widely in their focus and application. Numbered among them are Ego Strength (Es), Prejudice (Pr) and the more diagnostically oriented MacAndrews Alcoholism Scale (1965).

While the major thrust of the MMPI is as an instrument for differential diagnosis, clinicians have endeavored to drop the traditional Kraepelinian psychiatric labels which are regarded as meaninglessly obsolete. Literal interpretation of elevated scores on single clinical scales is strongly discouraged. Rather, the emphasis is currently placed on score patterns and the numerical coding of profiles. Several books have been published to systematize and simplify MMPI diagnostic interpretation through coded profile patterns (Dahlstrom, Welsh & Dahlstrom, 1972; Hathaway & Meehl, 1951; Marks, Seeman & Haller, 1974).

The Wechsler Scales

At about the same time as the MMPI was gaining prominence, a very different kind of individually administered intelligence scale was being added to the psychologist's array of testing tools. This test, the Wechsler-Bellevue Intelligence Scale (Wechsler, 1939), was the initial version of two subsequent Wechsler scales very similar in format to the first scale for adults, as well as two forms for children and a preschool scale, all of which essentially parallel the adult tests.

Compared with the Stanford-Binet, a child-oriented scale, later extended to adult levels in somewhat procrustean fashion, the Wechsler tests are point rather than mental age scales. Items specially geared for either adults or children are not arranged by age levels as on the Stanford-Binet, but rather are grouped by type into subtests and ordered according to difficulty. Since the Wechsler scales are composed of Verbal and Performance subtests, separate Verbal, Performance, and Full-Scale IQs can be obtained. Furthermore, apart from estimating intelligence, study of the subtests from the standpoints of both intertest and intratest patterning can sometimes be meaningful in the diagnosis of various emotional disorders and brain damage. The Wechsler scales have been the subject of extensive clinical and research use. Numerous publications have appeared about these scales, including a great deal of work on short forms (Matarazzo, 1972), the latter with the goal of developing a quick screening instrument for intelligence. The revisions of the adult and children scales of the Wechsler primarily reflected an ongoing research effort to improve the representativeness of the normative standardization samples and additionally to refine item content.

World War II and Postwar Testing

At the start of World War II and once again facing the pressing need to screen and classify large numbers of recruits for the military, clinical psychologists already had some very substantial diagnostic tools. Unfortunately, however, formal clinical psychology training programs had not yet been established. This resulted in a dearth of individuals among the approximately 1,500 psychologists in the armed forces who had sufficient background training to use these instruments in actual clinical situations. There was no diminished need for psychologists at the conclusion of World War II. Rather, the opposite prevailed. The remarkable postwar growth of the Veteran's Administration (VA) clinics and hospitals decisively established a demand and role for clinical psychologists. Training issues were concomitantly addressed to a considerable degree with the inception of the United States Public Health Service funding for graduate training programs in psychology and the network of clinical psychology internships underwritten by the VA.

The professional activities of the clinical psychologist of the 1940s were mostly confined to psychodiagnostic testing. In the middle of this decade, Rapaport, Gill and Schafer (1945, 1946) published their classic two-volume work on psychological testing which had a major impact on the field. Rapaport and his collaborators articulated the concept of administering a battery of tests tapping diverse psychological functions, in lieu of a single test, to achieve a genuine understanding of the subtleties and complexities of the dimensions of personality. They endeavored to spell out the contributions of each test in a battery in the differential diagnostic process, drawing on psychoanalytic ego theory. Schafer (1948, 1954) added further dimension to differential diagnosis in two subsequent books on testing, the latter focusing explicitly on Rorschach interpretation from a psychoanalytic viewpoint. Still later, with Holt serving as editor, the Rapaport, Gill and Schafer volumes (1968) on diagnostic testing were skillfully updated and condensed.

After the enormous growth spurt of psychodiagnostic testing in the 1940s, interest in testing began to decline somewhat in the 1950s. Reasons for this decline have been offered from many diverse quarters (for example, Garfield, 1983; Goldstein & Hersen, 1984; Holt, 1967). Essentially, consequences of overselling the value of a very time-consuming activity were being felt. Furthermore, in the attempt to meet the inordinate demand for testers, a number of psychologists had received somewhat perfunctory training and experienced considerable uncertainty about their own testing competence. Test reports often contained a plethora of unwarranted speculations raising serious question about the reliability and validity of psychodiagnostic instruments. Meehl (1954), in an influential book on prediction, even argued that statistical or actuarial methods were superior to the judgmental processes employed by the clinician—a shocking assertion at the time.

Perhaps central to the lessened involvement in psychological testing, however, was the fact that testing was bound to a psychiatric taxonomy, in itself demonstrated, at the time, to be highly unreliable (Schmidt & Fonda, 1956; Zubin, 1967). In addition, it was a commonly held view among psychologists that testing, per se, was very restrictive and comparatively unrewarding, with typically no feedback on the usefulness of psychological reports from their recipients. Thus, psychologists successfully sought to expand their professional roles to include such activities as psychotherapy and community consultation which, in turn, further underlined the limited satisfactions that could be derived from testing. Furthermore, in the treatment sphere, behavioral therapy approaches were emerging, emphasizing coping with various behavioral problems rather than probing underlying conflicts, the domain of traditional psychodiagnostic testing.

Although testing activities were in some disarray, virtually every graduate program in clinical psychology retained their required courses in psychological testing. Also, assessment continued to be regarded as a relatively important activity to which clinical psychologists clearly devoted substantial time in their actual professional work (Garfield & Kurtz, 1976). Noteworthy, as well, was the remarkable stability of patterns of test usage over time (Lubin, Larsen & Matarazzo, 1984). In order of overall frequency of use across various clinical settings, the most popular instruments in a 1982 survey were: the MMPI, WAIS, Bender-Gestalt, Rorschach, WISC, Sentence Completion, TAT and DAP (Lubin, Larsen, Matarazzo & Seever, 1985).

Current Testing Trends

Recently, the indications are that not only is testing holding its own but, in fact, may be gaining an increasingly important role in the clinical psychologist's array of skills. This resurgence appears to be spearheaded by developments principally in two areas, namely, neuropsychological testing and computer-based test interpretation (CBTI).

Efforts to "test" the behavioral manifestations of brain damage can be traced back to the work of Kurt Goldstein in the 1920s. Goldstein's (1939) important book, *The Organism*, and his subsequent monograph with a colleague (Goldstein & Scheerer, 1941) spelled out his theories and procedures for assessing intellectual impairment occurring with brain damage. Goldstein felt that a key symptom was the presence of a deficit in abstract thinking. It was quickly recognized, however, that brain damage subsumed a broad spectrum of complex organic conditions with corresponding variable behavioral patterns, which, in turn, were influenced by such factors as age and duration of cerebral pathology.

The initial efforts made in the differential diagnosis of brain damage utilized already existing tests, in particular, the Wechsler scales and the Bender-Gestalt. Later, as psychologists acquired a greater degree of sophistication in evaluating organic pathology, systematic attempts were directed to developing comprehensive test batteries which tapped a wide variety of neuropsychological functions and could be administered and scored in a relatively standardized manner. The two best known batteries of this type in current clinical use are the Halstead-Reitan Neuropsychological Battery and the Luria-Nebraska Neuropsychological Battery.

The Halstead-Reitan has been developed and researched extensively over a lengthy period of time (Hevern, 1980; Reitan & Davison, 1974). The clinicians utilizing this battery typically include 11 tests which assess such factors as sensorimotor functioning and the presence of aphasia. In contrast to the Halstead-Reitan, the Luria-Nebraska ordinarily takes less than half the time to administer and is considerably more standardized in terms of content and administrative and scoring procedures. It consists of item rather than test units designed to provide more extensive coverage of possible organic pathology as well as a greater degree of specific localization of brain damage (Golden, 1979; Luria, 1973). The responses to each of the 269 items on the Luria-Nebraska are scored on a three-point normal to brain-injured continuum and then combined into areas to obtain total scores on such scales as motor functions, expressive speech, and memory. Despite this quantification procedure, it is to be recognized that the items composing this battery were selected on the basis of their qualitative clinical significance in diagnosis.

Computers began to be used in psychological testing shortly after they became available. Not unexpectedly, the first programs developed were for the MMPI and became operational some 25 years ago (Fowler, 1985). While the earlier CBTI systems for the MMPI drew largely on individual scale clinical interpretations and some fairly elementary configurational rules, later more sophisticated systems included, among other factors, actuarial-based interpretations (Lachar & Alexander, 1978) and demographic data to generate reports (National Computer Systems, 1984).

Piotrowski (1964) was the first to undertake the far more demanding task of developing a CBTI for a projective instrument, the Rorschach. Ten years later, a more quantitatively-oriented Rorschach interpretation approach was published by Exner (1974) based on the Exner Rorschach Comprehensive System. Exner emphasizes interpretation based on the structural features of the Rorschach expressed in various ratios and percentages. By contrast, Piotrowski includes content interpretation as an important aspect of his system. The Piotrowski system is not now commercially distributed, while the Exner system underwent a period of revision and became a fully operational service in 1983.

Computer programs have been developed for interactive testing, providing automated administration of a variety of tests including the WAIS (Elwood, 1969). Neuropsychological testing has been an area to which particular attention has been devoted. After reviewing current computer programs designed to analyze and interpret neuropsychological test data, Adam & Heaton (1985) concluded, however, that programs now available do not achieve the same level of accuracy as human clinicians. They recommend that such programs best serve as "ancillary information sources for experienced clinicians."

In an overview of present applications and future directions of computerized personality assessment, Butcher, Keller and Bacon (1985) note that computer usage has gained widest acceptance in standardized test scoring and/or administration. They observe that in this role, which capitalizes on the computer's speed and accuracy, it essentially functions as a reliable, but unskilled, clerk. More recently, however, the computer has been put to more complex tasks such as producing interpretive psychological reports akin to those written by clinicians. Butcher and his colleagues believe, however, that the computer need not be confined to established assessment strategies. Rather, the potential exists in the future for utilizing the computer's adaptive capabilities and versatility to modify standard testing methods, as, for example, tailoring evaluation procedures to the individual examinee.

Not to be overlooked with respect to CBTI reports are some unresolved ethical issues concerning who is qualified to use such reports which are often distributed by mail-in services. A related problem pertains to the ready availability of CBTI software, in many instances to persons who lack appropriate professional testing credentials.

As mentioned briefly at the beginning of this chapter, the efficacy of psychological testing clearly interfaces with the reliability of psychiatric diagnosis. At this juncture, it would be meaningful to examine the development of the American Psychiatric Association's *Diagnostic and Statistical Manuals* (DSM-I, DSM-II, DSM-III and DSM-III-R).

DIAGNOSTIC AND STATISTICAL MANUALS (DSM)

DSM-I

Although the first edition of the American Psychiatric Association's *Diagnostic and Statistical Manual* (DSM-I) did not appear until 1952, it had been apparent for a number of years that there was a compelling need to develop a uniform nomenclature system in the United States. In the late twenties, for example, virtually every large psychiatric teaching institution had a classification system of its own. As a result, there was a plethora of diagnostic labels that effectively disrupted meaningful communication. As recently as 1948, the confusion that existed was manifested by three separate nomenclatures (Standard, Armed Forces, and Veteran's Administration) in general use in America, none of which complied with the international classification system of the time.

DSM-I was the first official manual of mental disorders to include a glossary describing the diagnostic categories. The influence of Adolph Meyer's psychobiological orientation that mental disorders reflect personality reactions to psychological, biological, and social factors was reflected in the use of the term "reaction" throughout the DSM-I. This manual limited itself solely to the classification of mental disturbances, excluding, for example, neurological diseases. It employed the name "disorder" generically to encompass a group of related psychiatric syndromes. All mental disorders were separated into (1) disturbances of mental functioning primarily having a known organic etiology and (2) a group consisting of conditions of more general adaptational difficulties in which any related brain function pathology was judged secondary to the psychiatric disorder.

In contrast to prior diagnostic usage, the term Mental Deficiency was applicable in DSM-I only to those cases where there was intellectual impairment without recognizable organic brain pathology prenatally, at birth, or in childhood. Other long-standing organically-based disorders of intellectual functioning were listed under Chronic Brain Syndromes.

DSM-I expanded the number and type of Schizophrenic Reactions found in other nosology systems to permit more detailed diagnoses, while reducing the number of Manic Depressive Reactions and grouping them with Psychotic Depressive Reaction into an Affective Reaction category. In addition, psychosomatic disorders were classified under Psychophysiologic and Visceral Disorders to capture the interaction between psychic and somatic factors implicated in these disturbances. Titles in Personality Disorders and Transient Situational Disorders were also elaborated and extended.

DSM-I nomenclature permitted the use of three qualifying phrases: with psychotic reaction, with neurotic reaction, and with behavioral reaction. These qualifiers were intended to describe the appearance of a major change in the clinical symptomatology of a diagnosed condition, occurring when further psychological symptoms are superimposed on the existing disorder.

DSM-II

The second edition of the *Diagnostic and Statistical Manual* (DSM-II) was published in 1968 by the American Psychiatric Association and revised the 1952 standards for recording and reporting psychiatric diagnoses. The nomenclature of DSM-I and the diagnostic system presented in the sixth revision of the World Health Organization's *International Classification of Diseases* (ICD-6) were not compatible. DSM-II attempted to bring American nomenclature more in line with international practice as reflected in ICD-8 which was also published in 1968.

Compared with DSM-I, DSM-II modified the names of many of the disorders as well as defining them differently. There were also changes in the organization of the nomenclature. The reporting of multiple diagnoses and related physical conditions was specifically encouraged and qualifying phrases were altered.

More explicitly among the changes, the term "reaction," which was thought to be somewhat restrictive, was removed from many diagnostic categories. Organizationally, in lieu of the three major disorder categories of DSM-I consisting of organic, functional, and mental deficiency diagnostic groups, DSM-II was divided into 10 categories. The basic distinction, however, between organic brain syndromes and all other conditions found in DSM-I was retained in DSM-II. A significant new diagnosis—Schizophrenia, Latent Type—was added for disorders previously designated unofficially as incipient, prepsychotic, pseudoneurotic, pseudopsychopathic, or borderline schizophrenia, and classified in DSM-I under Schizophrenia Reaction, Chronic Undifferentiated Type.

In DSM-I, Sexual Deviations, Alcoholism, and Drug Dependence were single diagnoses. To permit far greater specificity, DSM-II listed these three diagnoses as major headings, under each of which were listed a number of new diagnostic categories. While DSM-I did not classify acute reactions to stress of psychotic proportions under Transient Situational Personality Disturbance, DSM-II did explicitly permit psychotic disturbances that are viewed as reactions to inordinate environmental stress to be included in this category. The category, No Mental Disorder, which did not explicitly appear in DSM-I, was added to DSM-II as a "positive" diagnosis which could be reported.

By comparison with DSM-I where each of three qualifying phrases could be used with any diagnostic category as long as the phrase was not redundant with the disorder, DSM-II had seven different qualifying phrases, all but one, "in remission," linked to specific sections of the diagnostic manual. The remaining six DSM-II qualifiers were: acute, chronic, not psychotic, mild, moderate, and severe.

Although DSM-II was judged to reflect significant gains over DSM-I, it was not without its critics (Korchin, 1976). Among the major criticisms was the lack of comprehensive and explicit criteria for the various diagnostic categories as well as the significant symptom overlap among different diagnoses. Some dissatisfaction was also expressed over the absence of adequate coverage of a number of clinical problems, particularly those pertaining to children, adolescents, and the aged, for which the DSM-II diagnostic categories appeared unrealistically compacted. Further, the principles of classification seemed to be bewilderingly variable with some conditions defined by patient characteristics, others by behavioral symptomatology, and still others by etiology. Finally, the largely descriptive and loosely empirical nature of the DSM-II categories without theoretical underpinnings and their different "width," with some highly focused and others a rather sweeping group of disorders under one rubric, were regarded in some quarters as shortcomings.

DSM-III

In 1974, the American Psychiatric Association appointed a task force to begin work on the development of DSM-III. Concern was expressed that ICD-9, scheduled to become official at the very beginning of 1979, would not be fully suitable for use in the United States. Specific ICD-9 classifications did not seem sufficiently detailed for clinical and research application, while the glossary was perceived as not reflecting such important methodological advances as explicit diagnostic criteria and the multiaxial approach to assessment. The task force, therefore, embarked upon preparing a new classification and glossary consistent with the most current state of knowledge pertaining to mental illness and compatible with ICD-9. There was agreement at the time, among members of all the mental health professions, that DSM-II was both comparatively unreliable and rarely as useful as it should be.

After five years in development, two years more than had initially been anticipated, DSM-III was published in 1980. DSM-III represented a far more extensive undertaking than its predecessors in terms of planning, deliberation, number of clinicians involved, and field trials. According to Spitzer (1980), the prime architect of DSM-III, the most important modification accomplished by DSM-III is having specified diagnostic criteria for all disorders, rather than ambiguous, stereotypic descriptions. This, he felt, would greatly enhance clinician communication.

A second meaningful change in Spitzer's estimate was the multiaxial evaluation system, providing that, in fact, the optional Axes IV and V, dealing with psychosocial stressors and highest level of functioning, respectively, are found helpful and are used regularly with the clinical syndrome, personality, and developmental disorders, and with the physical disorders axes. While multiaxial systems were not new, this was the first one actually incorporated into an official classification system. Lastly, he felt that including the restrictive requirement of overt psychotic features at some time during the illness in the definition of schizophrenia was a major and very significant clarification.

Pointing to the much richer, more comprehensive, and detailed descriptions of the diagnostic categories, Spitzer also cited comparable efforts at organizational clarity. The format rigorously followed initially presents the core or essential features of the disorder, then the characteristics always present, and, finally, features commonly but not necessarily in evidence. In candor, he notes that after a dialogue with the American Psychological Association, a statement which was to be included in DSM-III indicating that the mental disorders in the manual were medical disorders was withdrawn as not being a contribution to the process of classifying and describing mental disorders.

There were other important features of DSM-III that differed from DSM-II. There were four times as many diagnostic categories of childhood disorders, mirroring the great increase of knowledge in this area. The label of Borderline Mental Retardation has been deleted, however, since these persons typically do not have marked difficulties in adaptive behavior. Organic mental disorders were no longer divided into acute or chronic based on a reversibility criterion, as in DSM-I and DSM-II. Rather, these disorders were classified much more precisely by the syndrome they cause and their etiology, if known. The substance use disorders section of DSM-III combined Drug Dependence and Alcoholism categories of DSM-II to emphasize the similarity in the maladaptive use of all substances of potential abuse.

In addition, the DSM-II categories of Schizophrenia, Simple Type and Latent Type, in which psychotic symptoms were absent, are not included in DSM-III, but were covered by the new severe personality disorder categories such as Schizotypal or Borderline Personality Disorder. The Schizophreniform Disorder of DSM-III generally replaced the diagnosis of Acute Schizophrenic Episode of DSM-II with the added stipulation that duration of the illness is less than six months but more that two weeks. In DSM-III, Schizoaffective Disorder, the one diagnosis lacking specific criteria because consensus was not achieved on defining it, was reserved for those situations where a differential diagnosis cannot be made between Schizophrenia and Affective Disorder.

The affective disorder classification was very likely the only sphere in which DSM-III may be somewhat simpler than DSM-II. In DSM-II, all major affective disorders were categorized as psychoses except those precipitated by stressful life events. Affective disorders in DSM-III were grouped together under the subclass Major Affective Disorder. Bipolar Disorder replaced Manic-Depressive Illness, Manic or Circular Type, of DSM-II, based on the rationale that virtually all individuals who have experienced a manic episode inevitably develop depressive episodes. On the other hand, the DSM-II Manic-Depressive Illness, Depressed Type, was considered a Unipolar disorder, and was classified as Major Depression in DSM-III. The neuroses nomenclature of DSM-II was dropped. The disorders found under this classification were grouped mostly together as Anxiety Disorders in DSM-III, with a few classed as Dissociative Disorders and Somatoform Disorders and the diagnosis of Depressive Neurosis or

Dysthymic Disorder placed in the Affective Disorders category. Post-traumatic Stress Disorder, which appeared only in DSM-I, was reincluded among the Anxiety Disorders of DSM-III.

DSM-II Sexual Deviations were termed Paraphilias in DSM-III, a subclass of Psychosexual Disorders. Another subclass is Gender Identity Disorders which cover Transsexualism and Gender Identity disturbances in childhood. Ego-Dystonic Homosexuality is substituted for the DSM-II category Sexual Orientation Disturbance, or Homosexuality, the former perceived as a more accurate description. A new category in DSM-III, Factitious Disorder, described individuals who simulate physical or psychological symptoms in the classical Munchhausen or Ganser Syndrome manner. Adjustment Disorder replaced the DSM-II category of Transient Situational Disturbance; in contrast to the latter, it excludes reactions of psychotic proportions.

As indicated earlier, Axis II was utilized to code Personality Disorders, ensuring that they are not ignored in the presence of a more floridly obvious Axis I disorder. The V codes of DSM-III supplanted the Conditions Without Manifest Psychiatric Disorder of DSM-II. The V code category was for conditions not attributable to mental disorder but still a focus of attention or treatment. Unlike the DSM-II category, a mental disorder may additionally be present. Marital Problem and Uncomplicated Bereavement are examples of V code conditions.

As was the case in comparing DSM-II with DSM-I, the advent of DSM-III marked considerable diagnostic improvement over DSM-II, though some substantial problems clearly remained. Schacht and Nathan (1977) pointed to the "enormous underlying complexity" of the multiaxial classification system which was masked by its apparent simplicity. They question particularly the ability of the clinician to use the rating scales of Axes IV and V in a meaningful fashion. Further, they recommend the inclusion of an additional axis for coding response to treatment, which they feel might help to classify the diagnosis in certain difficult situations.

Other issues raised by Schacht and Nathan, primarily from a conceptual standpoint, pertain to what they regard as an erroneous view of the relationship between organism and environment postulated in DSM-III which, in turn, impacts on the concept of organismic dysfunction. An explicit definition of psychological health against which to evaluate deviance, not currently found in DSM-III, would, according to Schacht and Nathan, deal with questions of environmental versus organismic preeminence in psychodiagnosis. Concomitantly, defining health would shape the diagnostic process to address the individual's problems and needs rather than thinking in terms of illness models.

The stigmatizing effects of attaching DSM-III diagnostic labels to certain behaviors not ordinarily regarded as psychopathological have also been criticized (Garfield, 1983). For example, a child who is "significantly below the expected level" and not functioning up to intellectual capacity in reading or arithmetic skills can be given new DSM-III diagnoses of Developmental Reading Disorder or Developmental Arithmetic Disorder, if evaluated by a psychologist or psychiatrist.

DSM-III-R

Contrasted with the difference between DSM-II and DSM-III, the revisions made in the latter to produce DSM-III-R are considerably more modest. In a three year period after the publication of DSM-III in 1980, a number of significant inconsistencies and ambiguities had surfaced which needed to be resolved. A work group was, therefore, appointed by the American Psychiatric Association, again chaired by Robert L. Spitzer, and charged with addressing these difficulties. DSM-III-R, published in 1987, essentially incorporates modifications derived from the wealth of clinical experience and research data accumulated since the appearance of DSM-III. Advisory committees of experts were utilized throughout the revision process to review proposals for diagnostic criteria and textual changes. In comparison to a small number of DSM-III codes not compatible with ICD-9 codes, all DSM-III-R codes were revised to legitimate ICD-9 codes as well.

The major thrust of DSM-III-R modifications entail: wording clarifications, criteria revisions to yield richer and more meaningful clinical descriptions, and, lastly, some regrouping of categories. The most prominent category changes occur in the Substance Use and Personality Disorders sections. Moderate revisions have been made in the Anxiety Disorders and Childhood Disorders categories and only comparatively minimal modifications in the remainder of the diagnostic classifications. Insofar as the multiaxial component of DSM-III-R is concerned, particularly noteworthy are the inclusion of new groupings of Developmental Disorders under Axis II and the revision of Axis V to incorporate a 100-point Global Assessment of Functioning scale. The latter now permits the clinician to rate psychological functioning in addition to the previously evaluated social and occupational functioning, on a hypothetical continuum of health-illness.

The focus of changes in what is labeled Psychoactive Substance Abuse Disorders in DSM-III-R is a significant broadening of the definition of dependence to encompass an array of symptoms which reveal a serious loss of control of substance use and sustained use of the substance in the face of patently adverse consequences. Most of the DSM-III cases of substance abuse are covered by the DSM-III-R categories, which also contain a residual classification for a disorder which does not meet the dependence criteria yet indicates a maladaptive pattern of use. Also covered in DSM-III-R but not found in DSM-III is inhalant abuse.

The primary revision for the personality disorders entails providing a one-sentence, broad description for each of the disorders. This is followed by a list of explicit behaviors so that no single behavioral manifestation is required for or sufficient for the diagnosis. Additional behavioral descriptors have also been provided for most of the diagnostic categories, while some confusing items have been removed. Noteworthy is the marked difference in the DSM-III-R concept of Avoidant Personality Disorder which makes it no longer mutually exclusive with Schizoid Personality Disorder. The former now corresponds to the clinical notion of "phobic character."

Changes have also been made in the diagnostic criteria in an attempt to clarify the distinctions among Histrionic, Narcissistic and Borderline personality disorders. In essence, the suicide item has been eliminated from Histrionic to afford more differentiation from Borderline, while an item pertaining to preoccupation with feelings of envy has been added to Narcissistic to distinguish it more clearly from the Histrionic diagnosis.

Most significantly, the hierarchic rule that an Anxiety Disorder is preempted by the presence of another mental disorder, such as Schizophrenia or Major Depression, has been removed in DSM-III-R. Panic disorder has been given more prominence and now is divided into subtypes based on whether or not agoraphobia is also present. To exclude transient anxiety reactions, the duration necessary for the diagnosis of Generalized Anxiety Disorder has been extended from one month to six months and the symptom list expanded to offer a more comprehensive description of the disorder. The stressor criteria for Post-traumatic Stress Disorder have been better defined to convey the notion that it is beyond the usual boundaries of human experience and would be markedly disruptive to virtually everyone. The range of symptoms have additionally been expanded for the diagnosis of Post-traumatic Stress Disorder to include those specifically applicable to children.

Under the rubric of Developmental Disorders, Mental Retardation, Specific Developmental Disorders, and Pervasive Developmental Disorders have been added to Axis II. In contrast to Axis I, therefore, all disorders coded on Axis II share an onset in childhood or adolescence and ordinarily continue into adulthood in stable form. The new subtyping of Conduct Disorder in DSM-III-R reflects a significant distinction between aggressive, antisocial behavior that is evident in solitary activity and antisocial behavior that occurs in a group situation with other children.

Among other modifications in Disorders Usually First Evident in Infancy, Childhood and Adolescence are criteria revisions to raise the threshold for diagnosing Avoidant Disorder of Childhood and Adolescence and Overanxious Disorder; to include older and abused or neglected children under Reactive Attachment Disorder of Infancy or Early Childhood; and to differentiate Oppositional Disorder, renamed Oppositional Defiant Disorder in DSM-III-R, from Conduct Disorder. The distinction between the DSM-III diagnoses Infantile Autism and Childhood Onset Pervasive Developmental Disorder was judged as lacking validity and as a result these categories are combined into the single DSM-III-R category of Autistic Disorder. Schizoid Disorder of Childhood or Adolescence is eliminated in DSM-III-R as it has been perceived only in the presence of symptomatology indicating a Pervasive Developmental Disorder.

Examining other important specific changes of DSM-III-R, among the Schizophrenic Disorders the paranoid subtype of schizophrenia in DSM-III has been redefined to emphasize its systematized delusional aspects, while DSM-III Paranoid Disorders have been renamed Delusional Disorder, reflecting a disturbance having greater breadth that mere suspiciousness. Other modifications among the psychotic disorders include: the elimination of the criterion that schizophrenia begin before age 45; specific diagnostic criteria for Schizoaffective Disorder—a disorder for which no explicit criteria were provided in DSM-III; and acknowledgment that a Brief Reactive Psychosis may persist for as long as a month, along with clarification of the criteria for this disorder in order to exclude culturally-sanctioned reactions.

The affective disorders have been given the more descriptive and accurate name Mood Disorders and have been reorganized so that the Bipolar Disorders and Depressive Disorders are each classified together. The criteria for melancholia have been revised and specification can be made that the Major Depression is of a melancholic type. A seasonal pattern of Major Depression can also be indicated.

The DSM-III diagnosis of Ego-Dystonic Homosexuality has been eliminated from DSM-III-R. The removal of this category was based on the reasoning that it conveyed the impression that homosexuality itself was a disorder and also that it has been infrequently employed clinically and in the scientific literature. Furthermore, it has been noted in the United States that almost all homosexual individuals experience an ego-dystonic phase with regard to their homosexuality.

There have been some significant appendices modifications to DSM-III-R. The detailed Sleep and Arousal Disorders classification which was found in an appendix in DSM-III has been simplified and included in the body of DSM-III-R rather than as an appendix. Among other sleep disorders, diagnostic criteria are provided for Insomnia Disorder, Dream Anxiety Disorder, and Sleepwalking Disorder. Three new diagnostic categories which have been proposed were judged controversial and deemed "needing further study" and are located in the appendices of DSM-III-R. They are: Late Luteal Phase Dysphoric Disorder (a more narrowly defined version of premenstrual syndrome), Self-Defeating Personality Disorder, and Sadistic Personality Disorder. Basically, they were assigned to an appendix because of some questions raised about their scientific potential for misuse. A number of professionals felt that the categories would result in the misdiagnosis of normal women as having mental illness (Late Luteal Phase Dysphoric Disorder and Self-Defeating Personality Disorder) or would be used in the courts to allow men who abuse women to escape legal punishment (Sadistic Personality Disorder).

Several other appendix changes worth noting are the inclusion of 18 defense mechanisms and their definitions in the DSM-III-R Glossary of Technical Terms and a new Index of Selected Symptoms included in the Diagnostic Criteria. This symptom index permits the clinician to locate, and review conveniently, all of the DSM-III-R disorders that have a particular symptom as one of their defining features.

DSMs, PSYCHOLOGICAL TESTING AND TREATMENT PLANNING

By virtue of the impressively higher reliability of the diagnostic categories of DSM-III and DSM-III-R in comparison to their predecessors, psychodiagnostic testing becomes a much more meaningful and viable activity. It is to be noted that DSM-III-R is an essentially atheoretical classification system. Its descriptive approach necessitates a reliance on symptom-oriented and historical data in the formulation of diagnoses. Although DSM-III-R does not preclude an intrapsychic or psychodynamic understanding of psychopathology, neither does it, for the most part, include criteria that are fundamentally useful to a psychodynamic perspective.

On the other hand, psychodiagnostic testing tends to be based on the premise that an individual's test performance reflects an internal state in terms of such factors as defenses, ego strengths, and inner conflicts, as well as the more proximal impact of current psychological difficulties and psychiatric disorders. Psychological test data are not necessarily atheoretical nor, for that matter, congruent with one specific personality theory. Although such data may contribute to an understanding of how an individual interacts with the world, test findings ordinarily do not provide a clear symptomatic and/or historical picture.

It is apparent, then, that DSM-III-R and psychodiagnostic testing have largely complementary roles as sources of information which can differentially delineate a mental disorder and offer a combined frame of reference for treatment planning.

Studies of psychiatric diagnosis have indicated improving, if somewhat variable, reliability over the period during which the three DSMs were developed. Reliability research using DSM-I and DSM-II revealed generally poor or, at best, fair reliability for most of the major diagnostic categories (Spitzer & Fleiss, 1974). The field trials for DSM-III involved 450 participating clinicians, conducting evaluations of nearly 800 patients of all ages in one of the largest reliability studies ever done. The results reported by Spitzer, Forman and Nee (1979) indicated good interrater reliability for most diagnostic categories, much above the levels achieved for DSM-I and DSM-II. In summarizing the overall reliability data on the DSMs, Spitzer (1980) gives reliability coefficients mostly in the .40 range, but occasionally around .60 for DSM-I and DSM-II categories like schizophrenia and depression, wile personality and neurotic disorders, at their highest levels, were .30 and .40. In sharp contrast, for a DSM-III study group of adults, schizophrenic disorders averaged .81 over two phases of field trials; affective disorders .76; and substance abuse disorders .83. The reliability was lower for childhood categories but substantially better than what was obtained utilizing DSM-II.

Not surprisingly, the frequency of requests for diagnostic "labels" in referrals for psychological testing appears related to the amount of effort directed towards enhancing nosological reliability at the time. One study (Dollin & Reznikoff, 1966) reviewed questions on a psychological testing referral form posed for a population of inpatients and outpatients by psychiatrists and psychiatric residents at a large psychiatric hospital. In 1956, only four years after DSM-I was introduced, a specific diagnosis was requested in 64 percent of the cases. By 1965, diagnostic enthusiasm seemed to have waned and in only 29 percent of the referrals was a diagnosis requested, a statistically significant decrease. In a 1976 replication of the prior study (Dollin & Phillips, 1976) in the same setting, the referral requests for a diagnosis had risen significantly to 53 percent. The authors interpret their findings in light of an apparent return to traditional diagnosis concurrent with the interest in the then ongoing preparation of DSM-III.

It is the confluence of psychological testing, the DSM-III-R diagnostic system, and ongoing work for DSM-IV, and their overlapping and unique contributions to treatment planning for the individual patient that is the focus of this book. The improvement of a diagnostic system to a point at which it is reliable and operational enough to guide differenital diagnoses and related treatment planning and encourage research is a quantum leap forward. We feel that this is such a major event that psychological testing used in the assessment of mental disorders cannot be the same as before. Thus, this book, while in the tradition of psychological testing in psychiatric hospital settings (Rapaport, Gill & Schafer, 1945-1946), is at the same time a different approach.

In contrast to the role traditionally played by psychological assessment, psychiatric diagnosis can now be made efficiently through information gathered in a more or less structured clinical interview, or with some of the semistructured interviews for the diagnosis of Axis I and Axis II conditions (e.g. Structured Clinical Interview for Diagnosis (SCID) or Personality Disorder Examination (PDE)). In that the current diagnostic system includes behavioral markers with a specific time frame (e.g. depressed mood for at least two weeks), this kind of data may be best obtained in an interview and is not tapped in tests that are a cross-sectional sample of behavior.

However, most importantly, the DSM diagnosis is necessary but *not sufficient* for treatment planning (Beutler & Clarkin, 1990). The DSM diagnosis provides a good beginning for focusing on feelings, behaviors, and symptoms that are troubling to the patient. But much more than this is needed to plan intervention. As an illustration of this fact, it must be recognized that two patients with the same Axis I and Axis II diagnoses may require quite different treatments in terms of setting, format, techniques, and medications.

What, then, is a relatively exhaustive list of information areas needed for comprehensive treatment planning? The relevant research suggests that the consultant needs information on the patient's symptoms and troubled behaviors. This is often, but not always, the focus of the patient presenting for help, the so-called chief complaint. The details of these symptoms in terms of the severity and frequency and impact on the patient's daily functioning are often captured in the DSM diagnostic categories. For treatment planning, however, the clinician must obtain information not only on the problematic behaviors and symptoms, but also on the patient's personal assets. As every clinician knows, a symptom or problem complex of moderate severity is quite different in terms of treatment and prognosis depending on whether it is a person with considerable assets or an individual with relatively meager strengths.

Not only does one need to know the target symptoms and behaviors that are problematic and the focus of change, but also one needs to know the source of these difficulties. Depression, for example, can be the end result of acute environmental stress or it can be the result of the individual's chronic and pervasive ways of conceptualizing the world. Furthermore, some symptom complexes appear to be relatively habitual and automatic ways of responding to the environment (e.g. panic attacks). The data suggest that in these situations, intervention directed at symptomatic habits may be the most efficacious method of intervention.

In other situations, however, it seems more profitable for treatment planning to conceptualize the problematic symptoms and behaviors as essential manifestations of underlying intrapsychic conflict. The assessment, of course, must provide information on both the behavioral level and the conflictual level. There are many tests which provide information along these treatment relevant dimensions (Clarkin & Hurt, 1988). It is precisely in these areas that are crucial to treatment planning that data from psychological tests can contribute most significantly to the clinical assessment process. In addition, there are also situations in which testing can be helpful in defining underlying organic factors and/or assisting in defining the functional level and capacities of individuals with such organic conditions.

SECTION

· I ·

AXIS I DISORDERS

CHAPTER 2

Disorders Usually First Evident in Infancy, Childhood, or Adolescence

A. EATING DISORDERS: ANOREXIA NERVOSA AND BULIMIA NERVOSA

Anorexia and bulimia are two eating disorders that are related but somewhat different symptomatic constellations involving the disruption of the routine of food intake. There is some indication that the symptoms of anorexia (e.g., the restriction of food intake with the subsequent reduction of body weight) are associated with fewer personality and interpersonal problems than bulimia (the usual intake of food, but its elimination by unusual means such as laxatives and vomiting). Disorders of food intake are more prominent among women, especially young women preoccupied with their appearance, all of which seems strongly influenced by the values of our culture.

ANOREXIA NERVOSA: THE CASE OF MS. C

Ms. C was a popular, bright young girl who had always done well in school. She was active in her new school, although her family had just moved to the area a few weeks before when her father had relocated because of his new job. She lost a very close race for head cheerleader of her ninth grade class, but her parents thought she got over it after a few days of disappointment. In truth, Ms. C was quite upset about the event and particularly so when she learned that the girl to whom she lost the election was later diagnosed as having anorexia nervosa.

Ms. C, now 15, had been trying to lose weight for the last year and a half. She and her 19-year-old sister had begun a program of vigorous exercise and severe dieting during the previous school year. Her exercise regimen had included up to four hours of long-distance running per day, along with morning and evening calisthenics and practicing her cheerleading routines.

Her weight had dropped to 82 pounds, some 40 pounds below normal for someone 5'7" in height. On two occasions in the last 18 months her pediatrician had become concerned enough about her weight loss and accompanying retardation of physical development (for example, Ms. C had never menstruated) that he had her medically hospitalized for weight gain. She passively cooperated with the intravenous feeding but simply returned to her old routine upon discharge.

Although Ms. C had been able to maintain weights slightly over 100 pounds in order to continue to run with the school's track team, her loss of the election caused her to redouble her efforts to lose weight. She had been restricting her food intake during the day and had been eating only at night. During the evening, she would spend hours in the kitchen preparing small amounts of many different kinds of foods. Now, she stopped eating entirely. As her weight began to drop rapidly, her pediatrician once again had her hospitalized and insisted that, on discharge, her parents take an active role in restricting her exercise, scheduling her meals, and preparing her food. At home, in response to this new regimen, Ms. C began to bite herself, pull her hair, and bang her head. Within a few days, she began to feel that her life was "worthless" and talked of suicide. Frightened at this turn of events, her parents brought her to a different hospital with an eating disorders program for psychiatric consultation and treatment.

On admission, Ms. C was described as an attractive but emaciated 15-year-old girl who looked quite a bit older than her 15 years. She was fidgety and restless during the admission interview, but her physical restlessness did not appear to interfere with her attention and concentration. She described her mood as "Okay" and admitted to periods of feeling "blue" or "depressed" on occasion. Her affect was described as irritable and she often made faces of disgust when asked to provide details of her experience. The examining clinician found no evidence of severe disturbances in Ms. C's perceptions or thinking. She knew she was underweight and "thin" and was aware of the medical problems this caused. She realized she was in need of treatment, but despite her repeated hospitalizations and her outpatient treatment, she claimed to have no idea what was bothering her. She simply stated that she felt better when she was dieting.

DSM-III-R Diagnosis

Axis I: Anorexia nervosa
Axis II: None
Axis III: Emaciation, bradycardia, lanugo, enlarged submandibular salivary glands and absent deep tendon reflexes

Axis IV: Moderate—Father had a serious heart attack six months previously; loss of election

Axis V: Poor—her dieting and exercise regimens had forced her to give up all her friends; her schoolwork had begun to suffer

Treatment and Hospital Course

Ms. C was placed on an initial treatment regimen involving fixed amounts of prepared foods served several times per day, daily weights, monitoring of her intake and output, and restriction of her exercise and activity. She tolerated this approach without the hostility and self-injury she displayed at home. However, she was unable to either gain or sustain her weight on this regimen and began her second week of the hospitalization on frequent oral feedings of a nutritional supplement. Regular foods other than fruit juices were eliminated from her routine diet and the amount of nutritional supplement was gradually increased to supply sufficient calories.

During the next six weeks, Ms. C was able to achieve her target weight range of 122-127 pounds. Her nutritional supplements were discontinued and she was returned to regular foods. She was enrolled in a full school schedule and did well in school. In her individual psychotherapy, she began to explore the reasons for her illness and came to focus increasingly on her mother's and sister's critical and teasing comments to her which she felt demeaned by and resented. However, she seemed detached and aloof in her social relations with peers and often needed a great deal of encouragement to be even modestly candid about her own thoughts and feelings.

Psychological Assessment

Psychological testing was postponed upon admission until Ms. C had achieved her target weight. With this achievement, her therapist requested an assessment of Ms. C's personality functioning and, in particular, wished to assess her capacity to utilize further insight-oriented psychotherapy. She received a WAIS-R, Bender, DAP, Rorschach, TAT, SCT and MMPI during the course of her psychological evaluation.

Ms. C evidenced no unusual behavior during the evaluation. She was pleasant and cooperative during the testing process, falling silent upon occasion when she seemed to experience some mild anxiety. Her intellectual functioning fell in the *Very Superior* range. She achieved a Full Scale IQ of 130 with verbal and performance IQs of 124 and 130, respectively. Subscale scores ranged from high average to very superior levels. Her best performance was achieved on a subtest requiring abstract reasoning (*Similarities*). She also performed at very superior levels on tasks measuring her understanding of ordinary social conventions (*Comprehension*), her ability to anticipate and plan appropriately in an interpersonal context (*Picture Arrangement*), her integration of visual-spatial materials (*Block Design* and *Object Assembly*), and a visual-motor task assessing new learning ability (*Coding*). Her weakest performances were given on those subtests requiring a wide range of factual data (*Information & Picture Completion*), use of words (*Vocabulary*) and easily deployed attention (*Digit Span*).

Ms. C's performance on the MMPI indicated some mild distress (*scale F*) combined with some depressive (*scale 2*) and anxiety (*scale 7*) symptomatology. The most prominent feature of her profile (*scale 0*) indicated a pronounced tendency for social withdrawal. Although her scaled scores all fell within the normal range, she endorsed several unusual items on the MMPI. These included "hearing very queer things" when with other people, feelings of unreality, and concerns that there is "something wrong with [her] mind," that people were trying to "steal [her] thoughts and ideas" and "making [her] do things by hypnotizing [her]." She also expressed the belief that she "deserved punishment for [her] sins" and that she was "a special agent of God."

Ms. C appeared to hold alternating and conflicting views of herself. Weight and physical appearance are given a prominent place in her reactions to herself and others. On the SCT she completed the sentence stems *I used to daydream about* with the phrase "being skinny," *my first reaction to her was* "She's skinny," *her reaction to me* "is she's pretty," *she felt she couldn't succeed unless* "she was thinner" and *I could hate a person who* "eats like a pig and stays skinny." Her efforts to achieve her goal of weightless perfection, however, have left her feeling guilty and ashamed. She reports being ashamed that "I starved myself," that she dislikes to "worry about my weight," that she was most depressed when "I weighed nothing," her conscience bothered her most when "she exercised obsessively," she was most dissatisfied when "I was skinny," and she feels sad about "my disease."

Her striving to achieve both physical and emotional perfection through control of her body shape has clearly failed. Although she worries that her "disease" has ruined the life of those in her family, she nevertheless finds home to be the safest haven from her troubles. Her parents are described in ideal terms, but even in the safe harbor of home, her conflicts continue. In her TAT stories, maternal demands are rejected (*cards 1 and 2*) and death by poisoning during a dinner party at home is the fate of one child (*card 18GF*). Her idealization of her parents appears to consist in part of a hope that they have not been exhausted by her constant need of them. She fears that she has been, like the man in *card 14*, "using too many outlets," "blew a fuse," and after opening the door "to get a little more light," is still "trapped in the dark."

Her attempts to hold on to the more comforting world of childhood are also evident in her figure drawings. Her self-portrait is of a young child, her hair up in ribbons, her body unencumbered by the appurtenances of adult sexuality. On the Rorschach, prominent child-like elements predominate. She sees very few well organized, whole responses and emphasizes animals in the content of her responses. Oral features are also conspicuous. She reports "an anteater" to the upper red details on *card II* because of "the long nose," a "bird's head" on *card V*, and "2 doves" on *card VI* because of the "beak," "a bulldog" on *card VII* because of "the mean black line through the face," and "a face" on *card X* with a mouth.

In the examining psychologist's report, Ms. C's reality testing was reported as largely intact. She was described as feeling alone and vulnerable, but with an interest in maintaining interpersonal relationships. The chief factors mitigating against the possibility of additional benefit to be derived from an insight-oriented therapy were her difficulties in accepting responsibility for her own actions and the absence of any evidence suggesting she was experiencing any significant distress.

Treatment Planning and Outcome

Ms. C remained in the hospital for an additional 2½ months following completion of her psychological testing. During that time, she was able to maintain her weight within her target range. As the psychologist had suggested, she was difficult to engage in individual psychotherapy, focusing her hopes for recovery on learning to ignore her continuing preoccupation with food and her caloric intake.

Her family psychotherapy met with greater success. She was able to discuss her guilt in criticizing her parents and her overattachment to them. Also discussed was her competition with her sister and her wish to be closer to her. Ms. C felt relieved at being able to express these negative feelings and her family was able to tolerate her expression of them. This resulted in her being able to develop a somewhat more realistic view of her parents and of herself.

Based on her in-hospital achievements, the hospital psychotherapist recommended she continue in individual psychotherapy with her present therapist, but on an outpatient basis, and with a reinstatement of her previous weight management plan which would include medical rehospitalizations for refeeding if her weight dropped significantly. As an alternative, given the prior difficulties with this regimen, the therapist suggested a residential placement where Ms. C could be more closely monitored.

Ms. C was not able to make satisfactory progress in her outpatient treatment and returned to her preadmission pattern of behavior. She shifted her entire eating period to the evening hours and returned to a strenuous exercise regimen to control her weight. Although she was able to maintain her weight within a few pounds of her hospital target weight, the reappearance of her previous maladaptive eating and exercise patterns, her continued preoccupation with food and dieting, and, finally, a return to her self-destructive behavior when her routines were interfered with resulted in her rehospitalization 10 months after her discharge. This hospitalization was brief and served as a retraining interregnum before Ms. C began boarding school. She responded well to the hospitalization and was able to accomplish the transition to boarding school where her family reports she has made a satisfactory adjustment.

EXHIBIT 1

AREA OF ASSESSMENT	CLINICAL EXAMINATION	PSYCHOLOGICAL EXAMINATION
I. Symptoms/Diagnosis		
Anorexia Nervosa		
—refusal to maintain body weight	Refuses to maintain normal body weight	None
—fear of gaining weight	Believes weight gain undermined her election success	Hopes to remain a child by retarding her physical development
—disturbance in body experience	None	Equates physical characteristics with psychological characteristics
—amenorrhea	Has never menstruated due to maturational lag related to weight	None
II. Personality Factors	None	Rigid and overcontrolled. Conflicted about her attempts to stop her maturation
III. Cognitive Abilities	Above average intelligence	Above average intelligence
IV. Psychodynamics	Conflicts with parents involving self-control	Guilt-ridden over her relentless pursuit of "physical perfection" despite its overvaluation
V. Therapeutic Enabling Factors	None	Active conflict regarding her symptoms, although there is no overt anxiety. Compliant with external structure
VI. Environmental Demand and Social Adjustment	Good academic record	Capable of goal-oriented behavior and high level of motivation
	History of stable friendships	Desires friendships and can relate to others

EXHIBIT 2

WAIS-R SUMMARY

Verbal Subtests	*Scaled Score*
Information	12
Similarities	18
Arithmetic	14
Vocabulary	12
Comprehension	14
Digit Span	12

Performance Subtests	
Picture Completion	11
Picture Arrangement	15
Block Design	14
Object Assembly	15
Coding	16

Verbal IQ	124
Performance IQ	130
Full Scale IQ	130

MMPI SUMMARY

F-LK: 02'7-813694/5:

RORSCHACH SUMMARY

Number of Responses	26
Rejections	0
Populars	4
Originals	0
Average R/T Chromatic	35″
Average R/T Achromatic	39″
F%	50
F + %	88
A%	58
H%	31
W:M	5:2
M:Sum C	2:2.5
m:c	3:2

RORSCHACH SUMMARY

VIII-X%		31
Fk + F + Fc%		54
(H + A):(Hd + Ad)		19:5
Apperception	W	19%
	D	61%
	d	8%
	Dd + S	12%

E X H I B I T 3

RORSCHACH SUMMARY

Response	*Inquiry*	*Scoring*
I. 6″		
1. Looks like a bat. Is that—	1. It was shaped like a bat.	drFA
2. A person—like a dancer. That's it.	2. The pointed toes and the skirt shape (*What about the pointed toes and skirt shape . . . dancer?*) How at the bottom it looked like toes and a skirt of a dancer. Looks like she's standing on her toes.	DMHP
II. 10″		
1. Looks like two Chinese guys. (*laughs*)	1. The whole thing (*Chinese guys?*) How they were kneeling with their hands up against each other.	WMHP
2. And a, like, ogre.	2. Right here just the face— the red. (*An ogre?*) The long nose and the horns made it look evil. (*Anything else?*) No—well the little eyes. (*Was it marked off by the red or did you see the ogre as red?*) It was a red ogre—devilish.	DFC(Hd)
3. And an anteater. That's it.	3. Like that. (*Anteater?*) The long nose and it was crawling on all fours.	DFMA
III. 14″		
1. A butterfly.	1. The red. (*Butterfly?*) The red was the butterfly. (*Was it marked off by the red or was it a red butterfly?*) It was a red butterfly.	DFCAP

RORSCHACH SUMMARY

Response	Inquiry	Scoring
2. A crab.	2. Without the blob—everything. (*Crab?*) Cause of the claws sticking out and the rounded body (*Anything else?*) No.	WFA
3. A seahorse. That's it.	3. One of these things. (*Seahorse?*) The long tail kind of thing and the hooked shape here.	DFA
IV. 7″		
1. Like a giant.	1. The whole thing. (*Giant?*) The two huge legs and feet.	WF(H)
2. A king.	2. It looked like a king—the head of a king because of the crown.	DFHd, Crown
3. A witch.	3. The hat and the pointed nose. (*Anything else?*) No. The hat and the pointed nose and the hat—where the lighter part is—one pointed nose.	DFC′(H)
4. A penguin. That's it.	4. The black and white and the beak. (*Black and white?*) Cause the blot was in black and white and the penguin is in black and white.	DFC′A
V. 51″		
1. A bat.	1. The whole thing. (*Bat?*) The wings and the little head.	WFAP
2. A bird's head. That's all.	2. The beak. (*Anything else?*) No.	dFAd
VI. 70″		
1. Some kind of like an insect, like a wasp or something.	1. That. (*Wasp?*) The long body and the wings.	DFA

RORSCHACH SUMMARY

Response	*Inquiry*	*Scoring*
(*Takes blot with hands to see, turns card*)		
2. Two doves. That's it. Amazed when I couldn't see the beaks.	2. The rounded bodies and the little beaks. (*Anything else?*) No. (*Beaks?*) See the two little openings—right there. (*That's the beak of each dove?*) Yeah like that, the mouth opening. (*Mouth openings?*) The little U shape.	drFA
VII. 4″		
1. A rabbit—a rabbit's head really—no the whole rabbit—now that I look at it a different way.	1. Right there—kind of a demented rabbit. (*Rabbit?*) The long ear and the little tails.	DFA
2. A bulldog. That's it.	2. Just this (*Bulldog?*)—Hm I don't know—the broadness of it—the little ears and the mean black line through the face (*Black line?*) When the bulldogs walk like this, the short little stubby arms. Wide and short. (*Arms?*) How it goes in.	DFM-A
VIII. 70″		
1. A puma.	1. The long body prowling and the rounded back, four legs.	DFMA
2. A Chinese fat face. (*Laughs*)	2. The long moustache and the slanted eyes.	diFcH
3. The Eiffel Tower. That's it.	3. (*And the Eiffel Tower?*) The painted building and the beams. Gorgeous. (*Painted?*) The color.	drFCArch.

Rorschach Summary

Response	Inquiry	Scoring
IX. 75″		
1. An elephant's head. That's it.	1. The pink part. (*Elephant's head?*) Two big ears and the eyes—(*Was the elephant pink or did you just use that to mark off the elephant?*) The elephant was pink.	DFC-Ad
X. 5″		
1. The seahorses again.	1. The green. (*Seahorses?*) The hooked shape head and the long body. (*Anything else?*) No.	DFA
2. Cockroach.	2. Where did I see it—this gray. (*Cockroach?*) The antenna and the little round body and the legs.	DFA
3. A wishbone.	3. The little orange. (*Wishbone?*) Just looked like a wishbone. (*In what way?*) Had the same shape.	DFAObj.
4. A face. That's it.	4. That whole thing. (*Face?*) The two yellow eyes—the blue lines like a moustache and the orange little mouth. (*Was the moustache blue?*) Yeah. And the wishbone looked like a mouth that way.	WF/CHd

E X H I B I T 4

THEMATIC APPERCEPTION TEST

CARD 1 (*Give me an example*) Yuk—A boy who wanted to play an instrument and he wasn't sure what he wanted to play and his mother used to be a violinist and she brought her old violin for him to look at and he's just sitting, trying to decide if he wants to play it. (*What's he feeling?*) Confused (*what happens?*) he decides he doesn't want to play it.

CARD 2 4″ There's a young girl who likes this guy a real lot and she's embarrassed about it and she wants to tell him but she's afraid to and he's really cute and strong and he works the fields all day and she wants to stay back at school—she delays going to school so she can talk to him but her mother's standing right there and he doesn't want her to get involved with him—she doesn't like him—the mother says he's just a farm hand and she can do much better but the girl ignores her and goes over to talk with him and they start to date each other. The end.

CARD 3GF 8″ This woman just finds out that her husband was killed in war. She's totally freaking out—she doesn't know how to control her emotions—she loved him so much and she doesn't know how she'll live without him. She cries constantly for about a week (*that's it*) (*what happens after that?*) she still misses him a lot—but she learns to accept it gradually—but she never forgets him.

CARD 5 OK there's a woman she lies all alone and she was sleeping one night and she heard a noise downstairs. She got out of bed to see if there was anything there—that's it (*you're sure?*) (*what happens?*) she found a burglar. (*What she feeling?*) Scared.

CARD 10 There's a father and a son who haven't seen each other in a long time—the boy was away at war and the war ended and he came back safe. The father was so happy that he hadn't been killed so they embraced for awhile (*that's it*) (*what was the boy feeling?*) homesick.

CARD 12F 6″ There's a young girl and it's her old mother's birthday and as a present she wants to give her a painted portrait of herself with her mother and there sitting in the art studio posing for a painter and he paints the picture and she gives it to the mother and she's very happy with it (*who?*) the mother.

CARD 12M 4″ This man is at his wife's funeral—wake—he's kneeling in front of her—praying for her he loves her very much and he misses her tremendously. No one will ever take her place in his life but he's going to try to continue his life.

CARD 13MF   The man and his wife are the characters and the man comes to wake up his wife and he finds her dead in bed. He's shocked and he starts to cry. (*What led up to this?*) She had a heart attack (*what happens?*) she just died unexpectedly—it was a total shock and he loved her very much and he was very disappointed.

CARD 14   5″   There's this man in this house all alone and he's using too many outlets and he blew a fuse all the lights went out and he was left alone in the dark. He went to the door to try to get some light (*that's it*) (*what's he feeling?*) alone (*what happens?*) he leaves the door open to get a little more light but he's still trapped in the dark.

CARD 15   4″   There's this sick man and it's about midnight and he decided to go into the graveyards. He's really crazy and he's thinking about digging up somebody's grave. He decides not to and just goes around and looks at all the graves in the middle of the night (*1′20″*). (*How's he crazy?*) Cause most people don't want to go dig up graves (*and sick?*)—I mean like sick crazy—a sick mind (*Blah—chews gum—sits immobile*).

CARD 18GF   Everybody's dying—this woman was with her son—and he had, and he just dies in her arms. Someone poisoned his dinner (*laughs*) they don't know who did it (*speaks mechanically*) because they had a big dinner party the night before—she's mourning his death a great deal and she's out to get whoever did it. (*That's it*) (*What happens?*) They never find who did it.

E X H I B I T 5

SENTENCE COMPLETION TEST

2. *She often wished she could* "walk to school alone."
4. *She felt to blame when she* "punched her brother in the face."
6. *I used to feel I was being held back by* "a strong force."
8. *As a child my greatest fear was* "being alone."
9. *My father always* "was great."
10. *The ideal man* "is like my dad."
12. *I was most depressed when* "I weighed nothing."
14. *When he turned me down, I* "felt worthless."
17. *Sometimes she wished she* "was pretty."
18. *Usually she felt that sex* "was gross."
19. *I could hate a person who* "eats like a pig and stays skinny."
20. *Her earliest memory of her mother* "was great."
21. *The ideal woman is* "like my mom."
22. *When people made fun of her, she* "felt ashamed."
24. *When I think back, I am ashamed that* "I starved myself."
25. *If I think the job is too hard for me,* "I quit."
26. *A relationship with a sister* "can be hard."
30. *Most men* "are ugly."
31. *When I have to make a decision, I* "get confused."
36. *Taking orders is* "being weak."
39. *Most women are* "chesty."
40. *After he made love to her, she* "felt guilty."
42. *When I am criticized, I* "feel rejected."
44. *She felt she couldn't succeed unless she* "was thinner."
45. *I used to feel down in the dumps' when I* "was underweight."
52. *Most of all I want* "to be normal."
53. *My sexual desires are* "nil."
54. *Her conscience bothered her most when she* "exercised obsessively."
55. *She felt she could murder a woman who* "was happy."
59. *His reaction to me* "is yuk!!"
61. *Sexual intercourse is* "disgusting."

SENTENCE COMPLETION TEST

63. *Whenever she does below average work, she* "feels guilty."
64. *She felt blue when* "she was hungry."
65. *I felt most dissatisfied when* "I was skinny."
67. *My first reaction to her was* "she's skinny."
68. *When they put me in charge, I* "messed up."
69. *I feel guilty about* "ruining my families lives."
71. *Her reaction to me is* "she's pretty."
72. *When she was punished by her mother, she* "was angry."
77. *When they told her what to do, she* "resented it."
79. *Her greatest worry was* "death."
80. *When she was spanked by her father, she* "felt ashamed."
81. *Most women act as though* "men mean the world."
82. *When I feel others don't like me, I* "get quiet."
84. *Most people are* "angry."
87. *I am afraid of* "death."
94. *When with her mother, she* "felt secure."
99. *I wish that my mother was* "with me."
100. *I feel sad about* "my disease."

BULIMIA NERVOSA: THE CASE OF MS. V

Ms. V, a single, white, 21-year-old college sophomore, had become increasingly worried about her health over the last year. She had entered outpatient treatment after returning home from her freshman year in college. During her freshman year, she went on frequent eating binges with her college roommates. After these eating binges, she vomited most of what she had eaten so that she would not gain weight.

She acknowledged that she always had been weight conscious and had begun dieting at age 15 because she was "chunky." Until her freshman year in college, she had vomited occasionally; periodically, she had abused diet pills, diuretics, and laxatives to help her lose weight. However, during the last year, she was binge eating and vomiting four to five times per day and taking 20 to 30 aspirins a day to "shrink my stomach" so that she could better control her appetite. It was this change that concerned her. Her stomach was constantly upset, she had a persistent "burning" in her esophagus, and she felt like she was "out of control."

Ms. V's parents became aware of her difficulties only when she entered outpatient treatment, since, to all outward appearances, she was enjoying college. She had completed the year with grades similar to those she had achieved in high school, maintaining a B- average. Her relationship with her boyfriend was a source of support for her and she actively participated in the school's intramural sports program. When she returned home, Ms. V hoped that her family would rally to her support. However, she found her parents' home to be filled with tension and apprehension. Her mother and father were constantly fighting over her father's drinking. Her father stayed away from home to work late at the office. At first, Ms. V's mother accepted this excuse since there was a financial crisis at Mr. V's company where he was chief financial officer. However, when he came home at all, he usually arrived smelling of alcohol and looking disheveled. Ms. V's mother suspected that Mr. V was having an affair. Mr. V denied his wife's accusations but confided to his daughter that he was having an affair.

Ms. V knew her parents' marriage had been unhappy for the both of them in the last two or three years. She was glad her father had "found someone else" but was uncomfortable keeping the secret from her mother. Ms. V's mother suspected that her daughter knew more about her father's activities than she was admitting. Ms. V had always been closer to her father than to her mother and Mrs. V attempted to get her daughter to tell her what she knew of her father's activities.

Ms. V kept her father's secret. She managed to regain some measure of self-control and returned to school. She soon learned that her parents had separated and that her mother had moved back to her parents' home where Ms. V's grandfather was seriously ill with heart trouble. She saw little of her mother and spent more time with her father. At the end of the semester, she learned that he and his company were under grand jury investigation for misuse of funds. Under the stress of her parents' separation, her grandfather's declining health, and her father's legal troubles, Ms. V once again lost control of her eating and returned to the pattern of bingeing and vomiting that had overtaken her toward the end of her freshman year. When she came home for Christmas vacation, she pleaded with her father to be admitted to the hospital and he reluctantly agreed.

At the time of her admission to the hospital, Ms. V was described as an attractive and fashionably thin young woman who arrived casually dressed and well groomed. She gave as her reason for seeking admission, "I feel that I need help to stabilize my health." She described her mood as "depressed and angry" and her affect was judged to be mildly depressed, but appropriate and within normal range. She gave no evidence of any disturbance in her perception or cognition other than to admit to some thoughts of taking her own life. When questioned about these, she denied any intention of acting on her ideas. She complained of difficulty concentrating and insomnia. Formal examination revealed no significant difficulty concentrating and her recent sleep problems seemed best understood in the context of her binges and vomiting which, while at home, had been carried out secretly at night.

DSM-III-R Diagnosis

Axis I: Bulimia nervosa
Axis II: None
Axis III: Rule out ulcer; irregular menses
Axis IV: Severe—separation of parents; severe illness of grandparent; possible indictment of father
Axis V: Fair—moderate impairment in her family relations; adequate but circumscribed social relations; no decline in school functioning

Treatment and Hospital Course

Ms. V was able to recognize the extent of her difficulties. She entered the hospital very motivated for treatment was admitted to a treatment program specializing in eating disorders. The program was a highly structured, behaviorally oriented program. Ms. V found the imposed discipline quite helpful and quickly adjusted to the routine of the unit. She was assigned a target weight range to maintain and began to learn how to maintain this weight on a well-balanced diet.

Her rapid adjustment to the treatment milieu confirmed her motivation for treatment. As the initial evaluation continued, attention began to focus on her difficulties in her family relationships. She expressed anger at her mother for what she felt was her failure to support her father and was surprised to find her mother supportive of her own hospitalization. She viewed her father, on the other hand, as someone whom she had always felt more in sympathy with and supported. She was hurt by his lack of support for her hospitalization and, following her admission, she found him resentful of her efforts to get well. In contrast to her father, her boyfriend was quite understanding of her desire for treatment and agreed to meet with the hospital staff to help them get a better view of her life at college and her relationship with him.

From information gathered from her mother and her boyfriend, the treatment staff began to form a broader picture of Ms. V. Her father's alcohol abuse was found to be of greater severity and extent than previously recognized. Moreover, his own father and an uncle had also been alcohol abusers, if not alcohol dependent, and his mother had committed suicide. Ms. V's own history raised questions about the possibility of a major affective disorder. There were periods in her life when, for several weeks at a time, she reported being somewhat incapacitated by feelings of depression. Usually, these periods were accompanied by feelings of guilt, tearfulness, and sleep difficulties.

The treatment team requested psychological testing not only to explore the contribution of a major affective disorder to Ms. V's present difficulties, but also, given her rapid adjustment to the more structured aspects of her treatment, to evaluate the possibility of entering her into a more insight-oriented psychotherapy.

Psychological Assessment

Ms. V was examined by the treatment staff's psychologist during the third week of her hospital stay. She was given the WAIS-R, the Bender-Gestalt, the MMPI, the Rorschach, and the SCT. She completed her testing in an efficient fashion, requiring just over two hours of time. The examiner described her attitude towards the testing as cooperative and formed the impression that she enjoyed the testing. Ms. V was pleased with her better performances and was obviously frustrated by her weaker performances.

On the WAIS-R, Ms. V's achievement on both the verbal and performance subtests indicated that her intellectual abilities were within the average range, with her performance scores somewhat better than her verbal scores. Her pattern of performance on the WAIS-R subtests indicated that her interactional style was one of adaptation and accommodation. Although her low *Comprehesion* subscale score suggests some difficulty in adopting and acting within conventional normative guidelines, her *Digit Span, Picture Completion* and *Picture Arrangement* subscale scores indicate a strong reliance on external reality to provide contextual cues to orient her behavior. This mix of features suggests that she is attentive to and easily influenced by her interpersonal surroundings. She seemed generally able to concentrate and there was no evidence of psychomotor slowing that would indicate a serious depressive disturbance.

On the MMPI, Ms. V did endorse several items suggesting some degree of depression was present and lending some support for the treatment team's concern. The depression subscale (*scale 2*) was scored at 79T, a clinically significant elevation, and one of only three scales scored in the clinically significant range. Also elevated and in the clinical range were the hysteria (*scale 3*) and paranoia (*scale 6*) scales. This 3-point configuration (2-6-3) reflected her difficulties in expressing her feelings, particularly hostile or aggressive feelings. Individuals with similar MMPI profiles are usually described as somewhat naive and unassuming and typically hold themselves responsible for the problems of others. Consequently, the treatment team's concerns regarding the presence of significant depressive features and accompanying feelings of guilt were seen as consistent with her overall personality makeup.

Ms. V's Rorschach protocol helped to illustrate her personality style but did not strongly support the possibility that Ms. V was very depressed at the present time. She gave a total of 40 responses and over 15 percent of these contained color as a determinant. Her productivity on the Rorschach was consistent with her perseverance on the WAIS-R. However, she produced a predominantly form-determined record and few well-integrated, whole responses, indicating her efforts to cling to the obvious and her difficulties in creatively exerting herself. Her only response to *card III*, one of her better whole responses and one of her popular responses, is of two people "trying to keep warm over a fire." This response reflects her need for external sources of encouragement and nurturance, factors critical for the maintenance of her own self-esteem. Her general concern regarding how she is viewed by others is also supported by the large number of shading responses (*cards I, IV and VIII*).

The remainder of her whole responses often involved humans or human details, including "two little kids playing on a see-saw" on *card VII*, and "faces" on *cards VII* and *IX.* The faces to *cards VII* and *IX* are poor form responses and the latter "face" occurs in an interesting sequence of responses to *card IX.* She begins by seeing a "Halloween witch, orange, and with a pointed chin and hat and laughing." She sees this face as a "mean face. These are the nostrils right in hers, the eyes and a long, mean mouth." She next reports something "melting and separating." The basically poor form quality of the responses and their somewhat fluid characteristics reflect her own fluid identity. She is uncertain about how her self-integrity and fearful of literally "melting and separating." She seems most secure if the environment is one filled with love and laughter (see also SCT 32) and most threatened if it is filled with meanness, requiring her to be distrustful of the behavior of other people.

On the SCT, Ms. V gives the most graphic indications that her own sense of self is intimately bound up with what others think and feel about her. She reports, for example, that *when he refused her, she* "made sure she knew that it wasn't because she was a bad person," that *when I am criticized, I* "listen and usually trust the opinion," and that *she felt inferior when* "she felt she wasn't as good as anyone else." Although these responses most likely represent long-standing trends in Ms. V's personality style (e.g. *as a child my greatest fear was* "not being loved"), they are currently exaggerated by family circumstances (*I am afraid of* "losing the people I love most" and SCT 45).

Her disappointment in her father is especially evident in her SCT responses. She is depressed and annoyed with her father and finds his affair confusing and threatening (SCT 9, 12, 34, 70 & 88). For Ms. V, her father's affair appears to seriously undermine her ability to see him as the "loving and caring man" (SCT 33) he was to her earlier in her life and she wishes that her father "wanted to be a father again" (SCT 96).

Equally confusing to her is her experience of her mother. She reports that *when with her mother, she felt* "both happy and sad" and wishes that her mother "stuck by feelings." Although angry and hurt by her parents' separation (SCT 100), at bottom, it is herself she most often blames for her problems (e.g. SCT 4, 6, 27, 43, 57 & 63). Central to her feeling of self-blame is her failure to communicate her own feelings (SCT 2 and 24), a skill she holds in high esteem (SCT 10 and 21). Finally, despite her feelings of disappointment, anger and self-blame, the SCT also gives evidence of her desires to succeed and to prove herself. She reports that *she felt proud that* [she] "recognized her problems and set forth to face them."

The examining psychologist reported that Ms. V's test results gave ample evidence of her difficulty in maintaining an adequate level of self-esteem and that depression and anger were feelings she struggled with in attempting to overcome her difficulties. The psychologist did not feel that these feelings were sufficiently overwhelming to Ms. V to warrant a diagnosis of a depressive disorder at the time of testing. However, because of her difficulty in adequately coping with these feelings without a high degree of directedness and environmental support, the psychologist recommended against a more insight-oriented psychotherapy at the present time.

Treatment Planning and Outcome

Ms. V's treatment team reviewed the results of her testing with the examining psychologist and developed a treatment plan focusing on her relationship with her parents, particularly her role as a go-between in maintaining her parents' marital relationship. She was able to understand that her eating disorder served as a distraction from her feelings of discomfort and emotional turmoil. She was able to see this discomfort as resulting in part from her role as go-between and recognized that her efforts to present each of her parents to the other in a positive light was an effort on her part to invent an idealized family constellation on which she could remain dependent.

To implement her treatment plan, separate weekly meetings, on alternating weeks, were arranged between Ms. V and each of her parents. This plan allowed her to deal directly and separately with each parent. In her sessions with her father, she was able to express her disappointment in him for failing to live up to her idealized view and later to address her resentment of his separation from the family. In her sessions with her mother, she was able to express her anger at her mother and explore how her previous inability to confront these feelings was related to her bingeing and vomiting.

As these sessions continued and Ms. V was better able to confront and explore her feelings for both her parents, she became concerned about maintaining control of her bingeing and vomiting outside the structure of the hospital's treatment program. She was encouraged by her treatment team to explore her newfound abilities by arranging for short leaves from the hospital. At first, these leaves were explicitly arranged around times and activities that did not involve an opportunity for her to eat while out of the hospital. She was able to enjoy these leaves and was relieved to find that impulses to overeat did not intrude on her enjoyment. As her confidence in herself increased, she was able to extend the length of these leaves so that meals away from the hospital could be included. She was reassured to discover that the strategies she had learned while in the hospital were equally effective outside the hospital.

Ms. V's confidence in herself continued to grow and discharge planning was begun. Initially, she wished to return home to live, but quickly realized that this was not in her best interest. She finally accepted the treatment team's recommendation to establish an independent living arrangement and, with the help of her boyfriend, found a small apartment close to her school which she could share. She was discharged at the end of a two-month stay, planning to work as a salesgirl until she was able to resume her studies at the start of the new semester. She continued in outpatient psychotherapy with her hospital psychotherapist. When contacted a few weeks after her discharge, she reported that she was doing well and enjoying her new job. Her parents had initiated divorce proceedings and although she was saddened by their inability to work things out between them, she accepted the fact that she and they would now pursue independent lives.

EXHIBIT 1

AREA OF ASSESSMENT	CLINICAL EXAMINATION	PSYCHOLOGICAL EXAMINATION
I. Symptoms/Diagnosis *Bulimia Nervosa*		
Episode binge eating	Consumes large quantities of food several times a week	None
Feeling of lack of control of eating	Reports feeling "out of control"	Vacillates between efforts at overcontrol and experienced lack of control
Vomits, abuses laxatives, diuretics, etc. to stop weight gain	Admits to abuse of laxatives, diuretics and diet pills	None
At least two binges per week for at least three months	4–5 binge/vomit episodes per day for most of last year	None
Persistent overconcern with weight	Vomits/purges to control her weight	None
II. Personality Factors	None	Inappropriate guilt; often feels responsible for things outside her control
		Very dependent on others for maintenance of self-esteem
III. Cognitive Abilities	Average intelligence Reports diminished concentration; intact on examination	Average intelligence Mild concentration difficulty
IV. Psychodynamics	Mediates conflict between her parents to alleviate her own dependency feelings	Idealizes parents and feels she contributes to their shortcomings
V. Therapeutic Enabling Factors	Motivated for treatment	Strives to put forth her best effort

AREA OF ASSESSMENT	CLINICAL EXAMINATION	PSYCHOLOGICAL EXAMINATION
	Rapid adjustment to the structure of the treatment milieu	None
VI. Environmental Demand and Social Adjustment	Has maintained academic progress	Difficulties in self-assertiveness and emotional expression
	Good relationship with her boyfriend	Seeks nurturing relationships
	Peer influence diminishes her self-control	Hypersensitive to external criticism

EXHIBIT 2

WAIS-R SUMMARY

Verbal Subtests	*Scaled Score*
Information	8
Digit Span	13
Vocabulary	11
Arithmetic	9
Comprehension	7
Similarities	9

Performance Subtests	
Picture Completion	11
Picture Arrangement	12
Block Design	9
Object Assembly	11
Digit Symbol	12

Verbal IQ	97
Performance IQ	106
Full Scale IQ	101

MMPI SUMMARY

F-K/L 263'71084-5/9:

RORSCHACH SUMMARY

Number of Responses	40
Rejections	0
Populars	6
Originals	0
F%	63
F + %	82
A%	40
H%	35
W:M	7:3
M:Sum C	3:3.5
m:c	3:6

RORSCHACH SUMMARY

VIII-X%		45
FK + F + Fc%		73
(H + A):(Hd + Ad)		22:8
Apperception	W	17%
	D	62%
	d	8%
	Dd + S	13%

E X H I B I T   3

RORSCHACH SUMMARY

Response	*Inquiry*	*Scoring*

I.

I have to find some sort of picture?

1. A profile of a German shepherd.	1. Shaped like a shepherd.	drF-A
2. A face, distorted, but . . . a jack-o'-lantern face.	2. The shape with the white eyes and mouth.	DF(Hd)
3. Legs and body.	3. Just the shape.	DFHd
4. This is also a person. The outer shading shows the clothes and it has a head.	4. Shaped like a person. It looked like it was wearing a dress from the way the shaded part looked.	DFcHP

II.

1. Heart	1. The way the red goes like that (*traces with finger*). Shape and color.	DFCAt
2. Dog	2. Shape	DFAP
3. Face with eyes, nose, and mouth. And this is the rest of the face.	3. Shape	DF-At

III.

1. Person. Whole thing looks like they are trying to keep warm over a fire.	1. Looks like it.	WMHP

IV.

1. Leg and shoe of Big Foot.	1. Shape only.	DF(H)P
2. Top view of a monster, a dinosaur or an alligator.	2. Shaped like a dinosaur or alligator.	DFA
3. Mushroom	3. Fine lines and shading.	dFcBt
4. If you flipped this over, these leg-type things, this could be one long thing, and this would be the spine.	4. Shaped like legs and the spinal column.	WF-At

RORSCHACH SUMMARY

Response	*Inquiry*	*Scoring*
V.		
1. A bat	1. Just the shape.	WFAP
2. A silhouette, on the side. There's a nose, mouth and hair.	2. Looks like nose and mouth. Shaded like hair.	DFcHd
3. Snails head with those slimy antennae	3. Shading makes it look slippery, like a snail's head.	dFcA
VI.		
1. This is definitely some sort of animal, a fish or something. Fins or wings on it.	1. Fins or wings make it look like an animal.	DFA
2. A head.	2. The shape of the head makes it look like a man.	DFHd
3. This whole dark area, a light bulb. There's the base and the part you screw in. A lamp without a shade.	3. Shaped just like a bulb, a lamp.	diF Obj
4. This is the moon, here in the dark part, the crescent, carve it out here and a face, an old man's face. Like in those books you'd see a face in the moon.	4. Shape	drF-Hd, Moon
VII.		
1. Two little kids playing on a seasaw and facing each other.	1. The ponytail sticking up.	WMNHP
2. Could also be a dog.	2. Way it's shaped and the snout over here.	DFA
3. Face	3. The eyes and cheekbones and mouth, big face, whole thing.	W(s)F-Hd

RORSCHACH SUMMARY

Response	*Inquiry*	*Scoring*
VIII.		
1. Animal on the side. These animals are climbing to top of peak and being pushed like over here but they'll make it up.	1. Face, legs and tail.	DFM A
2. Heart	2. Color and the shape, even though this is here. I see the shape forming even though it's not clear.	DFCAt
3. Water, ocean, moving kind of. It seems like it's expanding. Reminds me of H_2O.	3. Color. The way it shades the waves and ripples.	drcF.mF Nat
IX.		
1. Halloween witch, orange with pointed chin and hat and laughing.	1. The shape. Looks very much like it.	DM.F(H)
2. I see like a face but I'm trying to . . . a mean face. These are nostrils right in here, eyes and long mean mouth.	2. Shaped that way. A human face from the outline. (?) Just looks mean.	DF-H
3. This inner thing is melting and separating.	3. The way it's shaped and the shading.	dmFcF Obj
X.		
1. Bunch of bugs.	1. Shapes	WFA
2. Worm	2. Green and its shape.	DFCA
3. Scorpion	3. All the legs.	DFA
4. Cricket	4. I think that's the name of a bug, they're leggy.	DFA
5. Bugs with antennae.	5. Things sticking up, insects.	DFA
6. Snail or slug	6. The hump, its body is fat and curvy.	DFA

RORSCHACH SUMMARY

Response	*Inquiry*	*Scoring*
7. 2 doves facing each other and this is a music note they're singing.	7. Beaks and heads and wings, maybe color, maybe shape. They're kissing.	DF.FCA
8. Note (musical).	8. It just comes away from the kissing or singing doves and the shape.	DF Obl
9. Yellow things are canaries or birds.	9. Color and the shape, the feathered tail. (*Feathered?*) The way I picture it. It doesn't really look that way.	DFCA
10. White is a profile of a face on either side and	10. Shape of human face.	SFHd
11. Then the pink is also a face.	11. Shape. A person's face.	DFHd
12. If I look at the whole thing I see a butterfly. This could be the middle (draws line with finger) and the rest is wings.	12. The shape, it's not filled in or anything, the colors on either side, and the points up here are antennae.	WFC-A

E X H I B I T   4

SENTENCE COMPLETION TEST

2. *She often wished she could* "have an easier time communicating her feelings."

4. *She felt to blame when* "she failed to attempt her goals."

5. *When he refused her, she* "made sure she knew that it wasn't because she was a bad person."

6. *I used to feel I was being held back by* "my own hangups."

7. *She felt proud that* "she recognizes her problems and set forth to face them."

8. *As a child my greatest fear was* "not being loved."

9. *My father always* "made me believe that he spent all his time on his family."

10. *The ideal man* "should be honest, open, loving, and among others, have the quality of communication."

12. *I was most depressed when* "I learned my father had an affair."

19. *I could hate a person who* "is dishonest and deceiving."

24. *When I think back, I am ashamed that* "I couldn't communicate a lot of feelings I had."

27. *She felt her lack of success was due to* "her lack of self-esteem."

29. *I used to daydream about* "being a talented and well-known dancer."

30. *Most men* "get to a point in life when they feel that they only need themselves."

32. *Love is* "a beautiful and growing feeling."

33. *My earliest memory of my father* "was a loving and caring man."

34 *I was most annoyed when* "I couldn't understand what my father had done."

35. *When she thought of her mother, she* "felt badly."

42. *When I am criticized, I* "listen and usually trust the opinion."

43. *She felt she had done wrong when she* "realized she was taking her problems out on herself."

45. *I used to feel 'down in the dumps' when* "I thought about all the hurt my family and I were feeling."

57. *She did a poor job because* "she didn't try her hardest."

SENTENCE COMPLETION TEST

63. *Whenever she does below average work, she* "knows she could have done above average."
70. *When my father came home, I* "was confused."
87. *I am afraid of* "losing the people I love most."
88. *When with her father she felt* "like she didn't know what to say."
94. *When with her mother, she felt* "both happy and sad."
96. *I wish that my father* "wanted to be a father again."
99. *I wish that my mother* "stuck by feelings."
100. *I feel sad about* "my parents' separation."

DISCUSSION

We illustrated the testing results and related treatment planning of patients with eating disorders with the cases of two young women: Ms. C, a 15-year-old adolescent, who presented with symptoms of anorexia, and Ms. V, a 21-year-old college sophomore, who presented with bulimia. Both women were hospitalized on a behaviorally oriented treatment unit. It is important to note that on this unit, which specializes in the treatment of eating disorders, testing is not ordered until the patient has adjusted to the unit and eating habits and weight have been somewhat normalized. Thus, the testing results cannot be totally explained by initial stress on entering the hospital or gross malnutrition resulting from the eating disorder itself.

Ms. C, an energetic high school student who was active on the track team, took the insult of losing an election as cheerleader badly. Her disappointment magnified her obsession with weight into anorexic proportions. As the parents, with direction from the pediatrician, moved in to help her, she became more distraught and suicidal. Once admitted to the treatment unit, she quickly attained her target weight, and psychological testing was requested to evaluate her personality strengths and difficulties and her ability to profit from dynamic psychotherapy.

Intellectually, she tested in the very superior range. Symptomatically, she reported primarily depression, anxiety and social withdrawal on the MMPI. Despite her intelligence, the projective materials revealed a simple, somewhat dependent and regressed individual who wanted to avoid the assumption of adult roles and individual responsibility. Considering these aspects of her personality, she responded better to family therapy than to individual therapy but was hospitalized a second time before some substantial progress in overcoming her anorexia was accomplished.

Ms. V's symptomatic bulimia presented in the context of otherwise normal development. She was making satisfactory progress in college, obtaining marks that were representative of her high school work, and she had social skills that helped her to develop a relationship with a boyfriend and with peers. It would appear that a "coping" strategy of eating but avoiding putting on weight by vomiting became a pattern of bulimic abuse slowly but surely. There was, to be sure, considerable strain in her parents' relationship that developed coincident with her symptoms, but she was away at college and it is difficult to directly link her symptoms with the parental strife. However, the relationship between father and daughter seemed overly intense and exclusive of the mother.

The extent of the bulimia occasioned a hospitalization, and she was placed on a behavioral program. Testing was requested to explore the extent and severity of associated depression. The patient's adjustment to the unit, receptivity towards treatment, and test results all suggested that she could utilize her considerable strengths to obtain significant assistance from treatment. Concerning the breadth and severity of depression, on the MMPI the patient reported some symptoms of depression, enough to have a T score in the significant range. Her projective materials also suggested low self-esteem related to her depressive affect. Another prominent feature of her test protocol was paranoid ideation, suggested by the high score on scale 6 of the MMPI and the multiple faces and eyes perceived on the projective materials.

Ms. V was seen as reacting to considerable family discord, a situation in which she was triangulated, but with considerable personal strengths. She was not seen as having substantial personality disorder pathology. Her school accomplishments and social skills and social successes indicated that she is likely to make a good therapeutic alliance and further her own growth through good use of individual psychotherapy.

In comparing these two cases, Ms. V was more independent and had a wider range of strengths than Ms. C. Of course, Ms. V was older and her development more advanced than was Ms. C's at the time of hospitalization and testing. Given this difference, however, it did seem that Ms. V was more independent, less shy, and more able to leave the protection of the home base. However, Ms. V seemed to be more influenced by family conflict, whereas Ms. C was idealizing her family and found family meetings helpful in aiding a more realistic expression of her feelings towards them.

B. CONDUCT DISORDERS: GROUP AND UNDIFFERENTIATED TYPES

Conduct disorder is a diagnosis in DSM-III-R under the general heading of disorders usually first evident in infancy, childhood or adolescence. The conduct disorders are subdivided into group type (conduct disordered behavior as a group activity with peers), solitary aggressive type (individual aggressive behavior), and undifferentiated type (a mixture of solitary and group conduct disordered behavior). The defining characteristic of the conduct disorders is a persistent pattern of behavior in which age-appropriate norms and rules of conduct are violated. These behaviors, which break societal norms, include stealing, running away from home, lying, truancy from school, destroying others' property, using weapons and initiating fights, and cruelty to people or animals.

It certainly seems quite plausible that disruptive behavior which breaks society's rules may be motivated by quite different constellations in different individuals. This differential path to common conduct disordered behavior is one of the main reasons for psychological testing in these cases. One crucial assessment question is the possible absence of superego structures. It is common clinical wisdom that when conduct disordered behavior is related to a cry for help and depression in an individual who does have developed superego structures, the prognosis for treatment is much better than if these factors are not present.

CONDUCT DISORDER, GROUP TYPE AND
MIXED SUBSTANCE ABUSE

Mr. P, a 17-year-old student about to repeat the 10th grade, was transferred from a local community hospital where he was being treated for a sedative overdose. The overdose followed on the heels of his mother's exasperation at his continued drug abuse and her informing him that she was about to seek psychiatric consultation on his behalf. After she went to sleep that night, her son removed a bottle of pills from his mother's bathroom cabinet and took them "to get high." For the last year, Mr. P had "stopped caring about anything but getting high." He had stolen money from his mother to purchase drugs, had been arrested by the police for "joy riding" with some friends—using the cars of his friends' parents without permission, had set fires in an effort to get money from arcade games in order to purchase drugs, was chronically truant from school, and often came home bloodied from fights he'd had while high. He had returned home only a few days before after an absence of nearly a week. He said he'd "run away" but had returned home when he ran out of money and had no place to stay.

The previous summer, Mr. P's mother had gotten him into a drug treatment and rehabilitation program. He had remained drug-free for three weeks after completing the program, but when school started in the fall, he had quickly returned to his previous drug habits with a vengence. He began experimenting with hallucinogens, PCP, and heroin and was regularly using marijuana and Valium. He was especially fond of Valium since it helped him "not care" about things. Having developed a tolerance to the drug, he found himself in need of ever-increasing amounts and the cash to purchase it on the street. In the year prior to the onset of his drug abuse, Mr. P had maintained a B average. His average during the last two school years had fallen off to a D.

Mr. P was found in a semicomatose state by his mother the following morning. She had him taken by ambulance to a local community hospital where he was placed in intensive care to monitor his recovery. On the advice of his physicians there, Mr. P's mother sought admission for him at a nearby psychiatric hospital.

When admitted to the psychiatric hospital, Mr. P was casually but neatly dressed and was described as an attractive young man with striking green eyes and short, curly brown hair. He was oriented to time, place, and person and appeared to be suffering no untoward aftereffects of his drug overdose. He insisted that the overdose was not a suicide attempt, but did acknowledge that he had "stopped caring" about what happened to him and was nonplussed by his recent brush with death. Although he had accepted the recommendation for a psychiatric hospitalization, he gave as his only reason for seeking admission that "I have got problems." Asked to expand on this remark, he stated, "I want to go out and not take drugs." He admitted to feeling despondent over the last few weeks, but there were no other signs suggestive of depression. However, the examiner did note that his mental state during the last few weeks was difficult to assess in light of his chronic abuse of sedatives.

DSM-III-R Diagnosis

Axis I:	Conduct disorder, group type
	Mixed substance abuse, chronic
Axis II:	None
Axis III:	None
Axis IV:	Moderate—new school year and impending remarriage of his mother
Axis V:	Poor—marked impairment in his school functioning and moderate impairment in his peer relationships

Treatment and Hospital Course

Mr. P was admitted to a mixed adolescent and young adult unit where he very quickly made friends with the other patients and adjusted to the milieu with no difficulty whatsoever. As far as he was concerned, being in the hospital relieved him of the problem of managing his drug intake. He was placed on a schedule of random urine samples for drug screening and was enrolled in the therapeutic school on the grounds of the hospital. He was able to remain drug-free and attended all his classes where he did quite satisfactory work. During his first month in the hospital, occasional periods of dysphoric mood combined with a continuation of his desultory attitude towards himself, his treatment, and his school work led to a referral for psychological testing with a specific question regarding the possibility of a clinically significant affective disorder.

Psychological Assessment

Mr. P was referred for psychological assessment at the end of his first month in the hospital. His hospital psychotherapist wished to have the possibility of an underlying depression assessed and also asked for an estimate of the extent of his sociopathy. This information was requested in order to aid in determining if he would benefit most from continuing his inpatient treatment or if he might be more appropriately placed in a structured outpatient drug treatment program.

Mr. P received a WAIS-R, Rorschach, TAT and the Bender from the assessing psychologist. On the WAIS-R, he achieved a full scale IQ of 100 with verbal and performance IQs of 98 and 102, respectively. A consideration of his age-corrected subscale scores revealed that his performance on the WAIS was less consistent than these IQ scores might imply. His subscale scores ranged from low average to superior levels. His relative strengths were in those areas where concentration and attention to detail were required and his relative weaknesses were in those areas dependent on school-related past learning (i.e. *Information, Arithmetic* and *Vocabulary*). He was poorest on tests of practical and social judgment and visual-spatial comprehension.

On the Rorschach, Mr. P produced a total of 23 responses with no rejections. As he had been tested before, he made frequent references to his previous experience with the test. Several responses indicated his familiarity with the altered sense of reality engendered by his drug-taking history, especially his response to *card II* of something "breaking apart." A number of his responses began rather conventionally, but then were elaborated in idiosyncratic fashion. His human percepts were especially distorted, for example. On *card II*, he described "some sort of beast" with moustache and beard and a "big body and feet" from Fantasia. On *card VII* he characterized the "dancing girl" he saw as "weird." He seemed to be experiencing a somewhat peculiar world which he couldn't quite fully fathom, leaving him frustrated and angry, even out of control, at times, like the "nuclear explosion" and the "oil spurting out."

Many of his responses were seen in movement or with a sense of movement implied. Dancing (*cards II & VII*), flying and supporting and crashing (*card X*), exploding (*card IX*), and gushing (*card IV*) are all descriptions in the active voice and even the "skin as a rug" on *card VI* prompted him to observe that it "looks like when they kill a lion or something." Finally, his sensitivity to the shading in the blots, including shading in the colored areas (e.g. *cards VII & VIII*), taken together with the features already noted, mirrors pervasive inner distress and anxiety which he was endeavoring to control through action.

Mr. P carries through and expands on this theme throughout a notably unreflective TAT. Although he began conventionally enough with a story of a boy practicing his violin for a concert that night (*card 1*), he never again managed to relate a typical story involving a meaningful emotional relationship between the figures. Themes of grandiosity such as the "rich lady" on *card 2*, the appearance of Haley's comet on *card 14*, or the denigration of major political figures on *card 7BM* alternate with themes of remorseless exploitation or violence (*cards 13MF, 10, 4, 12M, 8BM* and *20*). Violence seemed to be the preferred response and criminality the preferred setting. Gangsters, other criminal activities, and wartime provided the setting for *cards 6BM, 12M, 8BM* and *20*. Even common misfortunes such as being laid off temporarily from a job resulted in contemplated mayhem (*card 4*).

Each of these stories was related in a bland, matter-of-fact manner, at best; in several cases, a more chilling undertone was apparent. For example, his response to *card 15*, which he found "morbid," was "I love it!"; the shooting on *card 8BM* left the shooter "Feeling satisfied"; self-defense was invoked to explain the shooting of a psychopath whose violence was courted in revenge for a close friend who was killed by the same man. Mr. P had perhaps the same theme in mind when he was asked for the meaning of *Strike while the iron is hot* on the WAIS and responded, "Get people in a more vulnerable period when they are more vulnerable to what you want."

The psychologist's report contained the observation that several of Mr. P's responses appeared to be delivered for their "shock value." Certainly, this is correct as regards their impact, if not their motivation. His attempts to distance himself from any troubling affects were seen, in overall context, as best understood as an attempt to avoid any painful situational stress. The absence of any emotional control, except to remain vigilant to what others expected of him, and the precipitousness of aggressive and sadistic impulses when thwarted left little reason to imagine that he would be amenable to psychotherapeutic efforts. His preferred mode of operation appeared to be a continuation of his substance abuse pattern as a means of providing a ready excuse for his more inappropriate behavior.

In summary, the psychologist formulated the case as one with primarily dyssocial aspects characterized by avoidance of feeling, absence of remorse, casual exploitation of others for immediate, personal gain, and an inability to empathize with or appreciate the rights of others.

Treatment Planning and Outcome

Mr. P continued to be well behaved, if uninvolved, during the next few weeks of his hospital stay. His individual psychotherapy sessions were characterized by a perfunctory compliance with the rules of attendance and conduct, but little of real value was accomplished despite increasing them in number from two to three times per week. His family sessions with his mother seemed more animated in that he apparently wished to return home and made many efforts to reassure his mother that he had finally recognized the error of his ways and intended to reform.

His mother remained unconvinced, but quietly so, and following the report of the psychologist's examination, his hospital psychotherapist attempted to place him in an outpatient drug treatment program. Although he was interviewed by the personnel of the program, he was refused acceptance into the program. The social worker who carried out the intake evaluation stated that Mr. P did not seem to sincerely wish to give up drugs and, in light of his poor motivation and his history of dyssocial behavior, she felt he was a poor risk for the program.

Upon learning of the outcome of this interview, Mr. P's mother became adamant in her refusal to take him home. Following a heated argument during a family session, Mr. P returned to the unit and cut his hand when he broke a window. He followed up on this outburst by quietly helping to plan a New Year party for the unit, for which he supplied "nonalcoholic" beer. Despite what had by now become routine urine screens, Mr. P returned from a pass seemingly intoxicated and the drug testing revealed recent alcohol and marijuana ingestion. Subsequently, he was caught cheating on his exams at school and a hunting knife was found among his personal possessions at the hospital.

Although several of these events prompted the staff to consider discharging Mr. P, he was retained each time as alternative discharge plans continued to be explored. He grew increasingly angry at the slow pace of his discharge and arranged to have himself accepted at a youth shelter from which he could return to his old school. Subsequent meetings with the head of the shelter, who felt able to support him in his wish to leave the hospital, managed to prevent an impulsive departure. Feeling somewhat supported in his own plans, Mr. P was able to make a good impression at an interview at a residential school in a distant state and was shortly discharged to this facility. He was able to stay out of trouble for several weeks but was caught sneaking back into the dormitory and was placed on closer supervision. At six months, he still remained on close supervision, but was not taking drugs and his school performance had been satisfactory.

E X H I B I T 1

Area of Assessment	Clinical Examination	Psychological Examination
I. Symptoms/Diagnosis		
Conduct Disorder, group type		
Six-month disturbance of conduct with:	Two-year history of difficulty with:	
Stealing without confrontation of victim	Stealing from mother's purse for drug purchase	Disrespectful of others rights
Often lies	Lies about school attendance, drug- taking	Uses drug abuse as an excuse for inappropriate behavior
Deliberate fire-setting	Sets fires at video game arcades	None
Often truant	Very frequently truant	Accepts no responsibility for his behavior
Often initiates physical fights	Often returns home bloodied in fights	Easily prone to aggressive or even sadistic acts
II. Personality Factors	Superficially charming and compliant	Overtly cooperative and engaging
	Able to profit somewhat from imposition of external structure	Complies with demands only when it does not interfere with his own wishes
III. Cognitive Abilities	Average intelligence	Average intelligence Attuned to external reality cues as guides to the expectations of others
IV. Psychodynamics	Disregards the rights of others and shows no remorse when they are perfunctorily violated	No regard for rights of others when they stand in his way
		No well-integrated capacity for tolerating painful affect; prefers immediate action

AREA OF ASSESSMENT	CLINICAL EXAMINATION	PSYCHOLOGICAL EXAMINATION
V. Therapeutic Enabling Factors	Able to contain drug-abuse habits to some degree with external restraint	Ability to focus on and recognize others expectations
	History of better than average school performance prior to drug abuse	No evidence of learning disabilities
VI. Environmental Demand and Social Adjustment	Noncompliant with the demands of others if they thwart his own desires	Generally unable to comply with the demands of others unless impulses are restrained
	History of being able to make and keep close friends prior to drug abuse	Quickly manages to engage with others on an immediate need-gratifying level

EXHIBIT 2

WAIS-R SUMMARY

Verbal Subtests	*Scaled Score*
Information	8
Digit Span	12
Vocabulary	7
Arithmetic	8
Comprehension	6
Similarities	8

Performance Subtests	
Picture Completion	10
Picture Arrangement	11
Block Design	11
Object Assembly	7
Digit Symbol	10

Verbal IQ	98
Performance IQ	102
Full Scale IQ	100

Rorschach Summary

Number of Responses	23
Rejections	0
Populars	5
Originals	0
F%	39
F + %	82
A%	30
H%	30
W:M	14:3
M:Sum C	3:1.5
m:c	8:5
VIII-X%	26
Fk + F + Fc%	39
(H + A):(Hd + Ad)	10:1

RORSCHACH SUMMARY

Apperception	W	61%
	D	30%
	d	4%
	Dd + S	4%

EXHIBIT 3

RORSCHACH SUMMARY

Response	*Inquiry*	*Scoring*
I.		
1. A bat.	1. Cause of the black and the way it's shaped.	WFC'AP
2. It just looks like an insect, a butterfly. That's all. Nothing else.	2. Just the shape. Two wings and the body. (?) Could be either really, if you just think about the shape.	WFAP
II.		
Oh no!		
1. This looks like something somebody would see when tripping on acid. Bugs me out, very weird.	1. The whole thing and the way it's drawn. Just the shape. It looks like it was all one thing and it looks like it's breaking apart. (*Anything else?*) No.	WmFAbs
2. And it kind of resembles a face.	2. Eyes, nose, looked like some sort of beast. Mouth, moustache beard. (*Beard?*) Just the position. (*Anything else?*) No.	W(S)F-Hd
3. Ever see that movie Fantasia? It looks like one of those dancers with a big body and feet.	3. Legs, fat bodies, eyes. (*Anything else?*) No.	WF(H)
4. A pit, maybe. If it were 3-dimensional it would be a bottomless pit or something.	4. That one wasn't too good. *I wasn't sure if you were seeing it in three dimension.* No.	SFPit

RORSCHACH SUMMARY

Response	*Inquiry*	*Scoring*
III.		
Oh my favorite (*sarcastic*). I can't understand who drew these and why they all look like bugs.		
1. Top view of a bug, arms, eyes, mouth. The red has nothing to do with it.	1. The shape.	WF-A
2. Two people with arms, legs, heads. I don't know what they are doing. They've got a bowling ball. And this could be like an alley going down there and these are lights.	2. (*Alley?*) It doesn't. None of these things look exactly like anything. I'm saying it's two people bowling so that's what it would ·be. (*Lights?*) They're hanging. (*Else?*) No.	WM.FmH, Obj P
IV.		
1. It looks like a tree.	1. Trunk going up and if it were filled in more then it would resemble a tree more. (*Anything else?*) Shape and line going up the middle.	WFPN
2. And a monster or one of those things like Godzilla.	2. Feet. This has nothing to do with it. I cut that out. Unless he's going to the bathroom. Well feet, claws, head.	WFM(A)
3. An oil—you know—when you have a hole in the ground and oil comes spurting out.	3. There's a hole in the ground and oil's just coming up. Ground oil pushing out and spilling out. (*Anything else?*) Black color.	WmF.C′FO.

RORSCHACH SUMMARY

Response	*Inquiry*	*Scoring*
V.		
1. They all look like insects of some sort. This one even looks like a bat, too.	1. The shape and color. It's black and bats are black.	WFC'AP
VI.		
1. It looks like when they kill a lion or something and use the skin as a rug. Or some kind of animal.	1. The whiskers coming out. The basic structure of the whole thing. Looked like they cut it open and spread it out. (*Skin?*) The way it's lying down.	WFAobj.P
2. Hmm . . . I never noticed that. It could look like a ship. Half the picture.	2. Smokestack, gun, a fire, like in a war.	WF-Obj, Fire
VII.		
I never saw this one.		
1. Looks like the side of a mountain. Just using half, is that OK? (*Yes. It's entirely up to you.*)	1. Tree here, cliffs, down here is a stream or a valley. (*Anything else made it look like cliffs?*) The color—like at night time—grey with fog or something.	DC'FN
2. Not counting the bottom. Indian ladies, with feathers, facing each other.	2. Just shaped that way. Looks like that.	DMH
3. This is weird. This half looks like a girl, arms, legs, dress, and big hairdo.	3. That's how it looked to me. Looks like someone in costume, dancing.	DMH

RORSCHACH SUMMARY

Response	*Inquiry*	*Scoring*

VIII.

This one is my favorite.

1. A mountain lion on some rocks and a reflection on some water he's peering into. This one is so perfect, it looks so much like that, it's hard to see something else.	1. Water because it's the same thing on both sides. (*Rocks?*) Cause that's what I want them to be. Well, the way they are drawn, with crevices. (*Crevices?*) Looks indented, the different colors, it's darker. (*Reflection?*) The way that it's the same on both sides.	WFM.cFA,N

IX.

1. A nuclear explosion. The mushroom cloud.	1. Blowing up here and this is the mushroom. (*Explosion?*) The color.	WmF.CF Explosion
2. Looks like a hippie with his eyes and long hair. Looks like sunglasses, if you take off the green and pink.	2. Just the outline—eyes, hair, sunglasses.	drF-Hd

Rorschach Summary

Response	Inquiry	Scoring

X.

This is the weirdest one of all.

Response	Inquiry	Scoring
1. It looks like something in a cartoon cause of colors. The blue is rock that this guy crashes through.	1. Looks like something I would see in a cartoon. The position of it and general form (?). It could be blue because it's in a cartoon.	DCFRock
2. It looks like a birdman creature sort of thing. Flying downward. This thing will break, this thing will clip on and he'll land in there.	2. Has wings. Looks like some green birdman-type creature. Has that shape.	DFM.FC(H)

(Anything else?)

Response	Inquiry	Scoring
3. Just two creatures holding this up from dropping down.	3. Just the shape. Some kind of hands here holding this thing up.	DFM(A)

EXHIBIT 4

THEMATIC APPERCEPTION TEST

CARD 1   I hate this one. Can I tell the same stories I told last time? The boy has a violin. He plays the violin. Right now he's studying the music. Not really, his mind is wandering. (?) To a girl. He stops thinking about the girl and practices. (?) He has a concert to perform that night and he's studying the music to make sure he gets it right.

CARD 2   A rich lady sitting in her room. The door bell rings and she wonders who it is and all of a sudden the maid comes in and tells her who it is. (?) It's the bill collector and she gets angry. (?) She pays the bill.

CARD 3BM   Kid is playing with his friends in his house and they are playing rough and running around. He hits his knee and he's holding it. He fell down right there on the couch and that's a toy gun he was playing with.

CARD 4   This looks good. A guy and his wife. Hey, what's this lady doing in background? As they went in their house, someone knocks at door and they open it and let the person in. It's some guy. This guy looks angry. This guy says I'm from so and so, the company where this guy works and he says "you are laid off for a week." He's walking out and his wife holds him back and says "don't worry, you'll be back in a week," so he doesn't go out and tell guy off and maybe hit him.

CARD 6BM   This looks like a gangster. Comes in, tells the mother the head of mafia, his father, is dead. They're both upset and he feels like: "I have to be one to tell her."

CARD 7BM   Two men at a political camp. The politician is speaking. R and B are there but they are humble. This guy is disgusted with what he saw. The other, sees his expression and asks him what's wrong. He says I'm angry and disgusted with how they presented themselves.

CARD 8BM   I hate this one so much. That's a gun. This teenager shot this lady or man. I'll make it a man. It's in gangster days over moonshine. Earlier in the night, he tried to take the bullet out and here he is beside his gun. (?) They are going to catch him. (?) Feeling satisfied.

CARD 10   Two kids are in a classroom, college. This good looking girl walks into the room. She's new. They think she's a knockout. I'd like to go out with her. One guy—he's leaning over telling his friend what he thinks.

THEMATIC APPERCEPTION TEST

CARD 12M   Are his eyes open or shut? A kid goes to war. He's fighting on the front line. He gets shot. Brought to hospital and he dies. The father comes over to shut his eyes and pray.

CARD 13MF   This looks nasty. Guy goes out, gets in a fight with his wife, and goes out to a bar, meets a girl. This girl gets around. They go back to her place and they go to bed. And he wakes up next morning with a hangover. He goes home and confesses to his wife what happened. (?) She'll forgive him 'cause he was drunk.

CARD 14   A guy comes home after work, gets a beer, sits down in front of the TV and watches the news. Soon Haley's Comet will go by and to get the full effect, he shuts off the light to watch for it. (?) He can't wait to see it. Excited. (?) Haley's Comet will pass by and he'll go to bed.

CARD 15   Oh my God, what's that? I'll make up a scary story! This is morbid, I love it. It is Sunday. Wait, I want to think. And this guy is driving along and he sees somebody on the road who looks like his daughter who is dead. So he goes to her grave and visits. He's mourning in front of her grave. It's very dark out and you can see he's worn out by all that has happened with his daughter.

CARD 20   This is Central Park in the city. This guy has had a few too many to walk in the park and he knows there is a psychopath loose. He wants to get the psychopath 'cause he killed a close friend of his. So he's walking. All of a sudden, he hears something and this guy with a knife says "I'm going to kill you." This guy calmly pulls out his gun and says "Let's go, I'm taking you to police." Psychopath runs at him and he shoots him. Police came, he's let go 'cause of self defense. Psychopath stays alone.

CONDUCT DISORDER, UNDIFFERENTIATED TYPE

Ms. A was "dropped off at the hospital" by her parents after she was returned to her home by the police. She had left home several days previously after stealing a neighbor's car and some money from her mother. She was arrested by the police, after a high-speed chase, in a city several hours away, where she had gone to visit friends. She ran away this time because her father had "grounded her" after she was fired from her last job as a hostess for stealing. Although only 17, she had not attended school since the beginning of the school year and had only completed the 10th grade.

This was not the first time Ms. A had run away from the family home, nor was it her first theft. Since the beginning of the present school year, she had refused to attend school. She had been staying home and "having fun." Her chief entertainment had been shopping with credit cards she stole from her mother and driving her father's car without permission. She had two jobs for a few days each but was fired from both for stealing either merchandise or cash from the register. She had been a "behavior problem" since the eighth grade and had been expelled from two boarding schools for chronic lying, running away, cheating, and poor academic performance. She had been seen in outpatient treatment several times, but had always refused to continue after a short time. Although she always promised to follow the rules at home and school, she was soon in trouble again. This time, after consulting with a prominent local psychiatrist with a specialty in conduct disorders, her father finally persuaded her mother to agree to having her hospitalized for treatment.

At the time of her admission, Ms. A volunteered that she was requesting hospitalization "because I want to try to make a better life for myself and be able to succeed in the outside world." Her mental status exam was unremarkable except for a noticeable apathy with regard to the seriousness of her behavioral difficulties. She expressed agreement with the view that her hospital stay would help her to "take responsibility" for her actions.

DSM-III-R Diagnosis

Axis I: Conduct disorder, undifferentiated type, severe
Axis II: Mixed personality disorder
Axis III: None
Axis IV: Mild—chronic family arguments and marital conflict
Axis V: Poor—no close friends; dropped out of school

Treatment and Hospital Course

Following her admission, Ms. A expressed feeling "trapped" in the hospital and focused on getting the hospital staff to "come up with some kind of treatment for me outside the hospital." She claimed that her parents had inappropriately hospitalized her "because I went to Cleveland" and she promised to mend her ways if released.

The efforts of the hospital psychotherapist to contact the parents were frustrated by their departure from the country. For several days, no one seemed to be able to contact them. During this time, Ms. A was on the phone frequently and eventually acknowledged that she was in contact with her parents several times a day. These conversations consisted primarily of her promising to follow her father's rules and pleading with him to get her released from the hospital. The hospital staff contacted the parents, who agreed to limit her phone contact with them and to support her staying in the hospital. Ms. A begrudgingly complied with restriction of her overseas calls to her parents, but gave out her mother's telephone credit card number to the other patients on the unit. When confronted about this by the hospital staff, she stated that her parents would just think the charges were her own and could easily afford to pay them.

Psychological Assessment

Although Ms. A evidenced few clinically significant signs or symptoms of an affective disturbance, her chronic history of impulsivity, behavioral dyscontrol and occasional tearful pleadings for release from the hospital led to a referral for psychological testing to rule out the possibility of a primary affective disorder and borderline personality disorder. She was examined by the psychologist during the second week of her hospital stay and received the MMPI, WAIS-R, the Forer Structured Sentence Completion Test, the Rorschach, TAT, Bender and DAP. The examining psychologist found the patient engaging and cooperative. She required little encouragement to put forth her best performance. She was examined on two occasions and although she kept both appointments, she did so on one occasion at the expense of a concurrently scheduled psychotherapy session which she "forgot."

Ms. A's WAIS-R performance indicated a verbal IQ of 114, a performance IQ of 126 and a full scale IQ of 120, placing her in the superior range of intellectual functioning overall. Her relative weaknesses were on the verbal subscales of *Information* and *Similarities*, but even here her performance was within the average range of functioning. Her relative strengths were on the *Digit Span* and *Picture Arrangement* subscales, which indicate an absence of anxiety and readily mobilized attention and concentration. She was quick and efficient on the timed tasks and, where possible, almost always received time bonuses for her productions.

On the verbal subtests, the efficiency of her performance was occasionally disrupted by her desire to demonstrate her personal feelings. For example, on the *Comprehension* subtest, she gave "feeling guilty" as a reason for borrowing money from a bank rather than from a friend but then went on to note that "I'd just feel uncomfortable." Later, on the same subtest, Ms. A gave "if you've got a chance, go for it" as an interpretation of the proverb *Strike while the iron is hot* and also said that to her this meant "take advantage of all that you can." Finally, reflecting both personalizations and a tendency for inappropriate playfulness, she gave as her first definition of *matchless*, a *Vocabulary* item, "That's me right now, I'm on match restrictions."

On the structured and semistructured personality tests (the MMPI and SCT, respectively), there was additional evidence of her general lack of anxiety. She reported no significant distress on the MMPI (*F scale*) and although showing a clear understanding of social norms (*K scale*), endorsed many items indicating difficulties in impulse control and a generally rebellious and nonconformist attitude (*scale 4*). Individuals with similar profiles are most often described as egocentric and shallow, do not profit from the consequences of their prior experience, and often have an unusually high tolerance of, and threshold for, punishment.

Although on the SCT she occasionally makes reference to these latter difficulties (e.g. *When I have to make a decision, I* "usually don't think about it for long enough"), she most often presents a picture of a happy, serious young woman with hopes and aspirations for a life of middle class success and conformity. Her life is marred only by the marital discord between her parents and she is quick to point out that although she feels "sad about my parent's relationship with each other," her own relationship with each of them individually is harmonious and fulfilling. She reports that *My father always* "made me feel like I was a special person, I was always his 'little girl'" and that *My mother always* "took care of my sister and I very well." By contrast, on the less structured TAT (*card 7GF*), she sees parents as insensitively deserting their child to go on a trip.

The themes of family disharmony and conflicting values serve as the touchstone for virtually all of her TAT stories. Most often, opposing loyalties serve to engender the conflict: self-fulfillment versus filial duty (*cards 2 & 12M*); honor and duty versus love (*card 6GF*); loyalty to friends or family (*cards 4 & 13MF*). Such crises are most typically resolved by breaking with the family (*cards 2, 3BM, & 12M*), which allows the central character to achieve great fame or wealth or glory, sometimes in an antisocial setting. Although these stories are presented as conflictual, there is less tension in them than might be expected. The underlying theme of abandonment, as previously mentioned, seems to provide more than sufficient motivation for the unabashed pursuit of self-interest and, as *card 3BM* makes clear, self-defense or self-protection provides sufficient rationale for justifying even the most heinous of crimes. *Cards 3BM* and *12M* are instructive in another sense. These two stories point out, in turn, the vindication that comes from determination in the face of family objections and lack of family support.

Ms. A's willfulness is equally in evidence on the Rorschach. Her aside on *card II*—"See, when I get one picture stuck in my head, I can only see one thing"—and her comment on *card VIII*—"I know [it] is impossible but that is the way it looks"—both illustrate her proclivity for responding with what first catches her attention. Her impulsivity occasionally impairs her reality appreciation, despite the general ability to view test stimuli along more acceptably conventional lines. This was reflected on the Rorschach where she combined incompatible concepts solely on the basis of their location in contiguous areas of the blot. On *card VII*, for example, she saw "cats crawling on the side of a flower."

Her overall emotional life may have a poorly integrated, explosive quality, as well as conspicuous dysphoric components like her Rorschach percept (*card II*) of a "space ship *blasting off* . . . in a black atmosphere." At the same time she feels enormously angry, dramatically revealed in the female figure she drew with a pronounced scowl and hands clenched, at an environment experienced as rife with shifting and contradictory behavioral demands on her. Males and associated sexuality may be especially unfathomable to her. In consonance with this confusion, her drawing of a man emerges as an androgenous-looking mannequin, but wearing a distinctly phallic-shaped tie. By comparison, her response to Rorschach *card IV* is a very destructive human-like "Big Foot eating a tree."

Treatment Planning and Outcome

In his report, the examining psychologist highlighted Ms. A's impulsive potential, despite an adequate understanding of conventional modes of thought and behavior, and the general absence of any evidence of either anxiety or guilt in her record. The psychologist also noted that she evidenced little likelihood of profiting from psychotherapy. Her need for more immediate gratification and the absence of any strong, internal motivation for change were described in this context.

Ms. A's psychotherapist struggled with whether or not to take her promises to remain well behaved at face value. Although she appeared to take some responsibility for her conduct when discussing these matters with him, there was little evidence in her daily life on the unit that she could be taken at her word. With the hope of establishing a greater atmosphere of trust and also of providing an opportunity to demonstrate her abilities to follow through on her commitment to a hospital treatment, she was allowed to come and go unescorted to her scheduled activities off her inpatient unit.

Ms. A was pleased at having won the trust of her psychotherapist and was aware that this had caused some friction between her and the other members of her treatment team. She reassured her therapist that this trust was not misplaced and that she would not directly disappoint him in this regard. For several days, she seemed to keep to her word. Little of consequence was reported regarding her behavior in the community and it began to seem that she might have finally come to terms with herself. However, within short order, the situation reversed itself when she failed to return from an activity at her usual time. Her psychotherapist, who was on vacation at the time, was notified of Ms. A's absence and her parents were contacted. They reported that they had not heard from her, but were not surprised at her elopement from the hospital.

Ms. A remained out of direct touch with her family for several weeks, although a general knowledge of her whereabouts could be gained from the trail of credit card receipts that flowed back to her parents' home. Finally, her parents reported their credit cards stolen and Ms. A was picked up by the police in a distant state when she attempted to use a credit card to make a large purchase. She was returned to her parents home when they refused to press charges and at last contact her parents were seeking another psychiatric admission for their daughter.

E X H I B I T 1

AREA OF ASSESSMENT	CLINICAL EXAMINATION	PSYCHOLOGICAL EXAMINATION
I. Symptoms/Diagnosis		
Conduct Disorder, undifferentiated type		
Six month disturbance of conduct with:	Three year history of difficulty with:	
Stealing without confrontation of victim	Uses family credit and car; steals on job	Places her own impulses and desires first before all else
Run away overnight, at least twice	Runs away to friends for several days and does not inform family of her whereabouts	None
Often lies	Lies about whereabouts	Offers whatever first comes to mind to justify her behavior, occasionally distorts reality
Often truant	Has refused school attendance for last year	None
II. Personality Factors	Awareness of ordinary social conventions	Prefers to flaunt authority
III. Cognitive Abilities	At least average intelligence	Above average intelligence
		Attentive to and easily utilizes social cues
IV. Psychodynamics	Chronic disregard for the rights of others; exploits the sympathy of others who offer help	Uses her knowledge of ordinary conventions and social privilege to promise and exploit others
	Feels no remorse for her past behavior	Takes no responsibility for her own behavior
V. Therapeutic Enabling Factors	Has used past treatment opportunities only to appease her parents	Claims appropriate ambitions

AREA OF ASSESSMENT	CLINICAL EXAMINATION	PSYCHOLOGICAL EXAMINATION
VI. Environmental Demand and Social Adjustment	Responds to limits by disregarding rights of others when her own impulses are thwarted	Will not tolerate for long any attempt to limit her behavior

EXHIBIT 2

WAIS-R SUMMARY

Verbal Subtests	Scaled Score
Information	9
Digit Span	13
Vocabulary	10
Arithmetic	11
Comprehension	10
Similarities	9

Performance Subtests	
Picture Completion	10
Picture Arrangement	15
Block Design	13
Object Assembly	12
Digit Symbol	12

Verbal IQ	114
Performance IQ	126
Full Scale IQ	120

MMPI SUMMARY

K'L/F: 4'836792115:0#

RORSCHACH SUMMARY

Number of Responses	12
Rejections	0
Populars	2
Originals	0
Average R/T Chromatic	9″
Average R/T Achromatic	4″
F%	33
F+%	88
A%	58
H%	8
W:M	10.1
M:Sum C	1:2.5

RORSCHACH SUMMARY

m:c		4:2
VIII-X%		33
(H + A):(Hd + Ad)		8:0
Apperception	W	83%
	D	16%
	d	0
	Dd + S	0

E X H I B I T   3

RORSCHACH SUMMARY

Response	Inquiry	Scoring

I. 2″

1. Like a sting-ray sort of.	1. Just the way it's going out . . . like the . . . Sort of just going like that. (?) And the little tentacles up there.	WFA
2. And a dog . . . the face of a dog.	2. These are the ears, the nose and then the two eyes here, and I don't know what these are supposed to be. These are just two extra . . . little white blobs.	W(S)FA

II. 10″

Oh my gosh (*laughs*).
Can I turn it upside down?
(*Yes*)

1. Okay, this is sort of a space ship blasting off, and this is the atmosphere.	1. This is the black part of the atmosphere, and this thing here is the space ship, and this is the fire that it's sort of blasting off with. (*Space ship?*) Just the shape of it. (*Atmosphere*) Although because when I saw the space ship that just sort of looks like the black of night or whatever. (*Blasting Off*) The way the ink is sort of splurted out and there's always fire when a space ship is taking off.	W(S)Fm.C′F-.mF Obj, Fire

RORSCHACH SUMMARY

Response	*Inquiry*	*Scoring*
III. 4″		
1. This looks like a mirror image of two people. Two women probably. No, two people. Should I tell you why? See when I get one picture stuck in my head I can only see one thing.	1. This is a person and that's a person and it's the view in the mirror because the same thing is sort of turned opposite. Head, nose, the body, the arms, the legs and the little feet. She's resting her hands on a toilet or something or a ball.	WMH, Obj P
IV. 6″		
1. This looks like Bigfoot eating a tree.	1. Because there are pictures in Colorado of Bigfoot and it looks like him. And because it looks like he had something coming out of his mouth and the picture in Colorado had something coming out of Bigfoot's mouth. (*Bigfoot?*) Yeah, it had big feet. Because it looked almost a little out of proportion but it would look mean because Bigfoot was not really that mean. (*Tree?*) Part looks like the roots down here.	WF(A),Pl
V. 5″		
1. It looks like a butterfly.	1. Because it looks like it had wings and it sort of had little designs on the wings. (*Designs?*) Here. Not really designs but little teeny smudges. And also the shape. It's sort of like a wavy-like line.	WFA

RORSCHACH SUMMARY

Response	*Inquiry*	*Scoring*

VI. 3″

1. A star with another star on top of it.

1. Because the bottom one was shaped like a star and so was the top little one. (*Else*) No. (*show me*) There's one there (*points*) and the top one is a little more deformed and it doesn't really look like a star. The like little sparks going out is like sort of the light just shining from it.

WFmObj

VII. 5″

1. This looks like a mirror image of two rabbits looking both like they're facing forward but looking back.

1. Because it looks like the long thing on top was an ear and their hands were sort of put in a rabbit sort of position like little paws sort of like that. I think their bodies were just sort of shaped like a rabbit. (?) Ears, face or the head, the paw and they're going down to the hind legs which are sort of blobbed together.

WFMA

VIII. 10″

1. It looks like a flower.

1. Because the shape and the colors. The pink and the orange colors and the shape, and sort of the stem and the leaves. The green leaves.

DCFPl

2. With two cats crawling on the side of it which I know is impossible but that is the way it looked.

2. It sort of looks like a cat with the body there with the legs and the tail and you can sort of see a little eye there, a little dark spot.

DFMA

Rorschach Summary

Response	*Inquiry*	*Scoring*
IX. 8″		
1. A pink mouse in a green jacket with orange pants.	1. The shape of the head and the big round ears, and that was pink. Then the green looked like almost a jacket because it had two arms going down. And then the orange pants just look like two legs with orange pants on. (*Mouse?*) Because head here and two ears. The arms going this way. The body of the jacket sort of going down, and the two legs there. (*where?*) Not really this part, no and this line.	WF/C(A)
X. 12″		
1. Umm, that just looks like a Picasso. Just bright colors.	1. Because it's just nothing. It's just splotches. (*Picasso?*) Because a lot of his pictures is modern art and I don't understand it and it just looks like paint thrown on canvas.	WCF Art

E X H I B I T   4

THEMATIC APPERCEPTION TEST

CARD 1 Right now the . . . what's he doing . . . he looks like he's trying to give her a violin. He doesn't know what's wrong with it. It's broken. He's confused. How do I lead up to this? (*Laughs*) His dog steps on it, I guess. This is hard. (?) And he went to class and he was put out of class because his violin was broken. Afterwards his teacher is going to come in and get him and tell him to play the tuba for today in class and send his violin to get fixed. But in the mean time he plays the tuba. (?) Confused because he wants to be in class and he loves his violin and can't figure out how to fix it.

CARD 2 Okay, right now this is a girl who comes from sort of a farming family and she sort of wants to break away from the farm life and become an educated person. Okay, before she talked to her parents about it and told them she didn't want to work on the farm. And by the look on her face, and her parents', they didn't agree. And she doesn't know whether she should go lead her own life or stay with her family. (*So they won't be angry with her?*) But she doesn't know which way to turn. Afterwards, um, she goes back and tries to talk to them and they say no way, you either farm or you go out on your own. And so she decides to go study and she becomes one of the first women to have a position in the American Government and she never hears from her family again. (?) She's torn between family and herself. (?) They are feeling sort of angry towards her. (?) To go get an education and try to do something more. She wanted to really be successful and do all she could with her life.

CARD 4 Um, okay. These two are married and he says he has to go leave home because, because. (*Why?*) Because. Oh gosh, this is so hard . . . because um, well . . . he's going to go with his friends and they have this big bank robbery planned and he couldn't turn on them now because it was the day of the big robbery and he had to go. His wife knows what he's going to do and she's trying to hold him back for the fear that he'll hurt himself, hurt other people, or get put in jail. Right before this, they were like arguing about it . . . and he stood up and stormed out and she went like running after him. And right after, he's going to turn around and say to his wife "you're more important than the bank" or something. (?) He really doesn't want to do it but he can't let his friends down. (?) And like it's the last hope to keep them together.

CARD 6GF Okay, the woman is surprised to see the man because she thought he was going to Europe for like the rest of his life and he just showed up at her house and she's like surprised. This is during the Second World War and they're in America but he's a Frenchman and he felt he had to go back and fight for his country. And she was all upset because she was worried he'd be killed fighting. And after he shows up, um, she asks why he's not in France and he says because it's not worth like losing everything I have in America. Then they live happily ever after in the United States. (?) Oh, the story changed. I decided to make it just for the war. (?) He's sort of determined and happy with this decision.

CARD 7GF Uh. Right now it's the nanny talking to the little girl. And her nanny is admiring the new doll her mother just gave her but the little girl isn't paying attention to anything the nanny is saying because she's looking off at a picture of her when she was a little girl which is on her mother's dresser. Oh, the nanny's reading a book! So instead of talking to her, she's reading the little girl a book. Umm, before the picture, the little girl's mother gave her the doll because the mother and father were going on a trip for about a month. And the little girl is just looking at the picture herself of when she was a baby and wondering when she was real small if her mother would never leave her. After she goes to bed, and she tucks in her doll and tells the doll that even when it gets older she'll always be there for it. (?) Of her when she was younger. (?) Thinking that she's never going to do to her doll what her parents did to her. (?) Europe.

CARD 13MF Okay, this is a depressing picture. Um, a man walks into sort of a dark room. Dark and dreary room. And he sees his wife lying on the bed naked and he bends down to look at her and she's dead. Um, he turns away and covers her eyes so that he won't see her. Before this happened, the girl was sitting alone in her room and her husband was a part of the mafia. And the husband defected from it because his wife didn't want him to be involved in it. And in retaliation, some mafia person came in and killed his wife. Afterwards, he feels very guilty because his wife had paid for his mistakes. Um . . . so he knows he can't get the police involved, so he just has his wife buried and goes and lives in the wilderness sort of far away for the rest of his life, sort of in isolation. (?) Feeling grief, and he feels that he almost caused his wife's death. (?) They strangled her I guess. (?) He was just a member (?) Just sort of sits in his log cabin and lives off the land and just thinks.

CARD 3BM Okay. Okay this is going to be a boring one. (Laughs) The woman was decorating the room. No I don't want to make it boring—cross that out. She is in a jail cell. And she tried to kill herself with a scissor lying on the ground but then she decided she had to pull herself together and get more strength. So she dropped the scissors and sort of just collapsed on the bed and started crying. Before this she was put in jail for a crime that she didn't commit and she had a sentence of 20 years. It became such a scandal and she was so embarrassed she never wanted to see anyone again because everybody thought she was guilty. This picture took place within like her 17th year. She just lost all hope afterwards. But then after the attempted suicide, she regained her strength and how to make her life go on. And she became a stronger person because of the whole incident. (?) Accused, she was accused of murdering her . . . a man that had actually tried to kill her (?) He was trying to rob her things. (?) Because things in the outside world were getting worse and worse and her family was still turned against her after 17 years and she realized she had nothing to go back to. (?) She's going to be so strong that she'll be able to survive with or without the support of her family and friends.

CARD 16 Oh my gosh—okay . . . why am I looking at this. Once upon a time, there was a man who crossed the road and bought some eggs and went home to make scrambled eggs and as he cracked one of the eggs, a chicken came out . . . a little baby chick . . . so he decided to keep it as a pet and raised the chicken and they lived happily ever after. I'm too tired to be creative. (?) A little shocked and then he was really psyched because this came to be his little buddy. (?) Because when I thought of chickens I thought of crossing the road.

CARD 12M Okay. This picture is the grandfather and his grandson. And the grandson is asleep when the grandfather comes in and sort of just blessed him goodnight. Before that the grandfather hadn't seen his grandson in many years and that night was the first night that the grandfather had come out to California. The father of the boy had come out to California many years before to mine gold but the grandfather felt his loyalty sort of towards the copper mines. No, toward the steel industry if it existed back then. So he finally comes out to California and sees his grandson and he's very proud of what a strong smart young boy he is. After, the next day, the grandfather decides to stay in California to get to know his son and grandson better and they all work together mining for gold, and they strike it rich and become millionaires.

EXHIBIT 5

SENTENCE COMPLETION TEST

2. *She often wished she could* become a famous broadway star.

9. *My father always* made me feel like I was a special person, I was always his "little girl."

12. *I was most depressed when* I was younger and my father hit my mother.

14. *When he turned me down, I* was disappointed for a while but then I moved on.

15. *Her new neighbors were* an English family with three young girls.

21. *The ideal women* would be intelligent, motivated, feminine, loving, and well-mannered.

29. *I used to daydream about* a huge, clear, calm lake with nothing but a daisy floating in the middle.

31. *When I used to make a decision, I* usually don't think about it for long enough.

33. *My earliest memory of my father* was when he used to throw me up and down in our library and then tickle me.

35. *When she thought of her mother, she* had only fond memories of their good times together.

43. *She felt she had done wrong when she* stayed out past her curfew and worried her mom and dad.

49. *People seem to think that I* am a cheerful and intelligent girl.

52. *Most of all I want* to make my parents trust me.

56. *At times she worried about* if she would forget to send her aunt a birthday card.

62. *Responsibility* is a vital part of maturity, and is necessary to lead a successful life.

73. *People in authority are* deserving of their position, so we must respect them.

100. *I feel sad about* my parent's relationship with each other.

DISCUSSION

The two cases we have chosen to illustrate the test battery of adolescents with conduct disorder involve a 17-year-old woman (conduct disorder, undifferentiated type) and a 17-year-old adolescent male (group type). In both cases, the disruptive conduct was blatant and could easily be assessed via history taking and interview methods. In both cases, psychological testing was called for in order to assess the possibility of depression and the relative strength of superego structures.

Most recently, it has become clear that adolescents, and even children, can and do manifest the classical signs of depression. The notion that depression in adolescents can be "masked" by acting-out behaviors which cover up the underlying depressive affect is still a clinically prominent one. It is quite possible that this latter clinical hypothesis was related to the test referrals in these two cases.

Ms. A. presents as a 17-year-old girl who was dumped at the hospital door by her wealthy parents. One gets the immediate impression from the history that her behavior is related to rage at her parents who ignore her no matter how outlandish her behavior becomes. She appears to be willing to perform any outrageous act (e.g., loaning her telephone credit card to the whole psychiatric unit) to get her parents' attention and the attention-getting quality of her behavior seems at odds with a truly psychopathic character. As noted before, testing was called for to assess the presence of depression in this context.

Testing revealed a bright young woman who admits to rebellious and nonconformist attitudes. Themes of family disruption and conflict were rampant in her TAT stories, almost a literal translation into projective material of what was going on in her daily life. The central character breaks from the family to achieve great success in an antisocial manner. There seems little doubt that a sense of deprivation and abandonment is driving her behavior. One might expect signs of depression in this context. Depression, in fact, might be a good prognostic sign as an expression of unmet needs. Unfortunately, this patient showed few signs of depression. For example, her score on scale 2 of the MMPI is within normal limits. Moreover, her superego structures are weak or nonexistent. Her prognosis, even with treatment, is quite poor.

Mr. P., a 17-year-old high school student, came to the attention of mental health personnel after a year of "getting high" on various drugs, climaxed with an overdose. This is an intelligent young man whose B average had plummeted in the year of drug abuse. The psychological testing was consistent with the history in that projective materials were filled with agitation and movement strongly suggesting an individual who approaches problems by action rather than by planning and/or thought. His TAT stories, like his personal life, are devoid of themes involving meaningful relationships between people. Not only do his stories bear the trappings of violence and crime, but he evidences enjoyment in the morbid and aggressive. Again, this record seems devoid of depression except for situational boredom, and there are no signs of superego concerns, or of tact and empathy in human relationships. Once again, the prognosis for meaningful treatment seems meager.

CHAPTER 3

Schizophrenias

A. UNDIFFERENTIATED AND PARANOID CHRONIC SCHIZOPHRENIA

Historically, there has been difficulty in arriving at a reliable diagnosis of schizophrenia due to the lack of clarity of the defining criteria. With the advent of DSM-III and DSM-III-R, the criteria are operational and reliable. The DSM-III-R schizophrenic is characterized by major disturbance in the following areas: content of thought (e.g. delusions), form of thought (e.g. loosening of associations, poverty of content of speech, neologisms, perseveration, clanging, blocking), disturbances in perception (e.g. hallucinations), affective expression (e.g. flat or inappropriate affect), sense of self (e.g. loss of ego boundaries, perplexity about one's own identity), volition (e.g. little or no self-initiated, goal-directed behavior, marked ambivalence), interpersonal functioning (e.g. withdrawal, emotional detachment), and psychomotor behavior (e.g. reduction in spontaneous movements and activity).

DSM-III-R provides criteria for identifying the following subtypes of schizophrenia: catatonic type, disorganized type, paranoid type, and undifferentiated type. In clinical practice, the catatonic subtype has become rare, and the majority of cases are of the disorganized type. A substantial minority are of the paranoid type (Pfohl & Andreasen, 1986).

Even those individuals who meet the DSM-III-R criteria for schizophrenia are a heterogeneous lot, and the recognition of subsets of schizophrenic patients is essential for treatment planning. Thus, it is probably not too helpful to offer a diagnosis of schizophrenia alone in a psychological report. Rather, one must address other issues relevant for treatment planning such as the number and nature of negative symptoms and positive symptoms, the presence or absence of paranoid ideation, and the quality of interpersonal relationships. The relative preponderance of negative symptoms (e.g. poverty of speech, poverty of content of speech, affective blunting, asociality, avolition, and attentional impairment) or positive symptoms (e.g. delusions, hallucinations, formal thought disorder, and bizarre behavior) not only provides useful prognostic information but also helps provide a focus for intervention.

The distinction between paranoid and nonparanoid subtypes is also relevant for treatment planning (Pfohl & Andreasen, 1986). The paranoid subtype is characterized by well-organized delusions, relatively well-preserved affect, minimal behavioral disorganization, and less likelihood of a family history of schizophrenia. The paranoid subtype is also less likely to show rapid deterioration. In contrast, the non-paranoid or disorganized subtype is twice as likely to have a positive family history of schizophrenia.

There is little collective data on the standard psychological test battery results in schizophrenic samples reliably diagnosed by DSM-III-R criteria. Just prior to the introduction of DSM-III, Exner (1978) summarized his data on a large sample of schizophrenics, diagnosed by clinical criteria, and found that the Rorschachs were characterized by evidence of thinking disorders, poor form quality, unusual verbal material, confabulatory thinking, and impaired perceptual accuracy.

SCHIZOPHRENIA, PARANOID, SUBCHRONIC

Mr. S, a 19-year-old Jewish adolescent, lived at home with his mother and aunt. He had not graduated from high school and had never been employed. He was brought to the hospital by his mother who had to have him certified as in need of mental treatment in order to arrange his admission. He saw no reason for his admission and gave as his reason for presenting himself at the hospital, "My mother brought me here."

He had been staying in bed all day and going out for most of the night for the last several months. He refused to give an account of this behavior to his working mother and to his aunt who is physically handicapped and draws social security disability. Recently, he was both verbally and physically abusive to his mother whenever she would persist in questioning him regarding his whereabouts. This abuse has led her on three previous occasions to attempt to take her own life, and she has even considered a combination suicide/murder in order to alleviate what she saw as both her and her son's suffering.

His aunt learned that he hung out in the neighborhood at night with a group of adolescents who smoked marijuana and hashish together. Two years ago, he had been asked not to return to his high school after being charged with smoking marijuana on the school grounds and vandalizing school property. He complied and simply dropped out of school. In response, his aunt pleaded with his mother to have Mr. S move out. At that time, he began behaving much as he had been in the last few weeks. His mother finally gave in to her sister's pleading and locked him out of the apartment. His exile from the family's apartment was brought to an end after three months when his mother visited him and found him living in filthy squalor.

When asked about his home life by the admitting psychiatrist, Mr. S admitted to some discomfort living at home. He found it difficult to be in the dining room because "there is too much wood around." He had also noticed changes in his hearing and had to ask his mother and aunt either to speak up or to speak more softly at times. He was polite during the interview and there was no evidence of the belligerence described by his mother. He was described as being of slender build and looking younger than his 19 years.

The examiner found no direct evidence for hallucinations although at first it was thought that his "hearing problems" might be the result of auditory hallucinations. Delusional material was elicited when he was questioned about the link between his discomfort and the wood in the dining room. He maintained that the presence of too much wood stopped his teeth from growing. Additionally, there were noticeable paranoid elements in his thinking insofar as he attributes his family's bringing him to the hospital as their way of "getting back at me for being lazy." He acknowledged that he and his mother fought a good deal but saw this as entirely her fault. Formal examination of his cognitive abilities provided evidence of some difficulty in concentration, but otherwise his mental status exam was considered to be unremarkable.

DSM-III-R Diagnosis

Axis I: Schizophrenia, paranoid, subchronic
Axis II: None
Axis III: None
Axis IV: Mild—chronic fighting with his mother and aunt
Axis V: Very poor—marked impairment in both social and occupational functioning

Treatment and Hospital Course

Although Mr. S's psychiatrist considered the diagnosis of schizophrenia most likely, he noted that both his mother and several of her relatives, including her sister, grandfather, and uncle, had all received psychiatric treatment for what appeared to be primarily depressive disorders. Consequently, he wished to delay the initiation of pharmacotherapy in order to have a chance to observe him in the hospital setting.

Mr. S was enrolled in the hospital school and gradually given a full schedule of therapeutic activities to help assess his abilities. Throughout his hospitalization, he generally cooperated with the plans made for him despite his concern that some of the sites of his activities, like his dining room at home, contained "too much wood." On the unit, he became friendly with some of the younger male patients, who generally treated him as a younger sibling, even when the actual age difference showed him as older than them. He enjoyed playing small pranks on the hospital staff, such as hiding out during hall checks and having food fights in the community dining room. As his four-month hospitalization was drawing to a close, he had done well enough in school to be scheduled for the General Equivalency Diploma exam and was considering future career plans as either "a Libyan terrorist or a pastoral counsellor."

Psychological Assessment

Mr. S was referred for psychological testing during the second week of his hospitalization to help establish his diagnosis. He accepted the need for the evaluation with some reluctance and was initially wary and somewhat guarded in his answers. He smoked nervously when given the chance to do so. As testing proceeded, he became more friendly with the examiner. He became more open and less constricted to the point where he was able to express his delight when he felt that his responses were taken favorably by the examiner. In light of the differential diagnosis, he was given a full battery of tests, including the WAIS, Rorschach, TAT, SCT, DAP and Bender.

His WAIS performance indicated that he was functioning in the *Average* range of intellectual ability with a full scale IQ of 101 and verbal and performance IQs of 112 and 87, respectively. His scaled subtest scores ranged from 6 on a pictorial test of discriminative judgment (*Picture Completion*) to 14 on tests of conceptual thinking (*Similarities*) and rote memory for numbers (*Digit Span*), demonstrating a high degree of intertest scatter. His highly variable performance on the WAIS and his especially poor performance on the Picture Completion subtest which required him to differentiate essential from unessential details indicated substantial impairments in his reality testing abilities consistent with a psychotic level of functioning. His impairment in reality testing was also evident on the Rorschach where he gave many poorly articulated responses with peculiar content and on the Sentence Completion Test which contained several contradictory self-statements.

Mr. S's retention of the capacity for abstraction and generalization as indicated by his relatively (and absolutely) high *Similarities* subscale score, taken in conjunction with his present impairment in reality testing, were seen as suggestive of delusional propensities. Additional paranoid elements in the test record included his frequent reference to "eyes" as the only feature supporting his perception of faces on the Rorschach and the attribution of menacing qualities to otherwise benign percepts. His preference for detail responses, including the use of small, idiosyncratic details, also were indicative of paranoid elements in his thinking. Finally, in his hypervigilant female human figure drawing, he drew the eyes closed and then carefully added the pupils of the eyes behind the closed eyelids.

There were also certain somewhat grandiose and expansive elements in Mr. S's test protocol that were consistent with his working diagnosis. He was unable to find space on a single sheet of paper for his Bender drawings and required a second sheet for the last two designs. On the Sentence Completion Test he reported feeling proud that he had "achieved his goal of education" (which he hadn't) and that his greatest desire was "to get married and have a good living" and that what he wanted most was a "good job with high pay." While these are certainly conventional expectations, they are clearly unrealistic. He noted that he hates to "go to school and work," and he felt that his boss "worked me a little too hard," an attitude which explains, perhaps, his history of unemployment.

Additional evidence from the test battery that was seen as consistent with Mr. S's diagnosis involved his understanding of and insight into ordinary human relationships. His low *Picture Arrangement* subscale score measuring anticipatory planning ability in a social context, his stereotyped and bland TAT stories, the absence of complete human and movement responses on the Rorschach, and his caricatured and bizarre human figure drawings all suggested a significant impairment in his relationships with others. He was especially ambivalent towards parental and other authority figures whom he represented as "loving," giving advice, and protective on the Sentence Completion Test.

In his Rorschach responses, however, which were much less susceptible to conscious control, cards often seen as reflecting attitudes towards male and female authority figures were seen as a "monster" and a "pig," respectively. Consistent with his paranoid stance in this regard was the unusual reference to the threat of unbridled aggression seen throughout the SCT (e.g. he could hate a person who "beats people up" and is afraid of "getting mugged while riding the train . . .") and Rorschach percepts of horned animals and alligators. A sensitivity to such threatening possibilities probably lies behind the vitiation of his female human figure drawing by omitting her arms while at the same time depicting her with clenched teeth. His inherently negative self-image and accompanying experienced vulnerability were mirrored in his clown-like male figure drawing with a silly hat but without shoes, as well as in his Sentence Completion item indicating that success cannot be achieved "without cheating."

In summary, Mr. S's test protocol seemed to support a diagnosis of paranoid schizophrenia. The findings of guarded, grandiose, and expansive elements in his thinking which he utilizes to defend against an underlying poor self-concept, impaired reality testing, poor social judgment, and empathic abilities were all consistent with the DSM-III-R diagnostic criteria for paranoid schizophrenia. It may be surmised that these difficulties were of fairly long standing in that there was little evidence suggesting the presence of anxiety. In this regard, his *Digit Span* performance on the WAIS was excellent, shading responses were virtually absent on the Rorschach, he relied on conventional, stereotyped methods of handling anxiety-provoking situations on the TAT and on the Sentence Completion Test, and seemed to be oblivious to the discrepancy between his aspirations and his abilities and achievements.

When he was made aware of these disparities, he seemed able to accept some responsibility for, and the consequences of, his lack of achievement. In one TAT story, the man worries that having lost his job he won't be able to provide food for his family. On the Sentence Completion Test he was ashamed that he "failed a few subjects." He went on to acknowledge that it was his own fault when "he failed" and he feels guilty about ". . . flunking and arguing." However, rather than addressing these difficulties directly by becoming "hardworking and ambitious" as he feels most people are, whenever he does a poor job he "gives up" or, as he reports in one TAT story where a husband is not in the mood to have sex with his wife, "go out and get drunk to forget his problems."

Although he remained hopeful about the future and seemed aware of the need to work towards his goals, there was evidence that he lacked the persistence or tenacity to fruitfully pursue them. In light of his multiple impairments, history of poor functioning, and diminished capacity to persevere, it was recommended some attention be given to bringing his aspirations more into line with his present abilities.

Treatment Planning and Outcome

On the basis of his performance on the battery of tests, Mr. S was given the diagnosis of subchronic paranoid schizophrenia and a trial of neuroleptics was initiated. In his individual psychotherapy, efforts were made to help him make realistic plans for his future in light of his illness and his resources. He made satisfactory progress while in the hospital and was discharged as improved. His prognosis was seen as guarded in light of his wish to return to live with his family and their continued denial of the severity of his illness. His mother expressed the view that she could "reach" her son and continued to harbor expectations for him that proved to be unrealistic. Nevertheless, his mother and his aunt did agree to accept the hospital's recommendation of partial day hospitalization and continued outpatient psychotherapy.

Mr. S remained out of the hospital over the next six years, but was never able to attain any level of independent functioning. His days continued to be spent in a partial hospitalization program and he continued on medication. Several efforts to stop medication led to increased aggressive outbursts and delusional preoccupations with attempts to influence him in a variety of bizarre ways. He was subsequently rehospitalized following a suicide attempt by his mother. At that time, his mental status exam and intervening psychiatric and psychological history clearly confirmed the earlier diagnostic impression of paranoid schizophrenia. Due to the long-standing nature of his illness and the severity of his impairment, he was given the diagnosis of paranoid schizophrenia, chronic with acute exacerbation.

E X H I B I T   1

AREA OF ASSESSMENT	CLINICAL EXAMINATION	PSYCHOLOGICAL EXAMINATION
I. Symptoms/Diagnosis		
Schizophrenia, paranoid, subchronic		
Bizarre delusions	Wood affects dental growth	Impaired reality testing combined with overly abstract thinking
Grandiose delusions	Career plans	Aspirations beyond abilities
Deterioration in school and self-care	High school dropout; Poor self-care	None
Duration six months—two years	One-two years of poor functioning	None
II. Personality Factors	None	Guarded but responsive to praise
		Little persistence or tenacity
III. Cognitive Abilities	Delusions	Average intelligence with cognitive disruption due to emotional factors
	Poor concentration	
	Impaired reality testing	
IV. Psychodynamics	None	Threatened by environment, especially women
	None	Isolation, idealization and projection as defenses against negative self-concept
	None	Affective controls inadequate
V. Therapeutic Enabling Factors	Cooperative to somatic treatment	Hopeful about future and believes therapy can help

AREA OF ASSESSMENT	CLINICAL EXAMINATION	PSYCHOLOGICAL EXAMINATION
VI. Environmental Demand and Social Adjustment	No friends Conflict with family	Inability to live up to social expectations Poor understanding of social relationships Markedly ambivalent towards parental and other authority figures

E X H I B I T   2

WAIS-R Summary

Verbal Subtests	Scaled Score
Information	10
Comprehension	12
Arithmetic	9
Similarities	13
Digit Span	14
Vocabulary	11

Performance Subtests

Digit Symbol	7
Picture Completion	6
Block Design	11
Picture Arrangement	7
Object Assembly	9

Verbal IQ	112
Performance IQ	88
Full Scale IQ	101

Rorschach Summary

Number of Responses	22
Rejections	0
Populars	6
Originals	0
Average R/T chromatic	22″
Average R/T achromatic	8″
F%	82
F + %	45
A%	77
H%	14
W:M	3:0
M:Sum C	3:3.5
m:c	0:1
VIII-X%	36
FK + F + Fc%	82
(H + A):(Hd + Ad)	9:11

RORSCHACH SUMMARY

Apperception   W   14%
D   73%
d   4%
Dd + S   9%

E X H I B I T 3

RORSCHACH SUMMARY

Response	*Inquiry*	*Scoring*

I. 2″

Looks like an inkblot.
Looks like it was made out
of ink.

1. And looks like it could be a butterfly. (*Pause.*) Looks to me like a butterfly, a butterfly, or a butterfly. Not too colorful. If it was more colorful it would look more like a butterfly but the shape makes it look like a butterfly. (*More than one thing.*) I can't see anything else. (*Returns card.*) I looked. It looked like a butterfly. What else can I say? What do you see in there?	1. The shape of it is like the shape of a butterfly. That's what it looks like.	WFAP

II. 11″

This one's a little more colorful. Has red in it.

1. Point of the head looks like an alligator.	1. That was on the last one, I don't remember. Don't ask me after it's over. I told you right away. You're writing fast enough. (*Alligator?*) The head was shaped like an alligator and it sort of had eyes like an alligator.	DF-Ad
2. And the back looked like a butterfly once again. And the middle, the head looks like an alligator. (*Middle?*) They didn't put anything there. And the tail looks like the back of a butterfly, a butterfly's backside.	2. Why didn't you ask me while I was looking at the picture? (*Pause.*) It was shaped like a butterfly. (*Back?*) Cause that's the way it was shaped like.	DFAP

RORSCHACH SUMMARY

Response	*Inquiry*	*Scoring*
3. And here I see a face. A face up top. And eyes on each side and, ah, ah, a funny shaped nose and silly mouth. Sad mouth.	3. Right. There was eyes on each side, not much of a nose and a sad mouth, like a frown.	D(S)M-Hd

III. 60″

(Leaves card on desk.)

1. I see black and red on a white board. And, ah . . .	1. *(A remark?)* No, I meant it as an answer. It's a white background with red and black on it. Like paint. Like red and black paint.	DCdesObj
2. Here I see a face on the side here and another face on this side here.	2. That it seemed to be a picture of eyes and nose.	DF-Hd
3. And here I see a butterfly. *(Butterfly?)* Yah, Right. Here's the butterfly. And that's it. Just a butterfly and nothing else.	3. The shape. The wings.	DFAP

IV. 9″

This one's kind of scary.

1. It looks like a monster *(Long pause.)* That's it. It looks like a monster. *(Reads back of card.)*	1. I don't know. *(Remind anything?)* It was nothing but a crummy blotch of ink.	WF(A)

V. 10″

1. This one looks like some sort of insect. Looks like a butterfly but not really a butterfly, looks like a bat. Shape of a bat, wingspan of a bat. Could be a bird. Not colorful enough to be a bird. Looks like a bat because it's black.	1. Bats are black and this is shaped like a bat.	WFC′AP

Rorschach Summary

Response	Inquiry	Scoring
(*Laughs; long pause.*) (*What do you see?*) See ink. Looks like somebody put an ink drop here and didn't really have any object of what they wanted it to look like.		

VI. 2'

Response	Inquiry	Scoring
1. Up here it looks like it might be a bird. The head of a bird. That's all.	1. The shape of it.	dFAd

VII. 7"

Response	Inquiry	Scoring
1. This looks like a butterfly.	1. Just the shape.	DFA
2. This looks like a pig. That looks like a pig.	2. Formed like a pig's head. That's all.	DF-Ad
3. Like maybe ram's horns over there. One of those two-way jobs.	3. Look like them. (*Two-way jobs?*) On either side of the head.	DFAd *Peculiar verbalization*

VIII. 11"

This one's more colorful.

Response	Inquiry	Scoring
1. It looks like an elephant. An elephant's trunk (*Pause*).	1. It was an elephant's trunk. (*Resemble?*) The shape.	diF-A
2. This one looks like, a, a, a butterfly.	2. The shape and the color.	DFCA
3. And this one looks like another kind of animal. I don't know the name of it.	3. You know, it had to be something so it had to be an animal. (*Animal?*) It's shaped like one. (*Particular animal?*) An animal I saw but I didn't know the name of.	DF-A

RORSCHACH SUMMARY

Response	*Inquiry*	*Scoring*

IX. 18″

1. Oh, now, this looks like, over here this red part looks like . . . a . . . a beetle with horns sticking out. And that's all I can make out of that one. (*Again?*) All right (*Long pause*).

    1. The shape.   drFA

2. Oh, yeah. A dog. A dog over here. That looks like a dog's face. And this one looks like a dog's face. A poodle. Not a poodle. I don't know the names of dogs but one of those dogs.

    2. Just looks like a dog.   DF-Ad

X. 12″

They're getting difficult.

1. This looks like one of them mean sea fishes. Maybe like a crab.

    1. Their shape and the eyes. (*Mean?*) The kind that bite you. Like a jellyfish. (*Mean?*) The way they looked. They're still right now.   DFAP

2. A deer. Here's a deer's head. A little picture there. Here's a deer's head.

    2. The shape of it.   DF-Ad

3. And, ah, (*Burps; apologizes*). Here, these are obviously eyes. That's all.

    3. Looks like someone's eyes.   DF-Hd

E X H I B I T 4

THEMATIC APPERCEPTION TEST

CARD 1 3″ It's a little boy and he's thinking about playing the violin. Looks like he wishes he knew how to play it. He looks like he wants to learn how to play it. He looks like he wants to take lessons, and perhaps he's thinking about who made it or how it was made. Maybe he'll pick it up in a little while and see if he can play it, see if he can make any music out of it. 1′24″.

CARD 3BM 6″ This guy's, ah, very sad. I see a gun lying down on the floor. He's threatening about killing himself. Probably because maybe he lost his job and his wife divorced him and has custody of the children and he has no money and no friends. (*Wait.*) And the gun is lying there and he's thinking about killing himself but he's thinking maybe he can work to resolve his problems instead of killing himself so maybe he still has something left to live for if he can find a new job and maybe work through his problems somewhat (*Wait*) and he comes to the realization that just killing himself won't help him any. He leaves the gun and doesn't kill himself and he gets up, come to think of it, it looks a little bit like a dress, so instead of husband and kids, wife and kids. She gets up, goes and talks to her psychiatrist and they give her some therapy and she gets better and learns to deal with her problems and goes on from there. 3′45″.

CARD 4 8″ 10″ Uhm, Man and lady are in love and, ah, man wants to take the lady, lady wants to go to the movies or out to dinner. Man wants to take her and says, "Okay, we'll go." Takes her out to the movies. After that they go for seafood and ah, after that they go dancing (*Sneezes*) and ah, uhm, he says, she says she wants some new clothes. He says, Okay, takes her to the store and buys her a new dress. She says, "Thank you for everything, I love you." They ride home in the car, watch a little TV and smoke a few cigarettes and chat and have a nice time. They say, "Well, it was a lovely evening and maybe we should do this more often." And they kiss good night and go to bed. 2′15″. Are mine corny?

CARD 6BM 11″ Uhm . . . A man and woman look sort of distressed and sad about something. They look upset and don't know what to say. Neither one knows what to say to each other because (*Wait*) they're so sad they're at a loss for words. They don't know what to say that could help the situation. (*Situation?*) Maybe they're, uh, uh (*pause*), um, he lost his job or something. (*Okay.*) Is that what happens? (*Your story.*) The guy lost his job and he's sad and upset and worried that he won't have food for the family. 1′58″.

THEMATIC APPERCEPTION TEST

CARD 7BM 6″. Looks like a father talking to a son. Looks like the father seems kind of, ah, pleased that his son is listening to him and, ah, he's telling him, ah, that his, ah, no, he's telling him . . . that . . . that, ah, his wife and children are coming along fine and that he doesn't have to worry that he didn't get the promotion on his job and that everything will be all right (wait). And the son says, the son's worried that his ambition, ah, he wants promotion for more respect and stuff and the father says that will come in time. Patience is a virtue and it will come in time. Son says, Okay, dad, I'll listen to you and we'll see how it works out even though it's not exactly what I wanted. 2′20″. (*Asthma attack*).

CARD 13MF I see a lady lying down in bed with no clothes on. She looks like she wants to have sex but her husband looks like he's not in the mood for it. (*Wait.*) And he, he's not, he looks like he's upset because he can't please his wife and he's going to go out and get drunk to forget his problems. (*Better*). Do you always show patients these kind of pictures? (*Yes.*) 58″.

EXHIBIT 5

SENTENCE COMPLETION TEST

6. *I used to feel I was being held back by* "my lack of confidence."
7. *He felt proud that he* "had achieved his goal of education."
9. *His father always* "loved him very much."
10. *A real man* "is educated."
12. *The worst things about women* "are their laughing habits."
15. *To get along in a group, you* "have to compromise."
19. *I could hate a person who* "beats people up."
20. *His earliest memory of his mother* "was very loving."
21. *I was most depressed when* "I was on my own."
28. *When they talked about sex, I* "don't listen."
38. *The kind of people I liked best are* "smart guys who know alot about politics and stuff."
42. *When I am criticized, I* "sometimes accept it."
44. *He felt he couldn't succeed unless* "he cheated."
61. *Sexual intercourse* "increases the population."
63. *Whenever he does a poor job, he* "gives up."
65. *I felt most thwarted when* "I was independent."
86. *I could lose my temper if* "I get beaten up."
87. *I am afraid of* "getting mugged while riding the train to Manhattan."
91. *Sometimes I feel that my boss* "worked me a little too hard."

SCHIZOPHRENIA, UNDIFFERENTIATED, CHRONIC

Until recently, Mr. L, a 17-year-old high school student, had been living in Florida with his older brother and sister in the family's home. His father wanted to move the family north in the hope that closer contact with his clients would help revive his faltering business as a medical supplies dealer. His children (Mr. L, his brother, and his sister) had agreed to stay behind so that their Florida house would be occupied while it was up for sale. Mr. L was happy to comply with his father's wishes. After his parents left, he dropped out of high school and spent his days loafing around the house and hanging out at a local beach by himself. Living this way was a relief and he was glad to be able to remove himself from school and the company of friends. Academic and social pressures were beyond him. For some time he had been experimenting with drugs, particularly hallucinogens, and now with the household income entirely at his disposal, he began to seriously abuse hallucinogens and marijuana.

One month prior to admission, his mother received a late night call from him. She said he had sounded "strange and frightened." Much of what he said to her she found incomprehensible. His father flew to Florida and finally tracked him down at the local beach where he had spent the last few nights. He was disheveled, poorly fed, and unable to give a coherent account of his activities over the last few days. The house was filled with dirty dishes, partially eaten food, and unwashed laundry. His older brother and sister had moved out two weeks previously, disgusted with the state of the house and unable to stop their younger brother from soiling it faster than they could clean it. His father learned that Mr. L's older brother was living with his girlfriend. Mr. L did not know the whereabouts of his brother and was surprised to hear that he had moved out. He agreed to return home with his father. At home, his mother found him distant and removed. Although he did not seem frightened, she still had trouble making sense out of much that he said. Mr. L went with his mother to consult a local psychiatrist who recommended that he be hospitalized. Seeing that he did not improve at home and given no assurances that he would improve with outpatient treatment, his parents finally decided to have him hospitalized.

His mental status examination at the time of admission revealed a poorly nourished, disheveled young man with long hair. He stated that his reason for seeking admission was that "I think I've got a problem of incoherency. I like to laugh." Although polite and willing to answer questions, he felt little anxiety about his present condition and related to the examiner with a detached, distant air that made it difficult to gather any pertinent historical data. His accounts of recent events and of his own experience were generally presented in such vague and abstract terms that it was often difficult to determine whether his responses bore any relationship to the questions he was asked to answer. He was able to complete the more formal parts of the examination and did demonstrate some curiosity about why he was being asked to do certain tasks. However, when given an explanation, he seemed not to comprehend what he was told and smiled at the examiner with an air of detached puzzlement. He acknowledged that he had recently experienced both visual and auditory hallucinations, but given his extensive, recent use of hallucinogens, it was impossible to determine if these phenomena had occurred outside the context of his drug abuse.

DSM-III-R Diagnosis

Axis I: Schizophrenia, undifferentiated, chronic
Axis II: None
Axis III: None
Axis IV: Mild—parents moved to a new city
Axis V: Very poor—marked impairment in both social relations and academic functioning

Treatment and Hospital Course

Mr. L's initial weeks of hospitalization involved a thorough medical workup and extensive efforts to gather additional information from his family regarding his personality and functioning over the last few years. In light of his extensive drug abuse, pharmacological treatment was delayed in order to provide a period of drug-free observation. Initial concerns were focused on the possibility of significant cerebral impairment related to his drug abuse and a prior history of electroencephalographic (EEG) anomalies. Computerized tomography (CT) and EEG studies were ordered by his treating psychiatrist. The CT results were reported as showing "considerable disturbance of white and gray matter patterns, especially noticeable in the frontoparietal region," suggesting "diffuse white matter disease." The electroencephalographic examination revealed a "diffusely abnormal EEG without focal features." In reviewing his past medical records, his present EEG findings were reported as showing no significant change from the results of the examination of a few years ago.

His hospital psychiatrist was able to learn that Mr. L had a family history of mental illness. Both his paternal grandmother and his older brother had received hospital treatment for "depression." No other family member, including his other five older siblings, was reported to have received any psychiatric or psychological care. His parents and his siblings all described him as a distant and seclusive individual who had always kept to himself and seldom participated in family affairs. Periodic concerns about his poor academic or social functioning had prompted the family to seek psychiatric consultation for him on two previous occasions. However, his lack of interest and the absence of any positive findings had discouraged the family from insisting that he pursue any extended course of treatment. He had always been pleasant, if distant, and his parents had most often felt that he, like his older siblings, simply wouldn't "come into his own and blossom" until later in life. They had been aware of his drug abuse, but not of its magnitude, and hadn't considered it a significant problem. They had not been aware of his dropping out of school; on learning of it from his brother, they had attempted to dissuade him from it.

During the initial period of observation, Mr. L continued to report auditory and visual hallucinations which he found entertaining and comforting. He spent most of his time in his room and involved himself with other patients or activities only upon direct request of the hospital staff. He was cooperative with, but puzzled by, these requests and would occasionally offer a mild complaint about having to participate in such activities since, as he saw it, the staff "didn't understand what my life is about."

After the first month of hospitalization, with no discernible improvement in his clinical state, his hospital psychiatrist decided to begin a trial of antipsychotic medication to determine if his hallucinations could be alleviated. He agreed to the trial, but the only positive effect he could report at the end of the next month was that the medication helped him to sleep better at night. There was no other change in his mental state. A repeat CT scan failed to confirm the earlier findings of disturbance in white and gray matter patterns although his EEG remained diffusely abnormal.

Psychological Assessment

In light of his medical findings and his failure to improve on medication, the hospital staff requested a psychological consultation to assist in differentiating between a schizophrenic syndrome and an organic syndrome. They also requested assistance in helping to formulate additional treatment goals for him. He was given the WAIS, Bender, Rorschach, TAT and SCT in order to evaluate the interplay of intellectual, cognitive, and emotional factors and their contribution to his present clinical state.

Mr. L approached the psychological evaluation with much the same attitude reported during his initial mental status examination. He arrived for testing dressed in a somewhat slovenly manner and although he was cooperative and polite, he was not always attentive. Questions and test instructions had to be repeated occasionally because he "drifted off" into his own thoughts. He stated that he enjoyed the testing because it gave him "something to do."

On the WAIS, Mr. L achieved a full scale IQ of 95, with both verbal and performance IQs of 96. Despite the similarity in his IQs, inspection of the range of subscale scores reveals extremely variable functioning. His subscale scores ranged from the mentally defective (*Comprehension*) to superior (*Block Design*) levels. His good verbal and nonverbal concept formation abilities are inconsistent with the possibility of a diffuse cerebral impairment. He possessed a good fund of general information and demonstrated superior abilities to analyze and synthesize visual designs. His social judgment, on the other hand, was grossly impaired. He concluded that if he found a sealed and stamped letter in the street that "I'd send them off a temporary note just to let them know the letter was sent, so they would get a return letter"; bad company was equated with "unsocialized youth" who could make one irritable; taxes are paid because of the "fanfare of commodities"; child labor laws are needed "to infuriate you . . . to keep the principle of the working man's life in order so the youth can't take over"; to find his way out of the forest "I'd use my own instincts."

His peculiar language and fluid and idiosyncratic thought were pervasively in evidence on both the Rorschach and TAT. He began the Rorschach by describing the "coming together of a mass with two hands stretching out" and also described the lower half of the internal detail of *card I* as a woman because "it looked like it was a dress on her, the outer part. Call it the outskirts." *Card III* was described as "an informal setting for a head." *Card VIII* seemed to him to be "a lion stepping across a stone path, I guess, kind of in a continental way. It signifies a ferocious beast all over the continent."

On the TAT, his already tenuous hold on reality completely evaporated. By the 10th card, he told the following story to *card 7BM*, a card with an older male figure in the background and a younger man in the foreground. This card typically elicits stories regarding the older man giving advice to the younger. Mr. L's story contained some of these elements: "You know, I can tell you 'You're right,' and I can tell you 'You're wrong' and you just sit there. You can look as hard as you want but I know you want the same information, no less and no more. You can find your way outdoors if you like, but right now you're here in prison. If you want to make it on your own, you've got to be able to stand up for yourself and speak the truth. All I can say is that I'm mad at all of you. Why did you pick on me? That's all." It was impossible to tell what private meanings he had drawn from this card and inquiry on the part of the examiner did not clarify them.

Mr. L's strongly metaphorical and at times allegorical approach to both the Rorschach and TAT was pervasive. His metaphors and allegories, unfortunately, often obscured what he had perhaps set out to clarify. His responses gave the impression that there was more depth than meets the eye, but Mr. L found ordinary speech a poor vehicle for conveying all that he thought and experienced. He could not struggle through the layers of meaning he dimly perceived, he could only allude to the many impressions which he glimpsed as they briefly passed by.

During the course of the examination, he agreed that others would certainly have difficulty understanding him. He was aware to some degree of the peculiarities in his thinking and in his speech, but he was not troubled by this. He simply recognized that others did not think and feel as he did.

He also made it clear that he had no desire to rectify the difficulty. The Sentence Completion Test provided an opportunity for him to record his responses to common, everyday situations. Even in this reality-oriented context, he retained his idiosyncratic modes of expression. He wrote that *he often wished he could* "relate true to knowledge"; *he felt proud that* "he understood"; *mother was all right when* "I know her"; *after he told them how he felt, he* "knew them"; *most of all I want* "to be." Absent from the SCT is any sense of volitional action (e.g. *when they told him what to do* "I looked on"). In its place he has substituted an intellectual state of merely being where an ostensible transcendent knowledge has its own rewards and is sufficient. Such abstruse intellectualization appeared to be his deepest desire (he noted, for example, that *love is* "auspiciously intellectual") and seemed to be sought for its ability to release one from tension. He used to feel down in the dumps when "I was tense" and noted that *the cause of his failure was* "tension."

Mr. L's peculiar and idiosyncratic thinking, his inability to differentiate perception and association, his convoluted intellectualized manner of distancing himself from reality, and especially his acknowledgment of and lack of concern over this difficulties were thought to be more in keeping with a functional rather than an organic interpretation of his difficulties. The absence of anxiety, turmoil or sustained efforts to remedy these difficulties suggested these problems were of long standing and although perhaps enhanced by his recent hallucinogen abuse, were nevertheless indicative of a chronic condition. As there was no indication in the test record of any desire to deal with and alleviate his problems, the examiner was unable to suggest any therapeutic goals which could be used to form a treatment alliance with Mr. L. It was recommended that, in light of his impaired social judgment, he be placed in a protective treatment setting where he could be given an opportunity to engage in some productive work that would not overly tax him emotionally. The psychologist also suggested that he be strongly encouraged to abstain from any further drug abuse.

Treatment Planning and Outcome

Mr. L and his family were informed of the outcome of the psychological evaluation and accepted the recommendations of the hospital treatment staff. Arrangements were made to discharge Mr. L to a rural, residential care facility where he would be able to spend an hour or two each day engaged in small jobs to help in running the facility. He and his family visited the facility prior to his discharge. He found the facility quite acceptable and looked forward to living in a quiet setting where he could "relate to the plants and animals." He continued to take his medication with the understanding that it would help him to remain in touch with things outside himself.

At the time of his discharge three months after his admission, Mr. L was given a guarded prognosis. However, he had no difficulty with the transition and settled comfortably into the routine of the new facility. Several months later, he wrote that he was glad to be living a useful life and contributing to his own upkeep. He had made a friend at the facility with whom he enjoyed discussing various ways in which knowledge could be acquired. He seemed content with his present life and he has not returned to the hospital.

EXHIBIT 1

Area of Assessment	Clinical Examination	Psychological Examination
I. Symptoms/Diagnosis		
Schizophrenia, undifferentiated, chronic		
Prominent hallucinations and incoherence	Persistent hallucinations for three-four months	Impaired reality testing
	Speech persistently vague, ellipitical and impoverished	Peculiar language, syncretistic and loose thinking
Deterioration from previous level of functioning	Dropped out of school; grossly impaired self-care	Poor hygiene
Duration of illness (including prodromal phase) of six months or more	Social withdrawal and isolation with marked impairment in role functioning and hygiene; vague speech followed by active symptoms	Absence of anxiety despite recognizing his impairments
II. Personality Factors	None	No capacity for sustained effort
III. Cognitive Abilities	Adequate fund of information; impaired judgment	Average intelligence grossly impaired judgment
IV. Psychodynamics	None	Sweepingly dependent on an intellectualized approach
V. Therapeutic Enabling Factors	Cooperates with plans made for him	Functions best with high degree of external structure
VI. Environmental Demand and Social Adjustment	Dropped out of high school; no work history	None
	No social relationships and uninterested in them	No interest in social relationships

EXHIBIT 2

WAIS-R SUMMARY

Verbal Subtests	*Scaled Score*
Information	12
Comprehension	2
Arithmetic	9
Similarities	11
Digit Span	10
Vocabulary	9

Performance Subtests	
Digit Symbol	6
Picture Completion	7
Block Design	13
Picture Arrangement	9
Object Assembly	11
Performance Score	46

Verbal IQ	96
Performance IQ	96
Full Scale IQ	95

RORSCHACH SUMMARY

Number of Responses	18
Rejections	0
Populars	6
Originals	1
Average R/T chromatic	35″
Average R/T achromatic	20″
F%	39
F + %	56
A%	28
H%	44
W:M	4:5
M:SumC	5:2
m:c	1:3
VIII-X%	33
FK + F + Fc%	39
(H + A):(Hd:Ad)	10:3

RORSCHACH SUMMARY

Apperception   W   28%

D   44%

d   28%

Dd + S   0%

EXHIBIT 3

RORSCHACH SUMMARY

Response	Inquiry	Scoring

I.

1. Hmm . . . I don't know. All I can see is it's the coming together of a mass.	1. (*Coming together?*) At first I didn't know what to think of it, but then I saw it as mountains. (*Mountains?*) Ah, just this, I just came from art therapy and I was doing some painting, and that's generally how I paint. (*Mountains?*) It was a quick glance and I happened to notice it. (*Coming together?*) (P) Ah, it's a coming together of a . . . well, the line was significant, I guess, thinking about it. Kind of like a center point.	DmF-Ldsc *Fab.comb.*
2. With two hands stretching out. The lines are significant, but it doesn't really relate to, ah . . .	2. (*Hands?*) Yeah. (*Stretching out?*) Uh-huh.	dMHd
3. Probably be a woman. That's all I can see.	3. (*Woman?*) Ah, just from the, ah, the lower point, the lower half looked like the lower part of a woman. But past that point, I really couldn't see that well. (*How remind?*) Ah, ah, just because it looked like it was a dress on her. The, ah, the outer, call it the outskirts (L). Womb of the woman. (*Certain?*) By her navel, can't fully read this.	DFHP *Peculiar verbalization*

Rorschach Summary

Response	*Inquiry*	*Scoring*

II. 7″

1. Ah . . . two Japanese ladies, in kimonos, with their heads down . . . ah, with their hands together. That's basically it. Probably be, I don't know, some sort of ritual if I'm not mistaken. Yeah. That should be it.

   1. 1.(*Japanese?*) The kimonos and the hair and the colors. (*Kimonos?*) Just the colors coming through. (*Ritual?*) Ah, just cause, you know, it was, ah, just because of their stance.

   WM-FCHP

2. You could call it a joyful, no, I don't know, I'd make it out as a bird. Where the hands come together, there's a bird. That's all.

   2. 1.(*Bird?*) The bird because of the beak. And because it was spread out like a plane but more in the shape of a bird.

   d(S)F-A

III. 45″

1. (*Smiles*) I don't know . . . the more I look at it . . . an informal setting for a head. Because, ah, it shows a lot of distinct qualities of people. I don't know, it's just . . . there are a lot of heads in

   1. (*Heads?*) Yeah. Ah, just from the distractive points. (*Distractive points?*) That's just from a line and how a jagged line forms a head. Kind of cartoonist (*Else?*) Nothing so distinctive. Except for the colors. They came together again. The same informality as the one before, just as distinctive.

   D(S)F-Hd
   Peculiar
   verbalization

2. It comes together with a bowtie and the distinction is that there is no head for the bowtie. I couldn't really get any more thoughts out of it.

   2. (*Bowtie?*) Yeah. And it's kind of left alone. (*Left alone?*) An, just cause it, I couldn't relate a head to it. Kind of Confounding a fearful thought that there's supposed to be a head there and there's no head there (L). (*Bowtie?*) Ah, ah, just it's distinctions. It just came together to me to look like a bowtie.

   DF Clothing
   Aut. Log.

RORSCHACH SUMMARY

Response	*Inquiry*	*Scoring*

IV. 10″

1. A giant mandrill. (*Smiles*) With two big feet. Ah, that's all I can get out of it really. Taking big footsteps, though.

1. (*Mandrill?*) Yeah. (*What is?*) One of those . . . it's an ape in South America. Colorful, too. They've got colorful noses but black. (*Remind you?*) Ah, just the . . . I saw a face. I like to see faces in pictures. I seen the face in it. Just from the top of my head, it came to me. And being of a massive size. Seems like it takes up the whole picture.

WM-FC′A

V. 43″

(*Shakes head, looks puzzled*)

1. Ah, two men playing a mandolin. Ah, side by side.

1. (*Men?*) Just cause, ah, the hair. Just because of the big shape of them. They look rather bold with their shape. Ah, playing a mandolin. (P) Could have been a flute, though. (*Mandolin?*) Ah, well, actually I thought it was a flute at first but then it came to me to be a mandolin. It seemed rather pleasant to me. The flute reminded me of a picture my mother painted. Ah, that's all I could get out of it except for the butterfly.

de(S)MH,Obj.

RORSCHACH SUMMARY

Response	Inquiry	Scoring
2. With a butterfly essentially in the background. That's it.	2. (*Butterfly?*) Well, actually I thought of it as a moth at first because it was gray, but ah, ah, it just, you know . . . (*Else?*) Yeah. (*What?*) Nothing else really. The picture's not too significant really. Didn't stand out too well.	WFAP

VI. 10″

Can I turn it any way I like? (*Okay*) (PP)

Response	Inquiry	Scoring
1. It's more like a lagoon-type picture. And it comes across as two island settings coming together at one point where the sun should be. But it isn't. Kind of a reflective type work. I don't know. It just hit me to turn it to the side, you know.	1. (*Lagoon?*) Ah, just, ah, a water-type setting. (*Water?*) Ah, ah, how did I think reflected? (*Explain?*) I seen a picture before that reminded me of it. (*Settings?*) Just cause of, ah, the black outline of the whole thing. (P) Uhm, just, ah, if I could point it out it would be more distinct. I see two islands coming together and I guess it made me think of where I used to live, in the Channel Islands there.	DcF.C′F-Ldsc *Peculiar verbalization*

RORSCHACH SUMMARY

Response	*Inquiry*	*Scoring*

VII. 23″

1. Two women with their bellies coming together. *(Bellies coming together?)* Yeah. Actually they should be pregnant. (P) Ah, that's all I can think of it.

1. *(Women?)* Ah, ah, just, ah, the out-stretch (*sic*) of their whole bodyies. Ah . . . (L) . . . ah, it just looks like their whole bodies coming together at the bottom. Like a slouch cause the bodies were kind of thin and then fat at the bellies. *(Pregnant?)* Just cause, ah, ah, just cause of their bellies in part and their stomachs coming together.

WMHP
Aut. log.

VIII. 50″

There I go turning it again.

1. It's a lion stepping across a ah, stone path, I guess. (P) Ah, kind of in a continental way, it signifies a ferocious beast all over the continent. Cause of the colors. Kind of like an atlas-type stuff.

1. *(Lion?)* Ah, just kind of made me think of a mountain lion on top of a boulder.

WFMAP
Contam

2. A path here.

2. *(Path?)* Like a path because of the shadow on its foot. Yeah. *(More?)* Ah, just kind of a, looked like it was on the run, with a lope. With spots below its foot.

DFc-Geo

IX. 48″

Try to think of it this way. Ah, it's colorful.

1. Ah, this is another like lagoon-type scene. This more than one when I look at it. (P)

1. *(Lagoon?)* Ah, just the colors, you know. I couldn't think of anything lengthwise or edgewise.

dr(S)CF-geo.

RORSCHACH SUMMARY

Response	*Inquiry*	*Scoring*
2. With a crab coming out of it this way.	2. (*Crab?*) Ah, ah, just 'cause it was round and it had feelers. At first I was trying to think of an astrological sign, Cancer.	DF-A

X. 25″

Response	*Inquiry*	*Scoring*
1. Kind of a Sgt. Peppers-type scene. But it comes out with, ah, a confrontation of some sorts. Looks like they're trying to head off, head off, ah, I don't know.	1. (*Sgt. Peppers?*) Ah, Sgt. Peppers. Just the colors coming together. And, ah, I don't know. (L) Maybe a face that was in the album cover. Oh yeah, I was thinking English-type, London bobbies. (*Bobbies?*) Ah, just the moustaches and their hats. Kind of English-style chaps. (*Head off?*) Ah, ah, I guess it just came together that their heads were together and they were looking for something together that they were turned away from.	DWFC-H *Confab.*
2. Then in other ways I can get a wrangler with spurs on, but the two times don't meet. That's about it, except I can see the place where they're protecting kids. I don't know, it's kind of abstract.	2. (*Wrangler?*) No, not a thing. (*Don't know now?*) Just an attitude. (*Protecting kids?*) Oh yeah. It was a, just two kids sitting down. Like youngsters. (*Kids?*) Just their restlessness, you know. Just fromthe projection point of view.	SF-Hd *Pec. verb.* *Confab.*

EXHIBIT 4

THEMATIC APPERCEPTION TEST

CARD 1 12″   I was wondering if this lesson wasn't made for me. I'd rather be outside playing than playing this violin. I don't know, I'm just bored sick, I have better things to do. Mom said I should play it but I still just don't have the ear for it. (PP) I don't know. That's about it. (*Come out?*) He's going to think it over. He's going to look at the violin, then look at the page, try to figure out the ends of it. (*Ends?*) Ends of it. How to get it over with. How to play it, I guess. Looks a little bit disturbed really. 3′.

CARD 13MF 12″   Just woke up this morning, and perceive myself to be an early riser. Wonder how I slept in my clothes. I know I'm tired but I couldn't have been that tired. All I had was one drink. Must have been 3 AM. Time to go to work now. Must leave, but should I wake up this lady? Or should I let her sleep? Well, I'll take my time. Get my head together. That's all I can think of really. 1′55″.

CARD 6BM 12″   Sorry that it ever happened. You tell me I shouldn't of, but I went ahead and did it. That loan you gave me was all the money I had. I don't know, I'll get by somehow. Hope you can make it your own way. Sorry it ever happened, but the money I used was my only risk, but it was a risk at getting myself in my own mode of living. Now we're both at a loss, aren't we? (P) Could have thought of more to say. (*Wait.*) (*Okay.*) That's all I have in mind. 2′14″.

CARD 7BM 20″   You know, I can tell you, you're right, and I can tell you you're wrong, and you just sit there. You can look as hard as you want but I know you want the same information, no less and no more. (*Wait.*) You can find your way outdoors if you like, but right now you're here in prison. If you want to make it on your own, you've got to be able to stand up for yourself and speak the truth. (*Wait.*) All I can say is that I'm mad at all of you. Why did you pick on me? That's all. 2′18″.

CARD 3BM 18″   Well, I might as well sleep right here. Looks like a cozy place. Too tired to pick up my keys. (*Wait.*) Seems like things are going to be different. Ah, might as well wake up and get my keys. Ah, not to mention I might as well get that book I was going to read. I'm too tired for all of this. Maybe I'll go back to sleep. 1′57″.

CARD 4 8″   No, don't leave yet. You're going to make it on your own, but just don't leave me yet. (*Wait.*) Might want to find your own time,

---

THEMATIC APPERCEPTION TEST

---

might want to do your own thing, but you seem ready to go without me. (*Wait.*) You're going to, ah, look for your own way, but why without me? Why can't I go? I see you're an adventurer at heart. (*Wait.*) Ah, but I guess I'm going, regardless, because I am an adventurer. That's all I can think of. 2'.

EXHIBIT 5

SENTENCE COMPLETION TEST

2. *He often wished he could* "relate true to knowledge."
5. *When she refused him, he* "left."
6. *I used to feel I was being held back by* "oppression."
8. *As a child my greatest fear was* "crying."
11. *A person who falls in love* "knows the meaning."
23. *Sometimes he felt that* "sex prohibited."
27. *The cause of his failure was* "tension."
32. *Love is* "auspiciously intellectual."
37. *I dislike to* "take orders."
40. *After he made love to her, he* "said hello."
45. *I used to feel "down in the dumps" when* "I was tense."
47. *When I fail, I'm* "awe struck (sic)."
50. *Mother was* "all right when I know (sic) her."
51. *After he told them how he felt, he* "knew them."
52. *Most of all I want* "to be."
57. *A man who masturbates* "better relate it."
58. *The trouble with marriage is that* "it (sic) not all together."
61. *Sexual intercourse* "relates."
65. *I felt most thwarted when* "I'm spectacled."
69. *I feel guilty about* "myself."
79. *His greatest worry was* "himself."
82. *When I try to get things off my chest, I'm* "uneasy."
93. *The worst thing a person can do is* "go crazy."

DISCUSSION

Our two cases of schizophrenia include Mr. S, a 19-year-old adolescent who lives at home with his aunt and mother, and Mr. L, a 17-year-old male who has been residing with his siblings. Both are quite young, about the age of the first episode of illness for male schizophrenics. Both have a mixture of the positive symptoms of schizophrenia, such as hallucinations and delusions, and the negative symptoms of schizophrenia, including social withdrawal and apathy. They differ, however, with regard to their subtypes. Mr. S presents with prominent paranoid symptomatology including ideas of reference and delusions of influence and control. Mr. L, on the other hand, more closely resembles the undifferentiated subtype. He seems rather diffusely disorganized and quite autistic in both his thinking and his social interactions. Nevertheless, for both these schizophrenic patients, the psychological testing is helpful in planning treatment interventions, especially around three areas of concern: reality testing, the presence or absence of paranoid ideation, and social skills, premorbid social competence, and quality of interpersonal relations.

The testing indicated that Mr. S was functioning at an average level of intellectual ability, but with great variability across different cognitive areas. He retained the capacity for abstraction, while at the same time his poor reality-testing ability interfered with accurate perception of details in the environment. Not surprisingly, the test data indicated an extensive impairment in reality testing at the time of testing.

Secondly, consistent with the diagnosis of paranoid schizophrenia, he did manifest paranoid thinking. He not only attended to details in the environment in an idiosyncratic way, but gave responses that suggested that he wished to mask himself and hide from his interactions with others. This suggests that in treatment planning one would have to go about developing a therapeutic relationship with this man in an extremely cautious, careful, and measured way.

Finally, treatment planning for schizophrenic patients always depends upon some assessment of the patient's premorbid capacity for human relations, both in terms of the potential quality of the patient's life and the potential for a trusting therapeutic alliance. Here, the test data are somewhat discouraging and suggest that this patient's customary capacity for and level of relating to others is poor. As noted previously, this is suggested by the low Picture Arrangement subtest score on the intelligence scale, his bland projective stories, and the absence of human and movement responses in the projectives. Thus, treatment planning for this young man with a chronic condition would emphasize a structured, but not intense, treatment program. The therapist would have to cautiously build a relationship with this suspicious and distant individual, going slowly from casual but regular contact to other modes of interacting with him.

The current thinking about schizophrenia is that it involves a vulnerability to cognitive overload, especially with stimuli of an intense emotional nature. This young man would very likely flee any intense contact and escape into isolation. It is most likely that, as he had in the past, he would accomplish this escape through illicit drugs. The issue of the management of his drug abuse is important and any attempt to keep him out of acute episodes must involve control of his substance abuse. Possibly a psychoeducational approach to this issue would be helpful.

Like Mr. S, Mr. L is a very disturbed young man who tends towards isolation and drug abuse. Mr. L seems to have been more involved in drug abuse than Mr. S, and the referral for psychological testing was focused on the nature of his cognitive impairment, including the hypothesis that his drug abuse had permanently compromised his cognitive functioning.

Once again, the testing revealed very poor reality testing. Mr. L's thoughts were characterized by loose and idiosyncratic associations. Helpful for treatment planning, however, was the fact that the nature of this cognitive malfunctioning was more consistent with functional rather than organic causes. His idiosyncratic productions were filled with metaphorical and allegorical meaning not readily understandable to others, but also giving evidence of vocabulary skills that seemed higher than his tested IQ. In contrast with Mr. S, frank paranoid ideation was absent. However, Mr. L seems enraged at his parents and other authority figures whom he sees as controlling. Mr. L's premorbid social competence and the quality of his interpersonal relationships are important to his treatment planning.

Unfortunately, the information gathered through his psychological assessment leaves many questions unanswered. At the time of the testing, he was so overwhelmed by his florid psychotic state that his verbal productions were often hard to interpret. He does refer to others in his world, a positive sign, but testing at a later date would probably yield a more valid indication in this area of concern. Management of this patient's extensive drug abuse would be central in maintaining some human contact with him.

B. SCHIZOAFFECTIVE BIPOLAR AND DEPRESSIVE TYPES

Schizoaffective disorder is a debated classification that comes and goes. While this classification was not present in DSM-III, it has been articulated with specific criteria in DSM-III-R under the general heading of Psychotic Disorders Not Elsewhere Classified. Thus, it is grouped with brief reactive psychosis, schizophreniform disorder, induced psychotic disorder, and atypical psychosis. According to DSM-III-R, this category is appropriate for individuals who at one point in time have met criteria for both a schizophrenic disorder and a mood disturbance and at another point in time have manifested psychotic symptoms without mood symptoms. The construct and discriminative validity of schizoaffective disorder is only tentative. DSM-III-R notes that in family studies the disorder bears a close relationship to schizophrenia.

Our two cases provide a comparison of a schizoaffective, bipolar type with a schizoaffective, depressed type. In contrast to other cases in this volume, the testing was called for to help solve a specific diagnostic dilemma: Was this patient schizophrenic or affectively disturbed? In other cases in this volume, we have noted that the DSM criteria were adequately addressed by the clinical interview and history, and psychological testing was utilized to address treatment planning issues not covered by the diagnosis itself.

Given the disputed nature of schizoaffective disorder, it is interesting to review the diagnostic criteria to see which ones would lend themselves to assessment by tests. There must be signs of affective disorder, either a major depression or mania, in the presence of schizophrenic symptoms. These schizophrenic symptoms would include psychotic behavior such as delusions, hallucinations, loosening of associations, or flat or inappropriate affect. In addition, the criteria note that schizophrenia itself has been ruled out; that is, the affective episodes have not been brief in duration relative to the duration of the psychosis. It is this latter duration criterion that cannot be decided by cross-sectional testing. Thus, we are looking for a battery which would include signs of psychosis as in schizophrenia plus prominent signs of mood disturbance.

SCHIZOAFFECTIVE DISORDER, BIPOLAR TYPE

Ms. N, 26 years old, single, Roman Catholic, and of Italian-American descent, had been in the emergency room of the local hospital about one year ago. She had been mugged and badly beaten while out late one night sixteen months ago, and was taken to the hospital with a fractured pelvis and a deep head wound. She remembered being "out of her mind" and had claimed at the time that she was a dog. She was therefore admitted to the hospital for observation and treated with antipsychotic medication which she found extremely unpleasant.

Now her parents had brought her to the hospital again. The doctors wanted her to take the medication again and to admit herself for another period of observation. She fled the emergency room in a panic and was escorted back to the hospital by the security guards. With the consent of her parents, the doctor petitioned for her to be hospitalized against her wishes and she was transferred to a nearby hospital that accepted involuntary admissions.

Ms. N was angry about the hospitalization. For the last few weeks, she had been preparing for her marriage to an elderly, widowed man whom she had "dated" off and on for the last two years. Her older sister had gotten married a few months earlier and was now expecting her first child. Although Ms. N's intended spouse was unaware of her marriage plans, she felt compelled to pursue them nonetheless. She believed she had been impregnated by the Holy Spirit and did not wish to give birth to the child out of wedlock. Over the last few weeks, as her parents had learned of the plans she was making and her reason for them, there had been many violent arguments and she had both verbally and physically abused her mother. She had formed the opinion that her parents were plotting against her to stop the marriage. She accused her mother and sister of adultery and attempted to exorcise them of "evil spirits."

Her family had seen her in similar states before. She was always going off on the spur of the moment in pursuit of some whim. This time, however, she seemed much more disorganized than usual. In the last week, they had been called by the police on several occasions when she had been found preaching against the sins of infidelity at a local shopping mall. Such behavior was clearly out of character for Ms. N, whose sexual life could best be characterized as one of casual promiscuity. She seemed to need very little sleep and often wandered around the house and the neighborhood at night. At times, her family had found her speech incomprehensible but she would refuse to slow down and explain her thoughts. Finally, they decided to take matters into their own hands. For years her parents had been trying to get their daughter to see someone for her problems. She had occasionally complied for brief periods, but these treatments had wrought little change. Now that things had gotten worse, they were prepared to have her hospitalized against her will, if necessary.

When seen at the hospital to which she was transferred, she was found by the examining psychiatrist to be an attractive, well-groomed, casually dressed woman who appeared somewhat anxious. Her speech was mildly pressured, but throughout the interview, she remained engaged with the psychiatrist and made good eye contact. The content of her speech was notable for examples of ideas of reference. She felt certain that much of what she heard on the television referred in some way to the sexual infidelity of her sister and mother and that she could avoid the impending punishment for her own similar transgressions by marrying and giving birth. She described examples of thought broadcasting and somatic delusions, but denied any hallucinations. Her affect was judged to be inappropriate at times. Her intellectual functioning, as judged from her fund of knowledge and abstracting abilities, the latter slightly circumstantial, indicated at least average intelligence and seemed consistent with her high school education and credit for some college courses.

DSM-III-R Diagnosis

Axis I: Schizoaffective disorder, bipolar type
Axis II: None
Axis III: None
Axis IV: No apparent stressor—no recent changes in her life
Axis V: Very Poor—marked impairment in both her social and occupational functioning

Treatment and Hospital Course

Ms. N was initially resistant to the idea of medication. She complied with the treatment only after hearing of her parents' wishes that she comply and learning that the hospital staff had deemed her a risk to herself and would proceed to treat her against her will if necessary. She was treated with increasing doses of a potent neuroleptic, but showed little improvement in her delusional symptoms. She was often active in a rather disorganized way, had great difficulty formulating plans and successfully executing them and easily became frustrated and angry at the smallest setback. Her emotional irritability and lability, as well as her rather entitled stance regarding others' rights, seemed consistent with a manic component to her illness. Consequently, during the second month of her hospitalization, the hospital staff considered adding lithium to her medication regimen.

While the diagnosis of schizoaffective disorder seemed to summarize her combined symptoms of cognitive and emotional disorganization and instability, the hospital staff continued to be divided over the issue of whether this was an exclusively affective illness, perhaps an atypical bipolar disorder, or an unadulterated schizophrenic disorder. In an effort to seek clarification of this differential, she was referred for psychological testing.

Psychological Assessment

Ms. N was seen by the examining psychologist at the start of her second month in the hospital and during the first week of her lithium treatment. She was given some of the subtests of the WAIS-R, the MMPI, Rorschach and SCT, and an abbreviated number of TAT cards.

During the examination, she expressed the hope that the examiner could "put in a good word" for her in order to speed up her discharge. Despite her wish to make a good impression so as to evoke the examiner's assistance in speeding up her discharge, she was restless to the point of distraction. She laughed often for inexplicable reasons and often sang to herself between tasks.

Her WAIS-R performance on the subscales administered indicated a pro-rated level of intellectual functioning in the *Average* range. However, her subscale scores ranged from *Borderline* levels to *High Average* levels of intellectual functioning. Her unevenness of functioning seemed likely to extend beyond the WAIS-R tasks at hand and was likely to be characteristic of her behavior in situations outside the testing situation.

Ms. N's efforts to present herself in a positive light (*K scale*), as well as her pressured and perhaps erratic behavioral propensities (*scales 8, 9* and *4*), were also reflected in her MMPI profile (K-FL 8'947-6/3150:2). She acknowledged her irritability and unusual experiences and idiosyncratic thinking (*scales 9* and *8*) while strongly denying any significant depressive symptomatology (*scale 2*). Her overall defensiveness (*K scale*) suggested her efforts to minimize these trends in her self-report and deemphasize the amount of distress she felt.

When asked to express herself in a less structured format, her idiosyncracies became more apparent. For example, her SCT contained a number of items with extraordinarily elliptical content. She reported that *she often wished she could* "have seen him"; *the ideal man* "is one with silver"; *the ideal women* "are these kind"; *I used to feel down in the dumps when* "I didn't receive any pictures"; *people seem to think that I* "am the postman"; *I could lose my temper if* "I knew otherwise"; *when I think of marriage* "I think of you." The sense of these responses is that she has something personal in mind that is very poorly conveyed by her choice of words—perhaps purposefully so.

In any case, there undoubtedly existed a poorly integrated sense of self as reflected in such contradictory experiences as her father always telling her "No," while her earliest memory of her father "is a good one" and when her father came home she "cried first, then laughed." Likewise, in reference to her mother, she reported that her earliest memory of her mother was "one of nastiness," but that when with her mother, she felt "quite good" and when her mother came home, she felt "relieved." An air of conflict and, as before, poor integration was also apparent in her sexual impulses. She notes on the SCT that she "closes her ears" when sex is discussed while at the same time describing her sexual desires as "somewhat untame."

On the Rorschach, she struggled to integrate contradictory associations which appeared in the context of fluid percepts. For example, her first response to *card II* involved "two little pantomime people" who, because of costumes which hide their human shape, might be people pantomiming seals or, alternatively, they might be seals dressed up as people. On *card III*, the looseness of her thinking, here manifest as a fluidity of perception, perhaps provides a clue to her vacillation and uncertainty. The percept of "pygmies in Africa . . . playing congos" is partially justified, and to her supported, by a later perception of the congos as "flaring nostrils . . . like someone's nose, maybe the nose of one of the African people."

As was her language on the SCT, her language on the Rorschach was marked by a number of peculiarities. On *card I*, she referred to "outside forms"; on *card II* she spoke of the "positiveness and negativeness of the drawing" to justify her perception of "a cat's face" and later referred to "a certain measure within the crab" to indicate a vagina percept. Additional examples included *card V* where she reported "two people leaning against each other very extremely," and on inquiry, "doing one particular act known as leaning" and, with considerable projection, describes the people as "underground type of people," meaning, she explained, detectives or criminals or "quiet people like nuns that slightly smell of secrecy"; *card VI* where the puppy dog "was very outreached"; *card VIII* where she finds "two eyes that looked like sunglasses"; *card IX* where a "space" becomes a "space-age movie" because "both sides of that, or part, were like retaliating, making way for what was going to come between those two sides."

This sort of elliptical and symbolic speech, often carrying a weight of meaning that is just out of reach of ordinary comprehension, illustrates the fragmentation of experience on which her delusional ideation might be said to rest. However, amidst this fragmentation, she could occasionally step back from the ongoing experience of fluidity and disintegration to acknowledge the unusualness of what she saw: for example, comments such as "wordy, very wordy" (*card I*), or references to her skills as an artist that helped her to see things in certain ways (*card VI*). Feeling as flimsy and vulnerable to destruction as the "tissue paper" she saw on several Rorschach cards, she vacillated between intellectual distancing reflected in her "geometric shapes" and espousing an innocent, childlike posture like the "angels" she saw on the first card of the Rorschach and children playing at a birthday party on the last card.

In her TAT stories, Ms. N carries over the same air of unusual novelty and wonderment that was evident on her Rorschach. She told a story to *card 15* of a man who "just had an encounter with a space creature" who is unable to decide whether or not to attempt to profit from "something very special" that was "revealed to him." Here, as on the Rorschach, a certain amount of idiosyncratic thinking and elliptical thought permeated her record. Her last story is told to *card 4* and in it, a woman is about to take her "big chance" to show the man that she loves him only to conclude that "he will give her the time of day." Somewhat more usual but slightly offbeat stories also appeared. *Card 3GF* prompted a story of a woman whose husband died when she thought he'd get better and *card 13MF* revolved around a rape and subsequent apology because "he realized the meaning of what he did."

In the examining psychologist's report, Ms. N's emotional lability, extreme counterdepressive tendencies, grandiosity, and sexual preoccupation were considered indicative of a manic state. When these features were taken in conjunction with the severity of her disorganized thinking and impairments in reality testing, the test evidence was reported as supporting a diagnosis of schizoaffective disorder, bipolar type.

Treatment Planning and Outcome

Partly as a result of the psychological consultation, Ms. N's pharmacological regimen was revised to include augmentation of her lithium treatment and her neuroleptic treatment was gradually reduced over the next month. Her clinical condition had noticeably improved by the end of the month. Although her mood remained somewhat labile, her delusional thinking had resolved and she was actively participating in several hospital activities. Her free time was primarily occupied with reading, which she enjoyed and seemed able to concentrate on for progressively longer periods. She came to see her delusional experiences as expressing her wish to "settle down" and lead her own life. During her psychosis, this had meant becoming a wife and a mother and her attempt to achieve these goals through an immaculate conception apparently had been a way of putting her life on a new footing unmarred by the sexual excesses of her past. As she slowly recovered from her psychosis, she was able to engage in more appropriate efforts to establish her own, independent life.

To help her consolidate her recovery, she was transferred to an intermediate care unit and, as her condition improved, she was enrolled in the hospital's vocational services program where she could receive training consistent with her goal of pursuing part-time clerical work upon discharge. As her condition further improved, she struggled to come to grips with the discrepancy between her parents' high expectations of her and her siblings' achievements and her own difficulties and more realistic aspirations. For a time, she considered living in a structured residential setting upon discharge, but her parents' vehement opposition to having her live "with those people" and her own wish to return to live in familiar surroundings ultimately decided the matter. At the time of her discharge, 5½ months after her admission, she had been accepted into a day hospital treatment program where she could continue with her vocational training. She returned to live at home and was involved in both individual and family psychotherapy with her hospital psychiatrist and social worker.

Over the next several months, Ms. N continued to slowly improve. She completed the training program at the day hospital and succeeded in acquiring part-time work as a typist. Her neuroleptic medication was finally discontinued. She continued to take lithium which she found helpful in containing her mood swings. At one-year followup, there had been no recurrence of her psychosis and she reported that she was making steady progress for the first time in her life. Her parents were also pleased with her progress and in addition, had become increasingly realistic regarding her abilities and difficulties.

EXHIBIT 1

Area of Assessment	Clinical Examination	Psychological Examination
I. Symptoms/Diagnosis		
Schizoaffective disorder, bipolar type		
A. Schizophrenia —grandiose, religious delusions	Believes she has been impregnated by the Holy Spirit	Poor reality appreciation and peculiar and fluid ideation
Mania—euphoria and irritability and:	Easily angered; has been assaultive	None
—restlessness	Unable to sit still	Restless
—pressured speech	Pressured speech	Pressured speech and verbosity
—grandiosity	Delusional impregnation	Idiosyncratic associations often having hidden meanings
—decreased sleep	Needs little sleep	None
II. Personality Factors	Maintains capacity and desire for relationships	Enjoys and seeks out others
III. Cognitive Abilities	Average intelligence	Average resources but present use is inefficient and compromised by affective instability
IV. Psychodynamics	Conflicted relationship with parents	Identity conflicts involving self and parental expectations. Vacillates between intellectual distancing and childlike compliance.
		Conflicts over sexuality as a means of expressing and achieving closeness and immoral behavior which invokes punishment
V. Therapeutic Enabling Factiors	None	Capacity for some self-reflection

AREA OF ASSESSMENT	CLINICAL EXAMINATION	PSYCHOLOGICAL EXAMINATION
VI. Environmental Demand and Social Adjustment	Extensive history of poor social adjustment	Cooperativeness compromised by suspiciousness and rebelliousness
	Seldom accommodates to imposed constraints	Difficulty accepting limits

E X H I B I T   2

WAIS-R Summary

Verbal Subtests	*Scaled Score*
Information	9
Comprehension	11
Arithmetic	7
Similarities	11
Digit Span	12

Performance Subtests

Digit Symbol	7
Picture Completion	6

Verbal IQ	101
Performance IQ (est.)	76
Full Scale IQ (est.)	87

MMPI Summary

K-FL/ 8'947-6/3150:2

Rorschach Summary

Number of Responses	48(-5)
Rejections	0
Populars	10
Originals	0
F%	44
F+%	88
A%	31
H%	31
Obj%	25
W:M	16:9
M:Sum C	9:8
m:c	5:8
VIII-X%	38
FK+F+Fc%	50
(H+A):(Hd+Ad)	22:8

RORSCHACH SUMMARY

Apperception	W	33%
	D	54%
	d	6%
	Dd + S	6%

E X H I B I T 3

RORSCHACH SUMMARY

Response	*Inquiry*	*Scoring*

I.

1. I see two outside forms. Two little angels and they're both kind of meeting each other—like this or holding onto each other's hands and they've got their knees—the thing in the middle—I really don't see—their feet are on a rung or something. Do you know what I mean?

1. Their wings primarily and, uh, their profile and they facilitate considering them angels for some reason. (*Facilitate angels?*) I think it's the fact that their wings are so—their wings are the main thing, and that makes them look like angels. If they weren't in profile they probably wouldn't look like angels.

WM(H)

2. It almost looks like a pelvis—you know like one huge pelvis of a woman and instead of these angels as the outline of a human being. Wordy, very wordy.

2. Just looking at the whole of it—the outer most parts— their shape. (*Huge?*) Did I say that? Oh not huge what I meant was contrary to seeing two little angels— the entire drawing looked like it was something.

WFAt

3. And the center—it looks like a woman wearing— something like from an 18th century gown with a very tight waist and she's raised both hands up and she's missing a head.

3. The pinched in waist or how could I put that? The waistline looking like a cor- set and uh how can I say the rest of her outfit also— like what's above and below the corset also. (*Head?*) All there was—was no collar but no head above the col- lar, however, there were two hands stretching up above the shoulder.

DMH

RORSCHACH SUMMARY

Response	Inquiry	Scoring

II.

1. I see like two little panto-mime people. And they're both going like this— they're touching their left or right hands together as they do a dance and they're wearing grey outfits, grey gowns and they've got two red hats on—like two little seals doing a dance.

1. They kind of look like seals too because the way their heads are bent over—the way seals tend to look— look like dressed up seals. (*Do you see them as seals or people?*) I would say dressed up seals really. Both of them equally. Feel strongly for both cases cause people doing pantomime—they can look so different any-way. Sometimes pantomime people do seem different— like they're different spe-cies of some sort. (*Dressed up seals?*) It has to do with their posture such as in the neck region they're kind of bending forward and also the way the entire body is postured—it makes them look like seals that have clothes on and if not seals—they look like two human beings imitating something like a seal.

WFM-FC'-FC(A), Clothing

2. I see a cat's face in the upper part of this blotch. How can I refer to this? Blotch or blot. (*Either*)

2. Well the upper part of the design has two white parts and the whiteness and the curvature of line make it look like a cat's face. It has to do with the positiveness and the negativeness of the drawing and not just the ink. Part of a picture can be the white spaces that you find in the drawing.

S(D)FAd

RORSCHACH SUMMARY

Response	Inquiry	Scoring
3. I see a butterfly in the bottom part of this and some kind of	3. The wings.	DFAP
4. seashore or like a crab or something—or some seashore animal besides a crab.	4. In that case—in the case of the crab—whatever was drawn in—yeah whatever was wherever the ink showed up—that was definitely considered part of the drawing but if you want to know specifically I saw two feelers coming out and I came to the conclusion that it looked like a crab because judging from the shape that the ink produced this was not a case of positive and negative like with the cat so it was his feelers and his shell which the ink showed for me and that's about it. His back shell or his vertebra or something.	DFA
5. Vagina down here in the lower part of this design— elements of—not the whole thing but parts of, innermost.	5. (*Parts of vagina?*) (*Pt. laughs*) There was a certain measure within the crab, it would have been let's say the spine of the crab and that resembled to me the part of the female known as the vagina, just the innermost part, like something from an anatomy book.	ddF-Sex,At. *Peculiar verbalization*

Rorschach Summary

Response	Inquiry	Scoring

III.

1. These look like two pyg-mies in Africa. And they're playing congos, got their rear sticking up in the air and they're bending down low to play their congo drums.

   1. I'll say Africans—it's more general—I'm not sure if pygmies could be Africans—too primitive people—could you say that? (*Primitive?*) The way the head was shaped, their postures and the fact that they had congo drums with them—the shape of the head was definitely what made me make up my mind cause it's different from what people's heads are shaped like.

   WMH,obj.,P

2. Butterfly.

   2. The shape and the red color.

   DFCAP

3. Looks like rose colored paper. The kind they make paper flowers out of—so that's the butterfly—it's both that and paper flower material and two red blotches on the side look like, well one of them.

   3. Just the light—the trans-parency of it or the light-ness of color, just looked both like a tissue in a way—light and fluffy, like a tis-sue. That is tissue paper that they use by the way, only it's colored.

   DFC-cF Obj.

4. Looks like a musical note or suggestion of a musical note.

   4. The stain and this roundish part here look like a note.

   DF Obj.

5. Also their congo drums look like someone's flaring nostrils. Seen as a whole looks like someone's nose. Maybe the nose of one of the African people. They definitely look African—I mean it's amazing.

   5. Maybe the kind of nose that is indicative of the race of the people. (*What about the blot made it look that way?*) The blackness of the ink in two circular shaped forms.

   DFC-Hd

RORSCHACH SUMMARY

Response	Inquiry	Scoring
6. The red butterfly in the center could also be a red bowtie.	6. The shape is the same as a bow tie.	DFC Cloth P

IV.

Response	Inquiry	Scoring
1. Look like two heels—two boots with, uh, heel touching the floor and the toe up in the air—toes, toe part up in the air.	1. The heel section and the toe section. The way the heel section part seemed to be dug into the ground and the rest was up in the air—it looked like a kick or something.	DMHd,Cloth P
2. Also see the letter M in here. And	2. It has the "M" shape.	DF Obj
3. I also see a giant person who's looking down from up where he is.	3. The fact that uh the fact that like when you look at him his head is so far away from where you are and you would be closest to his shoes and the rest of him seemed so far away. His lower part such as his boots were larger in comparison to his head.	WM(H)P

Rorschach Summary

Response	Inquiry	Scoring

V.

Phew!

1. Again I see two people and they're kind of two people leaning against each other very extremely—I mean the only thing touching on them are the shoulders and the head area.

1. What made it look like two people leaning—I don't know how to explain it. It just did, the bodies look like two humans and the bodies were doing one particular act known as leaning. (*What sort of people?*) Each was wearing a black cape or some kind of black outfit in the form of a cape and they may have been like underground type of people, like detectives, criminals or just quiet people like nuns that slightly smells of secrecy or anything like that (*patient laughs*) some kind of secrecy, doesn't matter who, something unspoken.

WM-FC′H
Peculiar
verbalization

2. I see an insect—some kind of a fly with big wings and I see two little antennae and two little feet on this fly. Do you have any idea when I might be discharged?

2. Well the wings looked like wings and, uh, anytime there are two short lines jutting out from something I always or very often tend to view them as antennae or little legs. The antennae or that part is a big thing in determining whether it's an insect or not.

WFAP

RORSCHACH SUMMARY

Response	Inquiry	Scoring

VI.

1. First thing I saw was uh violin. Next thing I see is

1. Um, the long neck, the upright position of it. It just looked very upright and prim and proper with the long neck and I associate prim and proper with violins. I mean I associate violins with those characteristics.

WFObj.

2. a puppy dog with his mouth all the way up. He could be looking up to his master or calling out.

2. (*Looking up or calling out?*) The only time a puppy dog is going to put his head up like that is when he's looking at someone a lot taller when he's sitting or if he's crying for some reason. He was very outreached. It was a position of outreach. His mouth really comes before any part, before the eyes too. (*Puppy dog?*) I've seen other puppy dogs that look like that picture before. I've seen that before and also the uh the hairs, the fur coming out from the jaw area. You know dog fur.

DFM-FcA

3. I see two profiles of the human head—two profiles—one on each side, of a human being with a long nose by the way.

3. Well the nose was very outstanding. I don't know, could I look at it again? I was just going, I was just generalizing from the outline of the forehead I noticed eyes, pronounced nose and probably chin that's what made it look like a profile.

DFHd

RORSCHACH SUMMARY

Response	*Inquiry*	*Scoring*
4. I see a highway with a line in the middle to show separation.	4. Oh I saw two parallel lines—two dark parallel lines with uh littler, very thin line in the center and I thought of some kind of highway as seen from an aerial view or photo. It's really two dark lines with the line in the center representing the dividing line—you know whatever they call that thing—	diFkRoad
5. I see the soles of two feet and the calves of those feet, of the person. And what else do I see?	5. (*Patient grimaces*) It was the shading of the feet, cause as an artist I know that there are certain parts of the feet that are lighter than others and I know that heels are lighter so I thought of heels.	dFcHd
6. I see a geometric shape. I don't know if you'd call it an octagon or what. It's the one with ten sides, not an octagon. It's the next one up.	6. Well I saw, I don't know how to answer this I saw many different sides, the sides you would see if looking at a hexagon let's say or octagon—they were symmetrically assembled to look like one large geometric shape. Don't even have to say large, not necessarily large, one whole geometric shape.	WFObj

VII.

1. Well I see uh vase with the front line across is missing. Like a vase with artistically (*patient sighs*) a horizontal line missing.	1. (*Patient laughs*) The shape.	SFObj.

RORSCHACH SUMMARY

Response	*Inquiry*	*Scoring*
2. I also see two women facing each other. I see two women doing some kind of a dance or in some kind of a funny pose.	2. Their profiles. (*Dancing?*) Position of their arms (*patient laughs*)	WMHP
3. And I think of a seashore animal also but I can't think of what I'm looking at, lobster or something. Also I see something sticking out of these women's head like feather coming out of the hat or something.	3. Something in the jagged edges of it that reminded me of that.	WFA
4. Rear end sticking up in the air like the moon— moonies—and with the rectum showing also.	4. (*Patient laughs*). Well, there are two very round surfaces you might say that made me think of a rear end. Also, the rectum seemed to be like a black hole. There was like a black hole in the middle of, in the middle, a slit.	DFC'-Hd
5. Also, I see two clown's faces.	5. The big noses, I think.	DFHd

VIII.

Oh God. Well here I see

1. two polar bears or what do you call that group of animals that includes rats and mice, (*Rodents?*) Two rodents, yeah.	1. They had the pelt and the shape of polar bears. (*Pelt?*) (*Patient sighs*) Oh the little (*patient sighs*) lines (*patient laughs*).	DFMAP
2. I see a geographical map and I see those rodents trying to climb some kind of structure. (*Patient sighs*)	2. The color green. It looked like a geographical map.	DC/FAP

RORSCHACH SUMMARY

Response	*Inquiry*	*Scoring*
3. I see that colored tissue paper that is used to make flowers and these animals have one leg up and another one stuck to some kind of substance. (*Patient laughs*) This could go on and on.	3. The color of the print—colors, namely pink and orange. (*Stuck?*) One of their legs was not with the other leg—it was left behind in some kind of trap.	WcF.CF Obj,A
4. I also see another face here. All right I think we have enough. It's very decorative. The whole thing that doesn't count as a statement does it? (*Patient begins singing to herself*)	4. There was a goatee and there were the two eyes that looked like sunglasses. Made good eyes and then I just filled in the rest. It was mainly the goatee and the eyes that made the face. (*Goatee?*) The way it hung down in the front.	DFHd

IX.

Oh brother.

| 1. Looks like a space, reminds me of a space, reminds me of a space age movie like a new movie of some sort, oh dear, let's see. | 1. The fact that both sides of that or part were like retaliating making way for what was going to come between those two sides, just looked like a big bubble coming in the middle of those two sides. Just looked like they were being taken aback by something that was happening. | WmF Movie *Confab* |
| 2. I see two ice cream cones. | 2. The shape of just, the round shape and the point of, the point of triangular shape together. | dF Food |

RORSCHACH SUMMARY

Response	*Inquiry*	*Scoring*
3. I see two beings trying to make contact with uh each other with their arms.	3. I see little not necessarily people. I mean you could see—it's like living organisms—like fauna but from the movie aspect it didn't have to be fauna, could be just shapes that are moving around and you get a new shape from them.	WFm(A) *Confab*
4. Um what do you call those little lanterns that you have to put oil in to get them going. Not oil lanterns but something like that. Well, I see something in here that reminds me of one of those lamps that we have, a little oil lantern.	4. The filter or flint, the wick made it, there was a part, there was a line in the center of the lantern which represents the wick.	DF Obj
5. I see a salt, a salt or pepper little you know, shaker and oh well I can go on and on but I'd rather not.	5. The shape of the outside of the salt or pepper shaker, the shape of the form that I saw.	dF Obj
6. I see two people meeting and they're exchanging either a candle or they're just meeting to talk and they're using a candle to help light their way.	6. I just thought that. It was two people since I have it on my mind to meet with someone and talk about important matters. I translated that to what I saw. Just what I had on my mind I don't know how to put it. Just looked like two little stick figures meeting over an important matter. Either exchanging the candle or having it out of necessity.	DMH,Obj.

RORSCHACH SUMMARY

Response	*Inquiry*	*Scoring*

X.

Oh boy I think of, uh

Response	Inquiry	Scoring
1. Merry-go-round.	1. There was one outstanding shape that dominated over the other shapes and it gave me the impression of something at a merry-go-round, it gave me the impression of something that would be in a merry-go-round. (*Merry-go-round?*) The colors and the shapes.	WCFsym. Obj.
2. I think of a children's birthday party. (*Patient laughs*) I think of children playing merry-go-round with their hands, they play merry-go-round with their hands, don't they? Children in a circle playing pocketful of posey or whatever those dances are.	2. Oh there was a lot of it, just looked like all the shapes and uh that would be part of an excitement that would be part of children playing those kind of games.	WM.CFsym., Obj.
3. chickadees. Yellow chickadees and I think of two	3. They were small and the color in the smallness and the exact color.	DFCA
4. crabs again. I see two	4. Not really just an impression, they reminded me of crabs but you wanna know why? They're just scattered and disorganized looking. (*patient laughs*)	DFAP
5. flowers. I think of the	5. They literally looked like two yellow little roses.	DFCPl

RORSCHACH SUMMARY

Response	Inquiry	Scoring
6. Eiffel Tower and what else.	6. It's pointedness and the grey color. By point I mean, literally headed toward the sky. Oh by the way I think also that it was the first thing on the top of the page. If it was found anywhere else it wouldn't have been.	DFC Arch. *Autistic* *Logic*
7. Two little worms like for bait, what do you call those?	7. They look like worms.	DFA
8. Seahorses like you find them on the beach. Yeah I see two seahorses here. They're teeny really small, OK that's it. Want me to show you everything. This is a bright round.	8. They definitely looked like seahorses. The shape and the size.	DFA

E X H I B I T   4

THEMATIC APPERCEPTION TEST

CARD 3GF   Her name is M she's very upset because she just found out that her husband died. She didn't expect him to. He was very sick and she thought he'd get better but he died. (*Laughs*).

CARD 4   Aaah. Lovers—um, this is her big chance to show him how much she loves him but she did know if she hopes that he'll give her enough time and attention to show it cause he's looking the other way. (*Feeling?*) She's feeling great cause she's with him (*Laughs*) (*Next?*) I think they'll get it together and he'll show her that it is worth the togetherness, he will give her the time of day. Let's put it that way. See that's a big moment for her.

CARD 13MF   He just raped this woman and I think felt sorry for what he did (l). It's a weird thing cause he realized the meaning of what he did and he felt very bad. (*Next?*) Process of—he'll apologize to her but he can't count on whether or not he'll accept the apology, naturally. I mean really.

CARD 14   Hmmm. (*Light inflection of tone*) He looks like he's yearning to go outside and merge with the rest of the world but he still has to deal with certain problems in the life that he's leading right now. But he's preparing to go out and mix with other people.

CARD 15   This is spooky. He just had an encounter of a space creature and he's trapped as to whether he's going to talk about it or keep it to himself. (*Feeling?*) He's feeling sneaky because he doesn't know whether he's entitled to know what he does but somehow something very special was revealed to him and he doesn't know whether he could profit from letting other people know it so he kind a feels trapped. (*Do?*) It's not for me to know or say what he'll do.

EXHIBIT 5

2. *She often wished she could* "have seen him."

9. *My father always* "used to tell me no."

10. *The ideal man is* "one with silver."

20. *Her earliest memory of her mother* "was one of nastiness."

21. *The ideal women* "are these kind."

28. *When they talked about sex, I* "closed my ears."

33. *My earliest memory of my father is* "a good one."

45. *I used to feel 'down in the dumps' when* "I didn't receive any pictures."

49. *People seem to think that I* "am the post man."

53. *My sexual desires are* "somewhat untame."

70. *When my father came home, I* "cried first, then laughed."

76. *When my mother came home, I* "felt relieved."

86. *I could lose my temper* "if I knew otherwise."

92. *When I think of marriage I* "think of you."

94. *When with her mother, she* "felt quite good."

SCHIZOAFFECTIVE DISORDER, DEPRESSIVE TYPE

Ms. R, a 22-year-old, single, Irish Catholic woman, agreed to her third psychiatric hospitalization in six years after attempting to throw herself out her parents' apartment window. Until the last month, she was doing well. Her last hospitalization was over two years ago and there had been no recurrence of her hallucinations, delusions or paranoid thinking. She had begun taking courses at a community college and was doing well in her day hospital treatment program and volunteer job. She was well-liked and seen as a productive member of the day hospital community and consistently had been given good reports on her job behavior and performance. She had been steadily dating a young man and both she and her parents described this relationship as a "warm and caring" one. She had been doing so well that three months prior to her rehospitalization, she had stopped taking her medication, with her doctor's approval, and had accompanied her family overseas to visit relatives, experiencing no difficulty despite the fact that the visit was prompted by the deaths of two relatives.

However, on her return, Ms. R and her boyfriend "broke up," much to her family's surprise. Within a few days, she became increasingly paranoid and despondent. She reported feeling that people were planning to harm her in some unspecified way and also told her family that she wanted to die. As she put it, "I've been feeling worse. I feel as if I'm so upset at home all I can think about is trying to take my life. I embarrass my family and I believe I shouldn't be around so I wouldn't embarrass them anymore."

When admitted to the hospital, Ms. R was described as a neatly dressed, attractive young woman whose manner was guarded. Her mood alternated between anger, anxiety, fear, and sadness. Her anxiety occasionally prompted inappropriate, nervous laughter. She admitted to auditory hallucinations, but would not describe their content. Her speech was at times incoherent and her thinking was described as loose and tangential. She acknowledged her suicide attempt, but added that "if someone would help me and I wouldn't have to be home with my family, I wouldn't want to kill myself." Her concentration, insight, and judgment were described as poor and her intelligence was estimated to be in the low average range.

DSM-III-R Diagnosis

Axis I: Schizoaffective disorder, depressed type
            Rule out Obsessive Compulsive disorder
Axis II: Dependent personality disorder

Axis III: None
Axis IV: Moderate—death of two distant relatives and recent breakup
with boyfriend
Axis V: Fair—Although functions well in highly structured setting,
has been unable to move beyond this setting; has a close relationship with a boyfriend, but otherwise no close relationships
except with family

Treatment and Hospital Course

Upon her admission to the unit, the staff rapidly learned of Ms. R's compulsive handwashing and showering and much attention had to be devoted
to structuring her time around her visits to the bathroom. She took hour-
long showers and made dozens of trips to the bathroom to wash her hands
if unattended by the staff. Her past difficulties in tolerating a number of
neuroleptics and a lack of previous response to either antidepressants, lithium, or electroconvulsive therapy persuaded the staff to reinstitute her
recently discontinued medication despite past problems with hypotension
when this neuroleptic was initiated. She did develop transient hypotension
but as she remained asymptomatic, no immediate change in her pharmacological regimen was made.

Her mental status, however, showed little change on the medication. She
did report feeling "safer" in the hospital and was able to reveal that her visual hallucinations consisted of seeing "dead bodies." She acknowledged that
she had auditory hallucinations, but would not reveal their content other
than to say that occasionally she recognized the voice as that of her cousin.
Her main concerns focused on other patients on the unit and her occasional
feelings that they "did not like her" and perhaps would hurt her. She could
give no reason for these feelings, but often looked scared and anxious. She
acknowledged that washing helped her to feel less anxious. At other times,
she presented as inappropriately cheerful and optimistic, but easily shifted
over into a mood of sadness and feelings of hopelessness when discussing
her present difficulties and future plans.

Shortly after her admission to an acute intake service, Ms. R was transferred to a longer-term treatment unit for additional treatment and discharge planning. The treatment staff there, after a brief period of
observation, felt that her dramatic fluctuations in mood and the appearance
of sleep difficulties, decreased appetite, and preoccupations with death and
feelings of guilt warranted consideration of a schizoaffective diagnosis and
requested psychological testing to help in assessing the relationship between
her psychosis and her affective symptoms.

Psychological Assessment

Ms. R was seen in consultation over a three week period during which she was examined by two psychologists using a wide variety of self-report, interview, clinical psychological and neuropsychological measures. She received some of the subtests of the WAIS-R, the Rorschach, TAT, and SCT, among other tests. In addition to the results of the present evaluation, the results of her evaluation two years previously during her second hospitalization were available for comparison, as well as standard academic achievement measures and other school records.

She had achieved a full scale IQ of 72 on her first WAIS-R testing at age 20 during her second hospitalization. With the exception of *Digit Span*, where she earned an average score, she achieved scaled scores of 4-5 on all other subscales. On subsequent retesting during the present hospitalization at age 22, she received scaled scores of 7 on the *Information, Arithmetic*, and *Similarities* subscales and scaled scores of 10 and 4 on the *Digit Span* and *Picture Completion* subscales, respectively. Her full scale IQ, estimated from these subtest scores, was 86, placing her in the low average range of intellectual functioning. This estimate seemed more consistent with her premorbid intellectual abilities as estimated from her school records and achievement testing and suggested that at the present time her intellectual efficiency was less profoundly influenced by her functional impairment than previously. Nevertheless, she maintained her earlier pattern of substantial intratest scatter, suggesting that her psychological difficulties continued to interfere with her intellectual functioning.

On the Rorschach, Ms. R offered a total of 18 responses, with considerable encouragement from the examiner. The record was remarkable for the complete absence of whole responses, a feature consistent with her generally limited organizational abilities. Her most consistent approach to the blots involved the perception of some edge or extruding detail, giving rise to a rather poor response justified on the basis of indefinite, minor features. For example, her responses to *card I* are "a frog," seen in the top part of the central detail, because of "the hands, the feet and the shape of the face" and "an alligator," seen in the lower portion of the central detail, suggested primarily by "the face, the way it came out. Long." She managed only two popular responses (*card II*, the "baby bears" and *card VIII*, the "tiger or cat") and one very unusual human response (*card VII*). The easily perceived, and popular, human figures on *card III* were seen by Ms. R as "chimps," in part because of their "brownish" color and their "hymen." Although the inquiry failed to elicit any clear perceptual support for the "hymen," she adhered to the association and related it to the "backside, back torso, right?."

Her overreliance on animal detail responses, poor (usually vague) form level, near total absence of any other determinants, and idiosyncratic associations and logic were consistent with a psychotic process. It was noteworthy that although she did not respond very much to color, which taps emotionality, she spontaneously characterized several animal responses somewhat inappropriately and incongruously as "beautiful" and "adorable," almost as if she were endeavoring to ward off dysphoric feelings.

Ms. R's TAT stories were most notable for their pervasive atmosphere of sadness and passive hopefulness. For example, her first story, told to *card 1*, focuses on the boy "thinking" which is "kind of hard on him. He's feeling sad and disappointed because he can't put it together." Despite these travails, she ends on a slightly optimistic note by indicating that "he's going to try to work on it and build his confidence and strength. He'll work on trying to remember what he has to remember." These themes recur on *card 2* where, again, everyone is "thinking" and she hopes for "something good" for the two women lost in thought. Acknowledging the same feelings in *card 3BM*, she concludes the story on a patently dependent note: "I hope someone will come and comfort her, I hope she gets over it, I hope she'll be alright." Although she manages to organize an affective theme for each of the cards, it is invariably disconsolate. This affect seems immobilizing since no one is described as taking steps to alleviate the vague but impending tragedy.

In her SCT, Ms. R makes it clear that effective action is beyond her capabilities. At bottom, she finds she lacks confidence in herself, a quality she wishes she had in greater abundance. As she notes, she often wished she could "gain self confidence" and attributes her lack of success to "her lack of confidence in herself." She feels unable to effectively persist in pursuing her goals. She "gives up" or "sometimes sigh[s]" if she runs into difficulty in getting what she wants. While she retains a desire "to succeed," she feels that she needs certain things from others in order to do so: "protection" from a lover; good cheer from her mother; the backing of those in authority; an abundance of "help and love," generally. These reactions of others affirm her own efforts and help her to achieve her own happiness by making "other people happy."

However, this receptive mode of relating to others thwarts her attempt to pursue her own goals. When confronted with opposition, she prefers to walk away. Yet, she worries about "losing my temper" since she feels guilty about "getting angry." The extent of her guilt and concern in this matter is perhaps best judged by her comments to the examiner during the TAT (*card 12M*) where she became concerned that the examiner might be either "scared" of her or "angry" at her since she felt she had a reputation among the staff and other patients as being "an angry person."

In the report, the examining psychologist noted her propensity to be easily moved by both affect and unrealistic fantasies and that in the face of her generally poor organizational abilities, a psychotic disorder with significant affective features was most likely. The examiner detailed her desire for warm, supportive relationships and indicated that this met her personal needs for direction and appreciation, as well as reflecting some realistic appreciation of her limitations. Unfortunately, her primary means of eliciting the support she needed required her to compromise her ingrained Catholic morality regarding sex and love. Thus, her active heterosexual life had left her with a burden of guilt she could not manage except through outright denial.

Treatment Planning and Outcome

On the basis of these results, Ms. R's treatment team elected to help her pursue her goal of separating from her family in order to encourage her efforts to establish an independent life for herself. Her family, as did the treatment team, harbored some reservations about her ability to function independently. She and her family were presented with a carefully formulated discharge plan involving a halfway house placement and productive employment in a structured work setting appropriate to her intellectual abilities.

Although Ms. R and her family were easily persuaded of the value of the plan, all agreed that additional effort would need to be directed at improving her clinical state. In an effort to do so, her medication was increased. This change, however, provoked the previously expected clinical problems with her hypotension. For the next few weeks, her treatment team attempted to find a suitable medication to little avail. She became severely constipated and was repeatedly worked up for various intestinal and abdominal pathologies, with no significant findings. She began to feel increasingly hopeless about her improvement and her anxiety and her attempts to control it with her compulsive washing both increased. Efforts on the part of the staff to restrict her access to the bathroom led to angry outbursts. She turned to a male patient on the unit for support and became involved in a clandestine sexual relationship which, when finally brought to light, left her feeling betrayed and guilty enough to make a suicide gesture.

At this juncture, she expected the treatment team to revise their discharge plans, but was astonished to learn that she had been accepted at both her favored halfway house program and job placement. Moreover, she found her family firmly resolved to help her pursue these plans and to support her in doing so in whatever way they could. A final change in her medication regimen began to bring about a satisfactory resolution of her psychosis. She was allowed to make several visits home where she began to feel the pull to return to her dependency on her family, but now witnessed their firm insistence that she do things for herself.

As her clinical condition continued to improve, the treatment team was able to work with her and her family to delineate appropriate responsibilities and expectations for her which she seemed willing and able to shoulder. Consequently, when it was learned that there would be an unavoidable delay in admitting her to her halfway house, she and her family were able to work out an interim living arrangement for her so that she could enter her job program. A followup contact several weeks after her discharge revealed that this interim arrangement was working satisfactorily.

EXHIBIT 1

AREA OF ASSESSMENT	CLINICAL EXAMINATION	PSYCHOLOGICAL EXAMINATION
I. Symptoms/Diagnosis *Schizoaffective disorder, depressive type*		
Schizophrenia— persecutory delusions with auditory & visual hallucinations	Believes other people wish to harm her; Claims boyfriend raped her; sees dead bodies; hears cousin's voice	Poor reality testing with prominent autistic and bizarre thinking; poor self-other boundaries
Depression— dysphoric mood	Is often sad or anxious	Preoccupied with sadness
—poor appetite	Poor appetite with mild weight loss	None
—insomnia	Has difficulty falling and staying asleep	None
—feelings of worthlessness and guilt	Feels she is a burden to her family and they would be better off without her	Feels damaged, ineffective and inadequate. Frustration stimulates anger which is projected
—wishes to be dead and suicide attempt	Wants to die and tried to jump out a window	Demoralized and sees self as unable to effect change
II. Personality Factors	Dependent and infantile personality features	Relies on others for support and guidance
		Remains passively hopeful although demoralized
III. Cognitive Abilities	Average intelligence	Low average intelligence
IV. Psychodynamics	Enjoys but feels guilty about her heterosexual activity	Sees her sexuality as necessary to her self-esteem and at odds with her self-image
V. Therapeutic Enabling Factors	History of compliance with past treatments	Relies on judgment of others when convinced they understand her abilities and limitations

Area of Assessment	Clinical Examination	Psychological Examination
	Aspirations are realistic	Realistic aspirations but doubts her ability to follow through
VI. Environmental Demand and Social Adjustment	Stable and consistent performance in structured settings	Able to use consistently applied limits and expectations
	Capacity for warmth in her relationships	Capacity for close relationships marred by fears of denigration

E X H I B I T   2

WAIS-R SUMMARY

Verbal Subtests	*Scaled Score*
Information	7
Digit Span	10
Arithmetic	7
Similarities	7

Performance Subtests

Picture Completion	4
Verbal IQ (est.)	86
Full Scale IQ (est.)	80–90

RORSCHACH SUMMARY

Number of Responses	19
Rejections	0
Populars	1
Originals	0
Average R/T chromatic	43″
Average R/t achromatic	43″
F%	37
F + %	74
A%	89
W:M	0:1
M:Sum C	1:1.5
m:c	2:8
VIII-X%	32
FK + F + Fc%	63
(H + A):(Hd + Ad)	11:8

Apperception	W	0%
	D	58%
	d	21%
	Dd + s	21%

E X H I B I T 3

RORSCHACH SUMMARY

Response	*Inquiry*	*Scoring*
I. 3″		
1. A frog.	1. The hands, the feet, the shape of the face. (*Else?*) No. The eyes, but I don't think so.	DFA
2. An alligator.	2. The face, the way it came out long, the nose, the feet and the shape of the body. The eyes. (*Else?*) The color and shading make it look like alligator skin.	DFc-A
3. Some kind of a deer. The face, the face of a deer. I don't think it looks like a deer, but related to a deer. No, I can't see a deer. That's all.	3. Where? I can't see it. Something about the shape. The ears are like a deer's ears.	dFAd
II. 98″		
I have no idea. I don't see anything to tell you the truth. (*Look further?*) I can't see anything.		
1. These are the only thing I can see, maybe a bear.	1. The ears, shaped like a cub, a baby bear. Really cute adorable like a baby bear, a pair of them. Small and fat and cute, you know?	DFAP

Rorschach Summary

Response	Inquiry	Scoring

III. 8″

1. Sea horse maybe. It's kind of ugly for a seahorse.

    1. I'd say the way it was shaped. (*Else?*) Sharp edges. (?) Color was red (?) No. On the sea horse there's like a long arm stretched but I didn't say anything because I didn't know if a seahorse has an arm. — DFCA

2. Chimpanzees I would say, kind of like monkeys. Two of them. That's all.

    2. The chimpanzees were shape. The hymen and the face. (*Hymen?*) Back side, back torso, right? (*Else?*) They're brownish. — DF-A,Sex

IV. 43″

Even if I do see things, I don't know what they are called.

(*Describe it?*)

I don't see anything in this picture.

1. There's something here but I don't know what it's called. The face of an animal . . . (*rubs blot with index finger*). I don't know what it's called. (*Any kind?*) A beautiful animal but I don't know what it's called.

    1. The black and white coloring like the coloring of a skunk. It's beautiful, but not a skunk. A goat maybe. I'm not sure what I saw. Maybe it is a skunk. It looks soft. (*Soft?*) Just looks nice. The colors look nice, like it feels nice, too. — dFC′.Fc,Ad

RORSCHACH SUMMARY

Response	Inquiry	Scoring

V. 42″

I really don't . . .

1. A seal or a walrus but I think it looks like a seal. The face and the shape of it, the way it has its head looking down. That's what I'd say. Can't think of anything else.

1. Just the shape of the thing. dFM-Ad

VI. 90″

Can't figure them out. Nothing in here.

1. I see a dog, face of a dog.

1. I'd say the nose, the way the face was shaped. The nose protruded. ddFAd

2. I see a man with a moustache. That's all.

2. The moustache made it look like a man. The eyes were nice and eyebrows. (*Nice eyes?*) The eyebrows. (*Else?*) No. (*Hums "Mary had a little lamb" to herself*) dFc-Hd

VII. 36″

Wow!

I don't see too much in this picture. (*Keep looking?*) Well, it

Rorschach Summary

Response	Inquiry	Scoring
1. looked like two people, one of them was holding onto something they were sharing. Two people, a man and a female, a male and a female.	1. They were faced backwards so you couldn't see their faces. One was holding onto a long stick or a handle. They were kneeling like in a prayer in a church. They were kneeling together, two people. (*Stick?*) A long candle or a stick. It wouldn't be a stick in church. A long candle. Maybe they weren't even in a church. I'm tired. Maybe I've been sleeping too much. That's horrible. (*Sleeping too much?*) Yes.	diMH, Obj.
2. I think I see a horse's head. Yeah, a horse's head right here. That's about it.	2. The nose, the color, the darker spot. And white coloring. Looked like a horse to me. Beautiful. (*Else?*) It was spotless, like the nose.	dFC'Ad
3. I see a dog, a puppy of a dog. The face of a dog, cute.	3. The ears flopping down, face like a collie. Beautiful. It doesn't necessarily have to be a puppy but it looked young. A lot of dogs aren't puppies but they look young. Looks furry.	drFcAd

VIII. 15″

1. I think this is some kind of tiger or jaguar. It doesn't have stripes or nothing, but it's like a tiger. That's all I can see. (*Keep looking?*)	1. The way it was stretched out and the length. That's all the legs, the shape of a tiger. (*Else?*) No. The face but the whole thing looked like a tiger to me, face and everything. They are beautiful, the shape of a tiger.	DFMA

RORSCHACH SUMMARY

Response	*Inquiry*	*Scoring*
That's all.		
There's two of them, of course. That's all I can see. The way it's stretched out is like when a cat stretches with legs stretched out.		

IX. 45″

I see animals, a lot of animals, but I don't know what they are called. That's all I can think of. (*Animals?*) Yeah, how many?

1. One, just one. There are two of them.	1. Just a face. (*Animal?*) Face, more like eyes. And the nose is the shape of a moose. (?) Just one eye and the color, the bluish color, is nice. (*Where might you see an animal like this?*) Don't know. I think I saw a picture of one in a book once. Nice coloring.	DFCAd

X. 48″

Wow! This has some crazy stuff in it. I don't know what it is. I really don't see anything.

There's nothing I see. Except I see something over here. I don't know what it is though. Wow!

1. Here and here I see a rabbit. Something like that. The ears come out of the top of this head protruding out.	1. The ears. (*Else?*) No, if there is, I don't remember.	DFA

RORSCHACH SUMMARY

Response	Inquiry	Scoring
2. Lobsters, some kind of thing with antenna here.	2. I saw antenna but I don't know if it was a lobster. I guess it was.	DFA
(*Keep looking.*) That's all I see.		
3. Maybe a dog, a poodle.	3. Looked like curly hair. It didn't look like a regular dog. Looked like a poodle. It just did. (*Else?*) It looked like a poodle to me so all I can see was curly hair. The face. The hair didn't look so flat (?) (*Laughs*) It wasn't the hair, it just looked like a poodle.	DFcA
That's all I see.		
4. And here are sheep. A goat, some kind of goat. Either sheep or goat. Some kind of goat, it's beautiful.	4. The goat because the color is black around the eyes. The coloring of the face, the fur. (*Fur?*) The coloring.	drFC'FcA
That's all.		

E X H I B I T 4

THEMATIC APPERCEPTION TEST

CARD 1 Looks like he's sort of given up—he's thinking and it's kind of hard on him he's thinking too hard and it's kind of hard right now (*Feeling?*) for me or for him. He's feeling sad and disappointed. (*Why?*) Because he can't put it together, get it together. (*Happen?*) He's going to try to work on it and build his confidence and strength. Work on trying to remember what he has to remember.

CARD 2 I remember this one. This lady is looking off in the distance thinking about something also. Another one is thinking. One is sad thinking about something that hurts. The other is thinking about something from a better point of view. The man is just looking off in the distance at the trees in same direction in the house—not the house but looking out that way. (*Feeling?*) Lady seems kind of sad, bothered. The other is thinking something happier and isn't bothered. (*Happen?*) What do you mean happen? I don't know, something good for both of them, all of them I hope. He looks like he has no problems. He might have problems, but nothing there.

CARD 3BM Ah. Poor baby. She's crying over—she's sad she's upset about something so she's bent over thinking about something, upset. She's sad, she's upset. (*Happen?*) I don't know I hope someone will come and comfort her. I hope she gets over it, I hope she'll be all right.

CARD 4 She's very pretty. This looks like a movie scene. Well they're very happy together she loves him. She may not look married but she is—he looks like he's going to be in a fight. She's holding on to him to keep him from getting in a fight. The way his teeth is looks like going to get into trouble. (*Feelings?*) She loves him a lot and he loves her too and he wants to go somewhere because he has to leave, he has something to do. Come to think of it the shading isn't too good his mouth, lips are closed. (*Happen?*) He's going to go. (?) She'll feel bad, sad because she wanted to hold him back and couldn't. He might get hurt or he might beat up on the person.

CARD 12M This might be a priest who's not dressed up who is putting a good word over her or blessing her because she's ill. (*Happen?*) Hopefully she'll be all right. Are you all right? (*Pardon me?*) Are you all right? (*Yes. Why?*) I thought you might think I'm angry and be afraid the word is going around the unit that I'm an angry person. (?) I don't know I'm scared I

THEMATIC APPERCEPTION TEST
---

just think you might be scared that I'm angry at you? Or maybe you're a little angry at me.

CARD 14   Well, I think ummm. . . . this person is in the dark and he wants light so he's opening up the window—wants light to come in, wants to see the light anyway because he's in the dark. (*Feel?*) He just wants light, to see the light, he's in the dark (*Happen?*) nothing really, he's going to open the light, get some light. I don't know why it's so light out and pitch dark inside.

EXHIBIT 5

SENTENCE COMPLETION TEST

2. *She often wished she could* "gain self-confidence."

11. *A woman who falls in love* "feels very protected and beautiful."

22. *When people made fun of her, she* "walked away."

25. *If I think the job is too hard for me, I* "either give up or do something different."

27. *She felt her lack of success was due to* "her lack of confidence in herself."

41. *If I can't get what I want, I* "sometimes sigh."

42. *When I am criticized, I* "feel bad."

60. *My mother always* "cheers me up."

69. *I feel guilty about* "getting angry."

73. *People in authority are* "helpful."

74. *I feel happiest when* "I make other people happy."

83. *More than anything else, she* "needed help and love."

87. *I am afraid of* "losing my temper."

DISCUSSION

The 26-year-old Ms. N was clearly psychotic in her fantasized romance and fertility with an unknowing older male and/or the Holy Spirit. This suggests a desperate yearning for an adult relationship with a male, and concomitant verbal and physical abuse against a mother whom she saw as thwarting this striving for independence. The hospital staff were deadlocked over whether this patient was suffering from schizophrenia or an affective disorder; psychological testing was requested.

Her behavior during the testing involved laughing and singing to herself, suggesting both mood and cognitive deficits. Her performance on the projective tests clearly illustrated her fragmented experience and perceptions, accompanied by elliptical speech and fluidity. In the cross-sectional testing it seemed clear that signs of a manic state, including affective lability, grandiosity, and sexual preoccupation, coexisted with severe disorganized thinking and impairments in reality testing. The testing was influential in redirecting the treatment toward greater attention to the affective symptoms.

In contrast to Ms. N's manic picture, Ms. R, another young single adult woman, presented with depression and psychosis. She, too, was referred for testing to clarify a complicated diagnostic picture. Her behavior included compulsive handwashing and showering in addition to frank psychotic material with visual and auditory hallucinations, but combined with prominent depressive features. These depressive symptoms seemed to arise on the heels of a significant and positive relationship with a boyfriend.

The testing revealed a woman of *Low Average* intellectual functioning. The tests were characterized by a depressed mood, a paucity of thought material which seemed consistent with depression and interpersonal themes of sadness and pervasive powerlessness and passivity. Psychotic thinking was suggested in her poor form level and absence of the ability to integrate percepts and focus on extraneous details.

One might ask how this record can be distinguished from psychotic depression. In this case, the results of the second examination, carried out after partial remission of her more acute symptomatology had been achieved, were very useful. Despite an improvement in her intellectual functioning, she remained quite prone to unusual and idiosyncratic modes of thought. At the time of the second testing, these could no longer be considered consistent with a concomitant disturbance in mood and were more consistent with the schizoaffective diagnosis finally offered.

CHAPTER 4

Major Affective Disorders

A. MAJOR DEPRESSION WITH MELANCHOLIA AND WITH PSYCHOSIS

Mood disorders in DSM-III-R are subdivided into bipolar disorders and depressive disorders. The depressive disorders are two: major depression and dysthymia. The major depressive syndrome includes some or most of the following symptoms for a minimum of two weeks: depressed mood, diminished interest or pleasure in most or all activitites, significant weight loss or gain, insomnia or hypersomnia, psychomotor agitation or retardation, fatigue or loss of energy, feelings of worthlessness and guilt, diminished ability to think or concentrate, recurrent thoughts of death and suicidal ideation or attempt. Since the individuals who become depressed are quite variable in strengths and weaknesses, and since the precursors to depression are multiple, psychological testing is often instrumental in further defining the treatment plans to fit the individual case.

MAJOR DEPRESSION, SINGLE EPISODE, WITH MELANCHOLIA

Mr. F, a 24-year-old, single, white male of Italian-Roman Catholic background, had moved to a new city to begin his graduate studies earlier in the fall. It was his first experience living away from home and he had trouble adjusting to a bachelor's routine. As a serious student, he resented his roommate's more lackadaisical approach to his studies. He had tried to accommodate his roommate's untidy habits and irregular hours and had even made an effort to be friendly to the seemingly endless parade of girlfriends who came by to visit. As his schoolwork began to suffer, he had retreated to the solitude of his own room where he hoped to ignore the distractions of his roommate and get on with his studies.

His school performance continued to demand more and more of his time. Increasingly distressed over his inability to excel in the classroom, he sought psychiatric consultation. After a few visits, the psychiatrist recommended a leave of absence from school and Mr. F returned home where he continued in an outpatient treatment with a local psychiatrist. He was bitterly disappointed in himself and was convinced that his family was equally disappointed in him. Although his psychiatrist encouraged him to get out of the house more, he was unable to face his old friends and spent most of his day at home.

Over the next few weeks, he became increasingly agitated and upset over his withdrawal from school and his psychiatrist recommended a brief hospitalization at a nearby private hospital for a diagnostic workup and initiation of pharmacological treatment of his anxiety and agitation. He was begun on a medication to help control his anxiety, but his guilt and distress continued to mount and his family agreed to let him return home against his doctor's advice. After several days of increasing agitation and sleepless nights, Mr. F and his family agreed to a hospital admission at a prominent local teaching hospital.

At admission, his agitation and distress were immediately obvious. When asked about himself, his report clearly revealed that in the last month he had experienced a pervasive disinterest in his usual activities, progressive social isolation, and a deterioration in his ability to function autonomously. His appetite had declined and he was not sleeping well. In a tense and worried manner, he attempted to give a clear account of his experience, but had difficulty concentrating, which he expressed as his difficulty in "thinking clearly." He was preoccupied with feelings of guilt and worthlessness and reported recurrent thoughts of his death. He could not rid himself of a nagging concern that he may be a homosexual. He had recently engaged in homosexual practices which he found "disgusting." Although preoccupations with his sexual orientation were not new, he had become increasingly self-conscious about the matter as his roommate had become involved in heterosexual relationships and his educational curriculum directly exposed him to sexual issues. He gave no evidence or history of hallucinations or delusions, but did express a fear that he was losing his mind.

DSM III-R Diagnosis

Axis I: Major depression, single episode, with melancholia
Axis II: None
Axis III: None

Axis IV: Moderate—beginning a new school year, revealing his sexual
            concerns to classmates
Axis V: Fair—good academic functioning but no close friends

Treatment and Hospital Course

Immediate management of his agitation and distress was attempted
with a neuroleptic and a benzodiazepine. This treatment regimen was
unsuccessful in alleviating his symptoms and he developed several non-
organic physical complaints. In the second week following his admission,
benzodiazepines were discontinued and he was begun on an
antidepressant. Despite adequate serum levels, he failed to improve and
two weeks later was referred for psychological testing. Following completion of the testing, Mr. F attempted to injure himself on several occasions, either by asphyxiation or electrocution, and was referred for ECT.
In the next seven weeks, he received a total of 19 unilateral treatments
and showed substantial improvement. He was discharged on a lower
dose of an antidepressant, with plans to live in a structured residential
setting where he would be involved in an outpatient treatment and
engage in a volunteer job.

Psychological Assessment

Mr. F was referred for psychological testing to help in establishing his
diagnosis and provide an assessment of his intellectual and personality
strengths and weaknesses. His failure to respond to antidepressant treatment, the slightly bizarre nature of his attempted suicide by electrocution,
and a persistent, intermittent and mild thought disorder provided the basis
for the diagnostic referral. The diagnostic differential suggested by the
referring therapist was between a major depression with melancholic and
perhaps psychotic features and a schizophreniform disorder. An intellectual
assessment was requested to ascertain if the patient had sufficient intellectual ability to undertake his graduate education. The assessment of his personality strengths and weaknesses was requested to aid in determining an
appropriate psychotherapeutic strategy once his acute difficulties could be
brought under control.

Although cooperative and motivated during the testing, he was clearly
distressed and anxious. He was aware of his difficulties in concentration
and of a decline from his previous high level of functioning in other
areas as well, and frequently sought reassurance from the examiner that

he was not "off the wall." His evaluation consisted of a complete WAIS, a Rorschach, TAT, DAP, a partial Bender (copy only), and the Object Sorting Test.

The test results repeatedly reflected Mr. F's acute anxiety and distress. There was considerable variability in his WAIS subscale scores, which ranged from low average to superior, with numerical reasoning among the lowest, a pattern which confirmed his concentration difficulty. A test which entails simple rote memory of numbers, and so requires less cognitive effort, yielded a better performance. Finally, there is evidence of muscular tension, a component of anxiety, in his reproduction of the geometric designs on the Bender.

The clinical history clearly revealed a recent, abrupt decline in functioning and was indicative of some strain between this young man's aspirations and his abilities. Although his verbal IQ of 122 suggested that despite his current distress, he had the intellectual ability to perform adequately in a postgraduate program, personality factors were clearly limiting his full employment of these intellectual abilities. This same inefficiency due to personality factors hampered his Rorschach performance, which was characterized by a paucity of complex, integrated responses, a restricted range of associations (A% and multiple determinants) and an overreliance on popularly perceived, unelaborated responses (P%).

Strong depressive themes and a considerable level of personality disorganization contributed most prominently to his inefficiency. His TAT contained stories about people who are "frightened by the complexity of life" and seek "refuge" in the security of family and home. Life in the larger world is fraught with danger, particularly the danger of having one's "imperfections" revealed. His awareness of his cognitive difficulties on the WAIS, perceived as "imperfections," provoked significant anxiety and contributed to an erratic pattern of subscale scores. However, the quality of his responses to the structured WAIS items as well as to the more unstructured Rorschach indicated retention of the capacity to adequately test reality despite frequent lapses in critical judgment and intrusion of fantasy material. Throughout the test record, there was abundant evidence of the toll taken by his efforts to adhere to reality constraints and, as suggested by the TAT, of a desire for a simpler, more trusting relationship with others, uncomplicated by the strife of adulthood.

The main psychological issues and personality factors which compromised his intellectual and emotional functioning seemed clearly related to the developmental tasks of early adulthood. He experienced conflict between his high need for nurturance and support and his desire for independence and achievement. The former threatened to shade into a passive dependency linked with a homosexual orientation, while the latter were at times confused with hostility and aggression. At either pole, his idealized view of the adult man as strong, ambitious, and competent, yet loving and sensitive to his family, was in danger of crumbling.

While struggling to integrate these aspects of himself, he apparently alternated between experiencing himself as "a robot" (Rorschach *card IX*) or as a small and insignificant animal (squirrels on Rorschach *card VIII*). His rigid self-control seemed designed to contain and blunt the threat of aggression he experiences, reflected, for example, in his Rorschach percept "someone with boxing gloves on." Yet, these efforts at denying its existence to himself and others left him filled with a loneliness that was "intense and agonizing." These concerns were heightened by the task of separating from his family and establishing an independent existence and identity. In achieving the goal of separation, efforts to help both the patient and his family to accept his ambitions and his limitations seemed likely to be rewarded.

Treatment Planning and Outcome

The results of Mr. F's psychological assessment were reviewed by his treatment team and, as a result, the patient's treatment plan was revised to include twice weekly sessions with his family. These family sessions were included to directly address the issues of separation and the family's denial of the patient's present limitations. Each family session was immediately followed by individual psychotherapy sessions to counter the potential for regression brought on by the discussion of these issues.

As a result of these changes in his treatment plan, the patient was able to sustain his improvement following ECT. Although he continued to struggle with feelings of depression and anxiety, these feelings appeared more realistically related to his immediate concerns and present limitations. His affect was generally better modulated and his feelings were more successfully integrated with his ideas such that he was neither isolating his feelings nor becoming overwhelmed by them.

The work with the family and the patient helped them to understand his need for continued treatment in a structured setting. Application to halfway house programs in his home area and to programs in the city where he had been doing his graduate study were made. At the time of the patient's discharge, he had been referred for continued individual and family therapy, was accepted at a halfway house program in the local area, and had obtained a tutoring position which would engage him in a few hours of work each week. He had not decided on whether to return to his graduate studies, but had agreed to continue to discuss this issue as part of his outpatient treatment.

E X H I B I T 1

AREA OF ASSESSMENT	CLINICAL EXAMINATION	PSYCHOLOGICAL EXAMINATION
I. Symptoms/Diagnosis		
Major depression, single episode, with melancholia		
Dysphoric mood and loss of interest and pleasure	No interest in any of his usual activities	Depressive themes and impoverishment of intellectual resources
Poor appetite	Eats poorly; has lost a few pounds	None
Insomnia	Difficulty falling and staying asleep	None
Psychomotor agitation	Paces, cannot sit still	Tense and restless
Feelings of worthlessness, self-reproach and guilt	Berates self for homosexual feelings and experiences	Feels unable to live up to idealized masculine image
Difficulty concentrating	Has trouble following conversations; seems distracted	Difficulty utilizing intellectual resources under moderately effortful conditions
Suicidal ideation	Has considered ending his life	Despairs of achieving his goals and living up to expectations of himself and others
II. Personality Factors	Ambitious, interested in mastery	Motivated by aspirations, achievement oriented
III. Cognitive Abilities	None	Above average intelligence
		Cognitive inefficiency due to acute distress
IV. Psychodynamics	Conflict over dependency/mastery	Ambivalent about success and the price it exacts
	Aggressive feelings consciously rejected but feels guilty	Wishes to be rid of baser human feelings

AREA OF ASSESSMENT	CLINICAL EXAMINATION	PSYCHOLOGICAL EXAMINATION
	Fearful of intimacy	Equates closeness with passivity and dependency
V. Therapeutic Enabling Factors	None	Intelligence
		Capacity for self-observation
		Achievement history and orientation
VI. Environmental Demand and Social Adjustment	Demanding educational environment and feeling of failure	Usually mobilized by demand given his high need for achievement
	Poor sexual adjustment	Desires for strength to compensate for underlying homosexual concerns

EXHIBIT 2

WAIS-R SUMMARY

Verbal Subtests	*Scaled Score*
Information	15
Comprehension	14
Arithmetic	12
Similarities	13
Digit Span	15
Vocabulary	13

Performance Subtests	
Digit Symbol	13
Picture Completion	8
Block Design	9
Picture Arrangement	8
Object Assembly	11
Verbal IQ	122
Performance IQ	98
Full Scale IQ	112

RORSCHACH SUMMARY

Number of Responses	19
Rejections	0
Populars	6
Originals	0
Average R/T chromatic	7″
Average R/T achromatic	7″
F%	42
F+%	79
A%	47
H%	32
W:M	8:5
M:SumC	5:1
m:c	6:0
VIII-X%	37
FK+F+Fc%	42
(H+A):(Hd+Ad)	13:2

Rorschach Summary

Apperception	W	42%
	D	42%
	d	0%
	Dd + S	16%

EXHIBIT 3

RORSCHACH SUMMARY

Response	*Inquiry*	*Scoring*
I. 2″		
1. The front part of a ship with oars on either side.	1. Shape.	WF-Obj.
2. Butterfly.	2. It's shaped like it.	WFAP
3. An animal that's on its front legs and its back legs are out.	3. (*Kind of animal?*) Not really a cow, like a goat or something. (*Goat?*) Just seemed that the back part was up kicking.	WFM-A
II. 10″		
1. I think I see the head of two dogs facing each other, probably puppies. That's it. Do you want more than one response? (*Whatever you see*)	1. Puppies looking at each other.	DFMAP
2. There's something—it seems like it's a jet or a plane going this way.	2. (*Jet or plane?*) Shaped like one and the red would be the smoke coming out the back. (*Smoke?*) It just was red and seemed like fire burning.	SFmObj DCF.mF Fire, Smoke
III. 10″		
1. This looks like two butlers facing each other and carrying dishes. That's it. (*Look longer*) That's it.	1. Wearing a tuxedo. (*Tuxedo?*) The way the front parts stick out and the back part was longer.	WMH, Cloth P
IV. 15″		
1. Looks like two boots that are leaned up against a wall, back to back. Here's one boot, the other, the heel and the toe.	1. Shaped like boots and they're leaning. (*Leaning?*) Looks like they are balanced there on their heels. They are tilting back a bit.	WFm Cloth

RORSCHACH SUMMARY

Response	*Inquiry*	*Scoring*
2. Another possibility would be an animal with wings and antennae over here. That's it.	2. (*Kind of animal?*) Sort of like an insect. (*Insect?*) The head part with the antennae.	WF-A

V. 5″

1. Again, it looks sort of like an insect with wings— here's the head, antennaes, two wings. That's it.	1. Just the shape.	WFA

VI. 10″

1. Seems like two people lying down with their arms up and yelling or talking . . . and they might be Indians if this is a feather coming out of the head. Here are the heads, mouths, arms, legs. The head is near me.	1. (*Yelling or talking?*) The way the mouth was open.	DMH,Obj.
2. This looks like a penis over here.	2. The way it's shaped.	diF Sex

VII. 5″

1. Again, it looks like two people, this time two women, facing each other, with their hair up, have ponytails that are up in the air. They must be mad because their jaw is out a little. Here's the hair, nose, jaw.	1. They're looking at each other and seem angry because of the shape of the jaw.	WMHP

RORSCHACH SUMMARY

Response	Inquiry	Scoring
VIII. 5″		
1. I see two animals, probably squirrels or beavers or something. Here are the legs, tails.	1. The shape of the figures. That's all.	DFAP
2. I see arms reaching out to them, here are the arms and the fingers.	2. (*Kind of arms?*) The arm part. (*Of?*) A person.	drMHd
IX. 10″		
1. I see like a robot—here's the head part, the body part, wheels on bottom.	1. It's shaped that way.	D(S)F(H)
2. The possibility that this is someone down here with boxing gloves on. (*Demonstrates*) Here are the eyes and the outstretched arms with boxing gloves on.	2. (*Boxing gloves?*) They just seemed to be very large in comparison to the rest of the body. They seemed to predominate and extend out.	D(S)M-Hd, Obj.
X. 2″		
1. I see two spiders here and here.	1. Legs of spiders.	DFAP
2. This looks like two lions over here.	2. They seemed to be proud, with the head up. (*Anything else?*) The front part of the body was very strong.	DFMA
3. This looks like two frogs. Am I completely off the wall?	3. The legs seemed to be outstretched.	DFMA

E X H I B I T 4

THEMATIC APPERCEPTION TEST

CARD 1   The parents of a little boy bought a violin for their son and wanted to give him lessons on this instrument. He would take the violin and sit at his desk in his room, close his eyes, and think of the day when he would be a great violinist. Through the years he spent many a day playing and enjoying the music he created with his violin. In time he became a great violinist and brought joy to all who heard him play.

CARD 3BM   The crippled girl sat alone often in the confines of her home. The tragedy of the accident she experienced years before had left her with a broken body and a broken spirit. The loneliness of her world was intense and agonizing. She would sit with her head buried in her arms and wonder why this tragedy was necessary. She wouldn't see the things that were happening around her but would isolate her feelings in the mattress that she was clinging to. The other people in her life tried desperately to remove the loneliness but were unable to penetrate her world of agony. She died on her mattress with her arms and her head buried in the graveyard of her room. (*How die?*) With a broken heart. (*Agony?*) Being alone (*Others try to penetrate*) she would just close herself off (*Why?*) she just couldn't accept herself and her imperfections.

CARD 4   The two children, the girl and the boy, grew up together in the small town beside the sea. Throughout the years they developed a fondness that was transformed into love. As they got older they sensed that they needed each other and decided to live in the cottage whose backyard ran up to the sea. They led a life that was difficult but satisfying and they were sustained by their love and by their devotion to each other. Their life was invaded by the cruelty and insanity of war. The husband was called to serve in the armed forces of his country and was asked to leave his home for far away lands. But his wife cannot understand his departure from her life and she attempted to stop her husband from leaving. The man was torn between the two worlds but decided that it was necessary for him to leave. He did return though and the tranquility and love in their lives increased even more.

CARD 6BM   The man woke up that morning and went on with his daily work and activity. The phone was used to contact associates for his very successful company. One morning the phone rang and his mother asked him to come to the home that he grew up in. His mother said that she needed him with her because his father had died. He came home and stood with his mother beside the bed of his deceased father. They stared out the window and his mother would cry and wish for the days that she spent with her husband. (*Son feels?*) Very sad.

CARD 7BM   The train moved slowly to its destination to New York, to Boston, from New York to Boston. The time seemed long for the two men who were anxious to return to their homes during the holiday season. They sat on the train and talked of their families who were awaiting their arrival at the train station. The other man had experienced a longer life than the young man who sat beside him. He saw in his companion a part which he had experienced 20 years earlier. He saw the uncertainty and the burden of responsibility in the young man's eyes. He assured his companion that he should enjoy all those things, his family, and life, that he had taken for granted during his own lifetime. The friendships, the disappointments, and the situations he had experienced when he was younger became very real to him as he listened to the words of the younger man beside him. He became more aware of his present and would return home with a greater appreciation of his family, and of his life.

CARD 10   The boy was frightened by the complexity of life and found refuge by his parents and the rest of his family. He would seek the reassurance and the power of strength that his mother and father provided. Those things that frightened him and made him seek his parents' reassurance, things that he eventually could cope with and understand. (*What?*) Just the complexity of life. I sort of thought about myself there. (*Who's in the picture?*) Me and my father, I guess. I don't know why I'm making such abstract stories rather than saying "a boy fell on his knee and ran to his father."

CARD 13MF   The man and the woman shared a small apartment in the heart of the busy city. Beyond the noise and confusion of life outside, they experienced a oneness in this love and devotion to each other. But fate could not be stopped even within the haven of their home and tragedy and death occurred. While they both slept through the night, he felt the coldness of her body and knew that she died peacefully. He went on with his life but no longer found the security and companionship in his lost partner.

MAJOR DEPRESSION, RECURRENT, WITH PSYCHOSIS

Mrs. D is a 47-year-old, recently divorced mother of a teenage son and a nine-year-old daughter. She has been hospitalized twice in the last two years. Her ex-husband has been carrying on an affair with his secretary for several years before their divorce. Even after the divorce, he denied Mrs. D's accusations of infidelity, telling her that she was "crazy." She tried to take her life on three previous occasions. Her two most recent suicide attempts were provoked by her despair over being unable to regain control of her ex-husband's affections. Her life had been devoted to her family and she had few interests or friends outside of her home.

Over the past month, she grew more depressed. She sent her son and her daughter to another state to live with her sister for a few weeks. She had trouble falling asleep and staying asleep. She spent much of the night pacing her bedroom. She cried frequently and was upset at the slightest inconvenience. She was eating poorly and lost 15 pounds over the last month. She was fearful of leaving the house and unable to keep her appointments with her psychiatrist or regularly go to work. She managed to call the psychiatrist periodically and in their last conversation told him that she had purchased a gun with the intention of using it to end her life if she didn't begin to feel better soon. Her psychiatrist persuaded her to come to the hospital despite her fears that she would be "poisoned by more drugs while there."

When admitted, Mrs. D was described as a "thin, very anxious, tearful, depressed woman who wrings her hands and becomes easily agitated." She was preoccupied with the idea that the hospital staff would hurt her, feeling that past hospitalizations had been harmful to her. She recognized that she was "nervous and depressed" and noted that "I haven't been sleeping well." She attributed her recent difficulties to her failures as wife and mother and alternated between an agonizing guilt over these failures and rambling descriptions of how her ex-husband and children had continually persecuted her over the last few years. She denied any present suicidal intentions, but made it clear that she felt she had few other options than to take her life.

DSM-III-R Diagnosis

Axis I: Major depression, recurrent, with psychotic features

Axis II: Dependent personality disorder with possible paranoid features

Axis IV: Moderate—conflict with her sons; recent divorce

Axis V: Fair—moderate impairment in social relations and occupational functioning

Treatment and Hospital Course

Mrs. D was admitted to an acute care unit with the expectation that she could be returned to her previously effective medication regimen and quickly discharged to the care of her referring psychiatrist. During previous episodes of illness, it had been established that she could not tolerate pharmacologically effective doses of many common antidepressants because of blood pressure problems. During her most recent prior hospitalization, she had been effectively treated with a combination of lithium and a monoamine oxidase inhibitor. The hospital staff reinstated this drug regimen, but despite several adjustments she remained tearful, depressed, and fearful that the hospital staff would harm her.

She was transferred to an extended care unit after one month with a recommendation for a reevaluation of her diagnosis and treatment plan because she had failed to improve. During the third week following her transfer, her hospital psychotherapist requested a psychological consultation. There had been some improvement in her depression but she remained preoccupied with her "failures" and continued to deny the severity of her illness.

Psychological Assessment

Mrs. D was given a WAIS-R, Rorschach, DAP, SCT, and Benton Visual Retention Test during the seventh week of her hospital stay. The specific referral questions included a request for a formal assessment of her intelligence, the severity of her suicidal ideation, and her capacity to utilize either a supportive or insight-oriented psychotherapy. While she cooperated with the examination, her manner was described as "obsequious" in that she was constantly concerned over whether she had given the examiner "what he wanted." Despite her desire to cooperate, it was necessary to extend the examination over 10 days as she tired quickly and would complain of fatigue and nervousness.

On the WAIS-R, Mrs. D obtained a full-scale IQ of 88 with verbal and performance IQs of 88 and 89, respectively. Her scaled subtest scores ranged from below average (*Similarities, Picture Completion* and *Digit Symbol*) to average (*Vocabulary*). Although evidencing only a modest degree of inter-test scatter, she invariably missed or received only partial credit for some of the easiest items on each of the subtests. This pattern of early misses raised questions about her intellectual efficiency and concerns about possible impairment of her reality-testing abilities. Her WAIS-R profile indicated that her performance was frequently disrupted by anxiety and that she had difficulty in making any sustained effort or in easily focusing her concentration.

Mrs. D's approach to the more unstructured tests in the battery revealed her intense needs for an orderly and predictable world in which affection and decorum were the mainstays of human relationships. When conflict erupted, she was left feeling annoyed, guilty and unable to cope. Her SCT responses traced this progression in the context of her marriage and divorce. She believed that *a woman who falls in love* "should know her man and love him just the way he is and not want to change him." Believing that *most men* "are honest, hardworking, and faithful," she seemed secure in realizing her daydream about "having a wonderful family of father, mother, and sons." Understandably, then, she reported that *I was most annoyed when* "my ex-husband was not truthful to me" and that *I could hate a person who* "lies and uses other people."

Surprisingly, she felt guilty about the divorce despite coming to believe that "I did all I could to make it work and it didn't work." This thematic progression suggested that she had few internal resources for coping with conflict. Instead, she relied on obedience to a hopefully benevolent external authority, a pattern adopted early in life (e.g. *When they told her what to do, she* "usually always obeyed because she wanted to please her parents."). Currently, she feels quite damaged by the events transpiring in her life, not unlike the "cat that someone ran over and the poor thing is squashed" which she perceived on *card VI* of the Rorschach.

Her lack of internal resources and her reliance on external structure were evident in her Rorschach responses. She gives five popular responses and nine easily perceived animal responses in a total record of 19 responses. Her percepts were most often highly congruent with the consensual reality of the inkblots (F+ = 88%), yet she repeatedly emphasizes the "fantasy," "exaggerated" or "cartoon-like" qualities of the blots to justify her percepts. These qualities were typically invoked in order to deal with her self-uncertainties as well as to distance herself from her emotional reactions to her percepts. Her emotionality may precipitate transient lapses in reality testing as demonstrated in her response to *card III*. She reports ". . . fantasy animals here. It looks like two chickens with the beak and the neck and one leg, and it almost looks like the leg has a high heel on, and I would say it would be two women chickens, because they got a little plume down here, so maybe they're excited about going out on a date—you know, how they have it on the cartoons. And this bow might represent their heart, each one's heart, that they're excited about what they're going to do."

Her need for emotional distance also appeared in the context of the perception of the "dangerous" qualities of her percepts. For example, on *card IV* she reported a monster "like Bigfoot because he has huge feet and a large tail and tiny arms and a tiny head." As she continued, she noted that the head is "like an alligator, so he could be dangerous" and summed up by saying that "so that's basically what I see this as—a cartoon monster, and I would call him Bigfoot." During the inquiry, she continued to rationalize and to distance herself from the percept by ascribing the origin of the percept to watching TV with her children when they were little, stating that "there was a monster similar to that on a Christmas show, a snow monster, and my son used to get afraid of that monster and we used to have to turn it off."

The somewhat paranoid sense of cold, ominous danger that permeates this response reappeared on *card VIII*. Two polar bears were seen as "trying to climb up the side of a glacier, a snowy mountain, to the top." In the inquiry, she responded that "immediately they resembled polar bears; not so fantasy-looking, like real polar bears . . . and it looks like they had a hard time getting up to the icy top." The response contained an implied success of the polar bears' effort. The Sentence Completion Test also revealed a focus on being successful. There were assertions of her desire for greater independence and the success hard work brings. She states that when she was completely on her own, she "became very independent," but ascribes her lack of vocational success to a "lack of hard work." She is ashamed that "I was not strong in my convictions."

Although she asserted that committing herself to such achievement goals and pursuing them with determination represent a viable alternative for her, they are presented more as attitudes likely to win approval than as motivating and sustaining beliefs. Her inability to integrate these two aspects of her self-representation—on the one hand, obedience and submission, and on the other, ambition and self-fulfillment—was apparent in her figure drawings. Both the male and female figure drawings are childlike representations drawn with smiling, open faces and arms, but with stiff and rigid postures. Her self-portrait lacks any sexual specificity despite the implication of adulthood derived from its larger size. The figure is presented with short hair and billowing, knee-length trousers, with buttons placed down the middle of the shirt and at the cuffs. Unlike the male and female figure drawings which are filled in with heavy shading reflecting apprehensiveness, her more idealized self is an open figure with only the short hair receiving any shading. The childlike qualities of the picture she drew of herself seem more in keeping with her wishes to be nurtured and directed; by contrast, the asexual but somewhat masculine qualities appear to be an attempt to honor her attitudes concerning ambition and self-assertiveness, but at the price of rejecting her femininity.

Treatment Planning and Outcome

In reviewing the results of the psychological testing with the hospital treatment team, the implications of her intellectual level, transient disruptions in reality testing in the context of psychosexual and aggressive thematic content, and reliance on external authority were the main elements of her assessment brought to bear on her treatment plan. Her pharmacological regimen remained unchanged in light of the depressive characteristics implied by her preoccupation with the divorce and her disproportionate guilt-feelings in relation to it.

In view of her history of reliance on external authority and her presently limited capacities to cope with internal distress, a supportive approach to her psychotherapeutic treatment was recommended. Within such a supportive framework, she was encouraged to develop realistic job aspirations in line with her intellectual abilities. She was also encouraged to widen her network of social supports and to share more equitably the burden of raising her two children with her ex-husband.

Over the next six weeks, Mrs. D's mental status continued to improve. She became less preoccupied with her divorce and her guilt ruminations as her depression resolved. Keeping pace with this positive development was a growing sense that the present treatment plan, in which she actively participated, was effectively designed to assist her and she gave up her concern that the treatment staff would harm her. She was, in fact, able to coordinate the care of her children with her ex-husband and felt reassured that she could rely on his help more than she had previously. She successfully negotiated a return to work with her former employer, who was able to keep her in her present position and provide the additional structure and guidance on the job that she needed.

At the end of her three month hospital stay, Mrs. D was discharged from the hospital and returned to the care of her referring psychiatrist. He found the recommendations made by the hospital treatment team useful and was able to provide for her care after discharge.

EXHIBIT 1

AREA OF ASSESSMENT	CLINICAL EXAMINATION	PSYCHOLOGICAL EXAMINATION
I. Symptoms/Diagnosis		
Major depression, recurrent, with psychotic features		
Dysphoric mood and loss of pleasure	Depressed mood and sad affect	Dysphoria related to divorce and mistrust verging on paranoia
At least four symptoms		
Poor appetite/ weight loss	Lost 15 pounds in last month	None
Insomnia	Initial, middle and terminal insomnia	None
Psychomotor agitation or retardation	Agitated, hand-wringing	Psychomotor retardation
Excessive guilt	Feels to blame for divorce despite objective evidence	Preoccupied and guilty regarding divorce
Impaired concentration	Easily returns to perseveration regarding mistreatment by husband and sons	Difficulty concentrating with impaired intellectual efficiency
Suicidal ideation/attempt	Past attempts and present ideation	None
Psychotic delusions of harm congruent with themes of personal inadequacy and guilt	Fears being poisoned by treatment staff	Transient impairment in reality testing in the context of sexual or aggressive themes
II. Personality Factors	None	Optimal functioning with high external structure
		Childlike need for nurturance and support
III. Cognitive Abilities	None	Low average intelligence
IV. Psychodynamics	None	Limited ability to cope with emotional distress

AREA OF ASSESSMENT	CLINICAL EXAMINATION	PSYCHOLOGICAL EXAMINATION
		Tends to externalize internal conflict; rationalization is a major defense
V. Therapeutic Enabling Factors	None	Responds positively to benevolent authority
VI. Environmental Demand and Social Adjustment	Feels unable to manage her children	Expects compliance with authority
	Few friends	None
	Recent divorce; conflict with ex-husband	Feels abandoned and betrayed by ex-husband

EXHIBIT 2

WAIS-R SUMMARY

Verbal Subtests	*Scaled Score*
Information	8
Comprehension	7
Arithmetic	10
Similarities	7
Digit Span	8
Vocabulary	6
Performance Subtests	
Digit Symbol	6
Picture Completion	9
Block Design	9
Picture Arrangement	8
Object Assembly	6
Verbal IQ	88
Performance IQ	89
Full Scale IQ	88

RORSCHACH SUMMARY

Number of Responses	19
Rejections	0
Populars	5
Originals	0
Average R/T chromatic	36″
Average R/T achromatic	7″
F%	42
F+%	88
A%	47
H%	26
W:M	8:2
M:Sum C	2:4
m:c	3:2
VIII-X%	53
FK+F+Fc%	42
(H+A):(Hd+Ad)	13:1

RORSCHACH SUMMARY

Apperception   W   42%
D   58%
d   0%
Dd + S   0%

EXHIBIT 3

RORSCHACH SUMMARY

Response	*Inquiry*	*Scoring*

I. 11″

1. It looks like it almost could be a cat's face. It that all you want, one thing? I think definitely it looks like a cat's face, when they are hissing, their ears go out and their back goes up, because he's afraid. I'd stick with that.

1. The entire picture just looks like, is a cat's face; a black cat that got frightened, the ears kind of go up like they do, and the mouth is kind of exaggerated, and that was my immediate thought was a black cat's face. (?) Just definitely the whole entire shape; the eyes, ears, nose; just a complete picture of a cat. (*Frightened or hissing?*) The exaggerated mouth and ears kind of sticking out rather than up, like cats usually are. It's an exaggerated picture, but that's how I'd describe it.

WFM.FC′Ad

II. 30″

1. I guess what I'd get out of this is two cartoon people touching hands, OK? What else do you want me to describe? They're exaggerated cartoon people because they have a pointed head, and stripes which would be their backs, and definitely an eye on each creature, and a little mouth and nose and a neck, with an exaggerated body, and each one is touching a hand, and as the body comes down, the red part would be a leg, and they have another leg in back, and the bump in the middle would be the tail.

1. Just the nature of it; it was more fantasy-type inkblot: I couldn't get anything realistic out of it, so it brought to mind cartoons for children.

WM(H)P

RORSCHACH SUMMARY

Response	*Inquiry*	*Scoring*

III. 36″

1. They're all so . . . All I do is see all these fantasy animals here. It looks like two chickens with the beak and the neck and one leg, and it almost looks like the leg has a high heel on, and I would say it would be two women chickens, because they got a little plume down here, so maybe they're dressed to go out, and this red bow in the middle, so maybe they're excited about going out on a date—you know how they have it on the cartoons, and this bow might represent their heart, each one's heart, that they're excited about what they're going to do.

1. (*Chickens?*) They just look like chickens to me, having watched so many cartoons with the kids, it just resembles chickens. (*Women chickens?*) Like leg had high heel and the plume, like they were dressed up to go out, the shape looks like a plume in each of their hands. (*Red bow?*) Represented each of their hearts, so their hearts were excited, they were going out. (*Hearts?*) Just the fact that they were dressed up and excited and it kind of had the shape of a heart, and they were connected, and sometimes I say I wear my heart on my sleeve, so that's how I use that.

WM(A)
DF Cloth
DFC Cloth P
Confab.

IV. 5″

1. I see nothing but cartoons (*Laugh*). Is that unusual? I know you can't say. This also looks like a monster feature, and I would say this is like bigfoot, because he has huge feet and a large tail and tiny arms and a tiny head, but a head like an alligator, so he could be dangerous. So that's basically what I see this as—a cartoon monster, and I would call him bigfoot.

1. Just because of watching from when the kids were little—there was a monster similar to that on a Christmas show—a snow monster, and my son used to get afraid of that monster and we used to have to turn it off. (*Anything else*) No, just the whole blot itself, like the story we used to watch.

WF(A) Fab.

Rorschach Summary

Response	*Inquiry*	*Scoring*

V. 7″

1. This looks like a butterfly, definitely, with the long wings and antennae and head, and a little part that comes out at the end of the butterfly. It's exaggerated, because it's not perfect like a butterfly, but it reminds me of a butterfly.

    1. The whole thing—a butterfly with the wings spread open.   WFMAP

VI. 3″

1. Oh God, here we go again with more animals. This is sad, but it looks like a cat that someone ran over, and the poor thing is squashed, and we've got the head with the little whiskers coming out, and the neck, and his whole body has been opened and smashed, and it reminds me of a cat that someone ran over—very sad.

    1. The head made me think it was a cat, and it being flattened out and opened up made me think it was in an accident and someone ran over it, because it wouldn't be in that shape if something hadn't happened to it but still alive.   WFM(A)

VII. 10″

1. Oh, gosh. (*Laugh*) OK, this one again looks like two women that are dancing. They've turned around to look at each other. You see the long hair fixed so it stands straight up, the puff of hair on the forehead, the nose, mouth, one hand. They're dancing from the side. This is like a theatrical play where they're dancing and they've kind of backed into each other and they turned to face each other. You can see one hand and one foot. Of course it's exaggerated, but basically that's it.

    1. (*Women?*) The heads— definitely very feminine looking heads. (*Hair?*) The way it was standing straight up, and puffy the front.   WMHP

RORSCHACH SUMMARY

Response	*Inquiry*	*Scoring*

VIII. 37″

Oh, wow! Hmmm. That's
in color. Hmm, let's see.
OK. Hmm . . .

1. OK, this to me looks like
two polar bears trying to
climb up the side of a glacier snowy mountain to the
top, which is the gray area,
the snowy area and you
definitely see four legs and
the shape of a polar bear
and the head, and on the
left one an ear. They're trying to climb up to the snow
peak, which is the gray
area.

1. (*Polar bears?*) Immediately
they resembled polar
bears; not so fantasy-
looking; like real polar
bears, and going up to the
gray area, the snowy
area.(*Why polar bears?*) Just
because I think of the real
cold, and it looks like they
had a hard time getting up
to the icy top, and the gray
area looks like snow, so
that's why I picked polar
bears.

DFMAP
DFC′Ldsc

IX. 25″

Oh, wow—I don't know if I
see anything. What hap-
pens if you don't see
anything?

1. The only thing I would say
is that it would be a very
exaggerated cartoon crea-
ture with a pointed head,
and eye, a mouth, and a big
long nose that comes out in
several kinds of pointers or
antlers, and it's got a funny
balloon-shaped body. I
really can't get anything
out of the other two . . .

1. (*How do you see it?*) Just as a
fantasy creature, like in a
cartoon, like from outer
space, that would run
around and do silly things.
(*Anything else?*) Just the
horns on the nose and the
pointy head; those remind
me of things that you see
on those outer space car-
toons that they watch, you
know, media.

DF(H)

2. The aqua and the pink;
they just look like blobs,
blobs of color. I can't say I
see anything in those.

DC Color

3. Also, as I look at it I see a
dust mop, with the handle
and the mop part.

3. (*Dust mop?*) The handle was
right there, and it was the
shape of a dust mop, and
they do some in various
colors, so it could definitely
be a dust mop.

DFCHObj.

RORSCHACH SUMMARY

Response	*Inquiry*	*Scoring*

X. 50″

Oh God, you got lots on here. Hmm, Oh God. OK. Hmmm.

Response	*Inquiry*	*Scoring*
1. I would say this is . . . real fantasy, OK, but it reminds me of summer, and	1. (*Summer?*) First of all, the bright colors, and the fantasy seahorses, crabs, and caterpillar, and summer is my favorite season; I think a lot of the pastels they used in the picture remind me of summer, and a lot of the things you see at the beach.	WCsym. Summer
2. the two pink objects could remind you of seahorses, and	2. (*Seahorses?*) The shape.	DFA
3. this blue out here on each side could be coral that you find at the beach, and,	3. (*Coral?*) The way it was kind of broken and spread apart, because the coral you find can be sharp and you have to be careful with it.	DFCoral
4. the gray up at the—again, as I said, this is more fantasy—could be, sometimes you see those crabs at the beach?	4. The sand crabs—the gray crabs at the beach resemble the ones at the top of the picture.	DF-A
5. And down here this green, green area could be an exaggerated fantasy caterpillar because it has two bodies but one head. So he's a fantasy caterpillar.	5. (*Caterpillar?*) The head and the coloring, and it looks like a caterpillar, and the two bodies made me say a fantasy caterpillar, and they do shed when they become a butterfly anyway, so . . . (?) So they lose one body and get another. (?) He's definitely a fantasy caterpillar, because you only see real caterpillars with one body.	DFCA

EXHIBIT 4

SENTENCE COMPLETION TEST

1. *When she was completely on her own, she* "became very independent."
3. *It looked impossible, so she* "tried even harder to accomplish the task."
5. *When he refused her, she* "felt very rejected."
8. *As a child my greatest fear was* "that something might happen to my father."
9. *My father always* "a very caring and loving man."
10. *The ideal man* "is one who loves you just the way you are!"
11. *A woman who falls in love* "should know her man and love him just the way he is and not want to change him."
12. *I was most depressed when* "my ex-husband took my children out of state just because I was in the hospital."
13. *My first reaction to him was* "that I will not let him get me depressed again. I will be strong and take legal action."
14. *When he turned me down, I* "was rejected after many reconciliations but I am now strong."
16. *Most fathers* "are very loving and protective of their children."
19. *I could hate a person who* "lies and uses other people."
20. *Her earliest memory of her mother was* "a very loving and friendly person."
21. *The ideal women* "is who loves and cherishes her children but shows them they have choices."
24. *When I think back, I am ashamed that I* "was not strong in my convictions."
27. *She felt her lack of success was due to* "lack of hard work."
29. *I used to daydream about* "having a wonderful family of father, mother and sons."
30. *Most men* "are honest, hard-working and faithful."
34. *I was most annoyed when* "my ex-husband was not truthful with me."
35. *When she thought of her mother, she* "thought of a very loving and caring person."
36. *Taking orders* "helps you in later life."
37. *I dislike to* "hurt people if it's not necessary."

SENTENCE COMPLETION TEST

43. *She felt she had done wrong when she* "didn't listen to the other person's sides of the story."

44. *She felt she couldn't succeed unless she* "started to put more effort into her job."

48. *When she failed the examination, she* "was angry because she didn't study."

55. *She felt she could murder a woman who* "wronged her. I feel you could never murder a woman."

62. *Responsibility* "I feel I am a very responsible person."

64. *She felt blue when* "the boy she wanted to ask her to the dance asked someone else."

69. *I feel guilty about* "divorce but I have come to believe I did all I could to make it work and it didn't work."

73. *People in authority* "are necessary to make jobs, schools, hospitals, etc. run in an orderly manner."

74. *I feel happiest when* "I am with my children and we are just enjoying each other."

81. *Most women act as though* "they must be independent and support themselves."

84. *Most people are* "nice and honest until they prove themselves different to me."

91. *Sometimes I feel that my boss* "makes a lot of demands on my personal life."

100. *I feel sad about* "break-up of my family but divorce is a fact of life and I am strong and I will raise my children and have a good and happy life with them."

DISCUSSION

While both Mrs. D, a 47-year-old, divorced mother of two, and Mr. F, a 24-year-old graduate student, experienced agitated, melancholic depressions severe enough to warrant hospitalization, the similarities end there.

Mrs. D was depressed over a number of months in apparent reaction to a clear stress, the loss of the attention and affection of her husband who had recently left her. A personal equilibrium that had been working prior to this stress was destroyed. She suffered some of the classical signs of depression with melancholia: disturbed sleep, frequent crying spells, and poor appetite with a loss of weight. At times her fears that others (including the hospital staff) would harm her reached paranoid proportions. She was not responsive to a brief hospitalization and reinstatement of her previously effective medication regimen. Thus, in the context of her failure to respond to acute treatment, she was referred for a more extended hospital stay. Psychological testing was requested to help assess her intellectual abilities and her capacity to utilize either a supportive or an expressive psychotherapy.

Mr. F also experienced growing symptoms of depression, including excessive guilt, psychomotor agitation, poor sleep, and disinterest in his usual activities. His thinking was disturbed, and he reported confusion and was preoccupied with being homosexual. Like Mrs. D, he failed to respond to a brief hospitalization and medication. It was in this context that psychological testing was requested. The chief referral question concerned the extent and severity of his thought disorder.

Thus, in both cases, the assessment of a patient with depression who did not exhibit the expected, positive response to acute hospitalization and medication formed the background of the referral for psychological testing. Developmental issues were more pronounced with Mr. F, as he was relatively young and preoccupied with sexual identity issues. Mrs. D was older, with a previous history of adequate functioning, including a connection to a husband and two children. In both cases, the referral question required a weighing of strengths and weaknesses in order to plan an optimal treatment for someone not responding to an appropriate medical treatment strategy.

Mr. F's testing revealed a bright (I.Q. of 122) but frightened and anxious young man with psychotic thinking and major dynamic themes involving his fear of the developmental tasks of young adulthood. His needs for support and nurturance conflicted with his desire for independence and autonomy. This conflict was reflected in his fear of homosexuality. Both of these test features led to the recommendation of a structured intervention, at least for the present, and family therapy to assist in a more planned and articulated emancipation from the family of origin.

In contrast, Mrs. D's test results revealed an I.Q. of 88. In unstructured situations, she relied on unimaginative responses, and seemed to possess little internal organization on which she could draw. Her thinking was less overtly disturbed than that of Mr. F. Her unconflicted and ego-syntonic reliance on external authority and structure, plus her relatively low-normal I.Q., led to the treatment recommendation of a supportive rather than an expressive psychotherapy.

In both cases, the symptoms of depression were clear and well evaluated before the referral for psychological testing. The testing was not used to diagnose depression, but to clarify the personality strengths and weaknesses, the defensive styles, the dynamic themes and preoccupations, and the intellectual resources of the patients. Especially unclear in both situations was the level of intellectual and cognitive functioning: present functional I.Q., and the extent and severity of thought disorder. This additional information from psychological testing in both cases led to modifications in the psychosocial intervention.

B. BIPOLAR MANIA: PRIOR TO AND DURING A MANIC EPISODE

Patients with bipolar disorder have experienced one or more manic episodes, and most have also experienced episodes of depression. Manic episodes are characterized by an expansive and elevated mood, accompanied by such behaviors as restlessness, talkativeness, flight of ideas, grandiosity, distractibility, and excessive involvement in activities that can be harmful and/or self-destructive, such as buying sprees and sexual indiscretions.

Differential diagnosis relevant to treatment planning involves distinguishing bipolar disorder from schizoaffective disorders and cyclothymia. Especially relevant to treatment planning are the personality features, both diagnostic (Axis II) and nondiagnostic. These features can assist in planning the format of treatment as well as predicting and sustaining functioning between episodes.

BIPOLAR, MANIC, WITHOUT PSYCHOTIC FEATURES

Ms. G is a 23-year-old, single Jewish woman employed for seven months as an actuarial trainee at an insurance company. Ms. G's family had encouraged her to take this job after she gained 25 pounds and became increasingly lethargic, spending all her time at home with her parents and five younger siblings watching television. With the continued encouragement of her family and friends and the impact of her work routine, she was able to begin to restructure her life. She began dieting and established a strict exercise program for herself which included jogging up to nine miles each day. Over the next four months, she set up a rigid routine of rising early to jog before going to her job. Upon returning from work, she would jog until dinnertime. Her evenings were taken up with a regimented exercise program she designed for herself.

In the month prior to admission, her by now rigid routine began to unravel. Her family reported that she became increasingly irritable and she began to have difficulty sleeping at night. Her activity level, previously quite high, began to vary from day to day. She briefly visited a former classmate and returned from the visit despondent at the barrenness of her life when compared to that of her friends. In the succeeding two weeks, periods of calmness and adequate functioning became more frequently punctuated with periods of irritability, agitation, and crying. Her mood was becoming more labile and her sleep more erratic. She stopped eating and was often restless, pacing about the house and unable to sit still. Finally, in the week prior to admission, she quit her job. She claimed that she needed the time to attend to several medical appointments, but never made any. Several days later she asked her father for help in contacting a female therapist. She had seen a male psychiatrist for several months following a previous psychiatric hospitalization, but had stopped seeing him after an argument about continuing on her medication. Her father did not follow up on her request.

In the two days prior to admission, she was involved in a physical altercation with one of her sisters who refused to run an errand for her. Ms. G described her mind as being in turmoil from this point on and her recollection of events was sketchy. As best she could recall, she ran next door to her neighbors and called the police, claiming that her parents had beaten her up. She was frightened of what was happening to her and late that night placed a call to her former psychiatrist. He was able to intercede with both the patient and her family and, after much discussion, the situation was resolved.

The next evening, she left the house without telling anyone where she was going and her parents, after returning in the late evening from a social engagement, began to search for her. She did not return home until the next morning, stating that she had spent the night in a local park with friends. Her father contacted these youngsters who denied knowing the patient and said that she sat by herself all night in the school yard talking to no one.

Ms. G's parents were able to persuade her to make an appointment with her former psychiatrist. Shortly before the appointment, however, she again wandered away from the house and spent the evening walking through the woods in a nature preserve near her home. She had been repeatedly warned not to venture into this area alone at night as it was notoriously unsafe. While there, she met a young man with whom she was found kissing on a street corner by her father. Finding her engaged in such reckless behavior, her parents were sufficiently concerned to bring her to the hospital to have her admitted, fearing for her continued physical safety if allowed to remain at home.

On admission to the hospital, she was described as a slim woman who, for a variety of reasons, was difficult to interview. She was preoccupied with her physical appearance and was constantly rearranging her clothes and her hair and staring intently at her hands and nails. When not preoccupied with her physical appearance, she gazed suspiciously around the room and seldom made eye contact with the interviewer. Her distractibility made it difficult for her to concentrate and she seemed to have a great deal of difficulty expressing herself, at times making motions as if to speak and being unable to do so. When directly questioned, she denied having any delusions or hallucinations. She was alternately tearful and anxious. She gave a disjointed account of her recent life and gave as her reason for seeking hospitalization that "I need help to come to terms with my sexuality and get better."

DSM-III-R Diagnosis

Axis I: Atypical psychosis
Axis II: Deferred
Axis III: None
Axis IV: Mild—quit her job; argument with her sister
Axis V: Fair—moderate impairment in both social and occupational functioning

Treatment and Hospital Course

A year prior to the present admission, Ms. G had been admitted to the hospital with much the same symptomatology. She had responded well during her previous hospitalization and was discharged as improved. She had continued to see a psychiatrist until they disagreed on the need for her to remain on medication.

When readmitted, an initial treatment plan was developed which focused on the reduction of her disorganization through individual, supportive psychotherapy and group psychotherapy. Family work was instituted with the goal of arranging alternative living arrangements following her hospitalization. The provision of a structured activity and diet plan was felt to be important to help her begin to reorganize her daily routine.

Over the next several weeks, she was generally cooperative with her hospital treatment plan and managed to make a modest recovery. Her grooming improved and returned to its former meticulous level. When engaged in structured activity, she was able to concentrate on the task at hand and to work towards successful completion. However, her perfectionistic strivings occasionally interfered with this and she continued to have difficulty in adapting to a more flexible approach. Left to her own devices without clear plans or goals, she still evidenced a noticeable tendency to become somewhat disorganized. Her most active treatment involvement was in her family therapy. Her difficulties in living at home and her need to separate from her family were the focus of her family work and led to discharge plans which involved her in continued outpatient treatment and living in a halfway house. She was referred for day hospital treatment as a transitional phase between the hospital and returning to full-time employment.

Psychological Assessment

Psychological testing was begun in the eighth week of Ms. G's hospitalization, approximately half way through her hospital stay. She was given the WAIS, Rorschach, Benton Visual Retention Test, and the Object Sorting Test in an effort to resolve the remaining uncertainty regarding her diagnosis. Although given an admitting diagnosis of atypical psychosis, the course of her illness, the nature of her symptoms, and the degree of her disorganization did not help the treatment staff in formulating a more precise diagnosis for Ms. G. In addition, the prior history of hospitalizations without psychotic symptoms led several of the treatment staff to raise issues concerning the possible diagnosis of a personality disorder. Additionally, it was hoped that the nature and degree of her continued disorganization in unstructured situations could be clarified.

Ms. G was cooperative with all testing procedures and was motivated to perform well. She arrived for each testing session meticulously dressed, each time in a different, well-tailored outfit. She gave more the appearance of a young businesswoman than of a patient in a psychiatric hospital. Her dress and manner gave the impression of someone carefully attuned to external appearances and with an eye for detail.

Ms. G's careful external preparation for the psychological examination seemed somewhat at odds with the irritable, restless, and distracted person described in the initial referral. There was some evidence of her former irritability during her examination. For example, on the WAIS Comprehension subscale, the item requiring an explanation for how one would go about finding one's way out of a forest prompted the facetious response, "Ask a squirrel. No, even I wouldn't be that stupid. You should just keep walking until you get to a clearing. You may find a lake or something. All the trees are what make you lost. I have to find open space."

An expansive and grandiose air also seemed partly to characterize her mood. In response to why people should pay taxes, she offered, "Sophia Loren didn't, she thought the rest in jail would do her good." To the Vocabulary subtest item *calamity*, she thinks of Calamity Jane and then remarks that, "I can make up something but I don't know. Someone who has a lot of spirit, involved in trickery, who knows how to outwit someone."

Her apparently fluid associative style as seen in her definition of *calamity* correlates with the clinical findings of her distractibility and racing thoughts. Moreover, in several instances during the psychological examination, and especially under time pressure or in the context of a more expansive mood, she seemed subject to unexpected errors or a perseverative fixation on details. For example, under time pressure on the Arithmetic subtest of the WAIS, she makes a subtraction error on an early item and resorts to writing out a second, later item on the palm of her hand and so loses the time bonus for her correct answer. Her Picture Completion subscale score on the WAIS is lowered by her fixation on irrelevant details. For someone so clearly attuned to external appearances, she is surprisingly unable to identify the missing arm in the reflection, the missing finger on the hand, and the missing eyebrow as the absent details in the sketches.

While these difficulties make only a minor contribution to her cognitive inefficiency under the structured testing situation provided by the WAIS, where she functioned on an overall average level with full scale, verbal, and performance IQs of 108, 109 and 104, respectively, they become major liabilities under the less structured conditions of the Object Sort and Rorschach testing situations. In each of the first seven items of the Object Sort test requiring the subject to choose all objects which "belong with" a stimulus object, her final assemblage of items is scored as loose. For example, she chooses the large spoon and knife, the toy spoon, knife, and fork, the real and toy pliers, screwdriver, cigarette and cigar, the pipe, the toy hammer, the corks, bell, matches, rubber stopper, white card, and piece of paper, the sugar cubes and the eraser as all "belonging together" with the stimulus object of the large fork. She gives as her reason for all of these items "belonging together" as the fork being an eating utensil, "so I picked the knife and the spoon. These are tools for eating so I picked the other tools. The rubber thing (stopper) is what you'd use to open things for dinner and the index card is for the recipe. The paper you'd use for the shopping list and the eraser is for if you made a mistake. The bell reminds me of the dinner bell. The cigars, cigarettes, and matches are for smoking after dinner which I associate with eating. The corks are for the wine after dinner and the sugar cubes are for the coffee." The loose concept of a meal, from the shopping to the cigarette and coffee afterwards, is highly unusual in such a context where most subjects tend to choose much narrower concepts for organizing the sort. Her overinclusiveness and her tendency to move freely from one association to the next while guided by a large, background idea is universally noted throughout the Object Sorting Test.

As with the Object Sorting Test, the Rorschach is interpreted by Ms. G as an opportunity to give free rein to whatever thoughts enter her mind as she is confronted with the perceptual ambiguity of the inkblots. She evidenced a high level of verbal productivity when she was given the Rorschach. In contrast to an average of 20–30 responses given by most individuals, she produced a total of 74 responses, usually initiating her responses rapidly, within 5–15 seconds of being presented the card. She tended to focus on details of the blots at the expense of organized whole responses, and many of her detail responses made use of unusual areas of the blots or of the white space. Her approach to the Rorschach was generally characterized by an alternation between an unreflective, overinclusive attitude and periods of preoccupation with endless details.

The personal idiosyncrasy of her response style is also noted in the absolute paucity of popular responses (3). However, animals, commonplace objects and plants comprised nearly two-thirds of her responses. When color and shading, which tap affective reactivity and anxiety components, respectively, formed part of the determinants of the response, there was a distinct preference for emphasizing these features as primary, with form characteristics secondary. Thus, 70 percent of these complex responses were scored with either color or shading as the primary determinant, at times with form reflecting reality appreciation which was somewhat uncertain.

When this latter observation is taken in combination with the content of many of her responses, the initial impression of a somewhat idiosyncratic but generally bland and unremarkable protocol requires some modification. Many of the responses are seen as decorative or occur in festive settings. A bell and a mask are seen on *card I*; white doves and a flower are seen on *card III*; *card IV* produces a rosebud and people with long, flowing veils; *card VI* contains a starburst and *card VII* another bell; *cards VIII* and *IX* both have flowers, with *card IX* having a parasol and a chiffon blouse with high collar and puffy sleeves as well; *card X* provides both fireworks and streamers. These responses typically occur in isolation rather than as part of a larger, more organized festive scene. They are reminiscent of her focus on external appearances and her fascination with detail, while at the same time demonstrating her considerable difficulty in properly appreciating these elements as parts of a larger, complex scene.

Her organizational difficulties might also be viewed from the vantage point of a pronounced emotional sensitivity and responsivity. She is easily threatened by an environment she often perceived as dangerous and destructive as reflected in her response of "a cat who's been electrocuted" on *card VI* of the Rorschach. In the face of such threat she sometimes retreats into an avoidant passivity. Nondescript leaf percepts presented on several of the inkblots represent this trend. She feels especially insecure and vulnerable with regard to establishing her psychosexual identification beyond surface appearances. On *card III* of the Rorschach, she could not determine the sex of the popular human figures, ultimately deciding that they were "half male and half female." Often feeling inundated by her experienced problems, she sometimes feels that she is in the "bottomless pit" she perceived on *card IV,* from which there is little hope of escape.

Treatment Planning and Outcome

Upon review of her test materials, the examining psychologist emphasized Ms. G's "magical and unrealistic thinking, peculiar, overprecise speech, suspiciousness, paranoid ideation, and hypersensitivity to criticism" as psychological test findings which compromised her capacity to function effectively in unstructured settings. Her awareness of these difficulties was perhaps behind her prehospitalization attempts to regiment and order her daily routine. Her emphasis on "superficial and external criteria" was seen as related to narcissistic elements of her personality functioning and might be seen as attempts to establish her identity by proclamation rather than by identification and integration.

Ms. G's treatment team was able to make use of these findings to emphasize with both her and her family the need for a structured aftercare program. They therefore focused the bulk of their energies on helping her and her family work through the need for her to move out of the house into a structured residential setting and attend a day hospital as intermediate steps to help her ultimately return to work and pursue a more independent living situation. Her attention to external appearances was an asset in helping her to gain acceptance at a halfway house and her reality testing and acceptance of her illness improved to a significant degree so that she was able to recognize the need for these aftercare plans. Additionally, she agreed to return to outpatient treatment with her former psychiatrist, who would also continue to work with the family.

The combination of the psychological test results and the brevity of Ms.

G's symptomatology prior to admission led to a single discharge diagnosis of schizotypal personality disorder. However, many elements of her psychological test results and her clinical symptomatology (ignoring its brevity due to rapid hospitalization) are characteristic of a bipolar disorder. Although she presented few clear-cut, classical features of bipolar patients during a manic phase of their illness, our review of her psychological test findings seemed most consistent with a diagnosis of bipolar disorder.

Following her discharge from the hospital, Ms. G did well for a time but was readmitted. At that time, the clinical picture had resolved and it was possible to make the bipolar diagnosis. She has since done well out of the hospital, remaining under psychiatric care with continuing pharmacological treatment but managing to return to full-time employment and moving from the halfway house to a supportive group apartment where her daily functioning can be monitored and further ameliorated.

EXHIBIT 1

AREA OF ASSESSMENT	CLINICAL EXAMINATION	PSYCHOLOGICAL EXAMINATION
I. Symptoms/Diagnosis *Bipolar, manic, without psychosis*		
Irritable mood	Fights with sister Crying spells	Irritable and expansive mood
Restless	Unable to sit still	Acts without deliberation under time constraint
Racing thoughts	Describes her mind as "in turmoil"	Uncritically overinclusive and perseverative
Distractibility	Gaze wanders; poor concentration; overconcern with minor matters	Alternately, focuses on minor details at the expense of a larger, more integrated view
Involvement in activities with potentially painful consequences	Goes to secluded area with stranger despite past warnings	Impulsive, swayed by her feelings of the moment
II. Personality Factors	Unpredictable and impulsive	Actions are inappropriate to larger social context
III. Cognitive Abilities	Average intelligence	Average intelligence
IV. Psychodynamics	Self-preoccupation and sensitive to rejection	Feels vulnerable and readily becomes absorbed in internal world
V. Therapeutic Enabling Factors	Ability to profit from structure	Performs best with a high level of external structure
	Desire to separate from her family	Lack of a cohesive identity hampers independence
VI. Environmental Demand and Social Adjustment	Few friends and difficulty sustaining relationships with others	Potentially affectively responsive but readily threatened and quick to withdraw
	Feels overprotected by parents but frequently relies on their assistance and judgment	Feels rather powerless in the face of external demands

E X H I B I T   2

WAIS-R SUMMARY

Verbal Subtests	Scaled Score
Information	9
Comprehension	13
Arithmetic	8
Similarities	12
Digit Span	14
Vocabulary	13

Performance Subtests	
Digit Symbol	14
Picture Completion	9
Block Design	12
Picture Arrangement	10
Object Assembly	10

Verbal IQ	109
Performance IQ	104
Full Scale IQ	108

MMPI Summary

FLK/ 2'437086-1/9:5

Rorschach Summary

Number of Responses	74
Rejections	0
Populars	7
Originals	3(−1)
Average R/T chromatic	6″
Average R/T achromatic	12″
F%	55
F + %	53
A%	34
H%	16
W:M	11:5
M:Sum C	5:4

RORSCHACH SUMMARY

m:c			10:14
VIII-X%			27
FK + F + Fc%			64
(H + A):(Hd + Ad)			22:15
Apperception	W	17%	
	D	53%	
	d	3%	
	Dd + S	27%	

EXHIBIT 3

Rorschach Summary

Response	Inquiry	Scoring

I. 5″

1. Looks to me like a bat.

      WFAP

2. Or a leaf. Has part of it missing.

  2. The way the edges were formed. (*Any particular leaf?*) Maple leaf.

      WFPl

3. Up on top I see two chickens.

  3. (?) Sections of ink blot that looked like two chickens. Feathers. (?) No, didn't say that. Yes, I did. The way it was designed.

      DFA

4. This part in here looks like a bell.

      DFObj.

5. This especially looks like a little creature with claws coming out of it.

  5. You could see a little tiny face with beady eyes . . . a bat-type face. Little parts coming out, looked like claws. (*Was it a bat's face?*) Looked like a little animal in bat/squirrel family.

      DFA

6. This part in here is sort of like an abstract design with negative and positive space contrasting it.

  6. Within the design there were open spaces. I always pay attention to contrasting sections. (?) Four white spaces helped to form shapes out of negative spaces.

      DC′F Art Pec.

7. If you turn it upside down, it's almost like a mask.

      WF Obj.

8. Very interesting. Five points, pointy lines and soft around edges. I think it would have more continuity if lines came to a point. These are too sharp.

  8. (*Soft?*) Part had pointy lines diverging from center and another looked softer. (*Soft?*) Wasn't a solid black. Different gradients in the tone.

      WcF Abs.
      Confab

RORSCHACH SUMMARY

Response	*Inquiry*	*Scoring*
II. 4″		
1. Looks like a pair of lungs.	1. They had . . . it was really an x-ray. Had x-ray, smoky look. I think x-ray shows up as white, not black. It's reversed.	DFkAt
2. Two faces looking at each other.		DMHd
3. An x-ray of a chest.		DFk X-ray At
4. A lamp shade.		SF Obj. O
5. Two eagles. Eagle heads.	5. Two eagle heads. The outline, the form. They weren't distinct. I made them out to be.	DFAd
6. A torch.	6. (?) Way it was shaped. Actually, if you don't mind, I think it looks like a penis. (?) The way it was shaped.	DF Obj DF Sex
7. A sea crab.	7. It had spidery things coming out of it. Pointy around the edges.	DFA
8. A zipper.	8. It had those lines in it. Looked like a zipper opening. (*Opening?*) Like it was halfway pulled down. It's broken. Way it came apart.	diF Obj.
9. A hole. (*Puts it at a distance and stares at it.*) You're drawn into this white spot in the center, like a parasol.		SF Obj.
10. Reminds me of cotton dolls, straw dolls.	10. Dress and body, no head. (*Straw dolls?*) No, more than outline.	SF(Hd)

RORSCHACH SUMMARY

Response	*Inquiry*	*Scoring*
11. Lizard or snake.	11. Same part that I called the penis. (*What about blot made it look like snake?*) Shape. May I see inkblot again? Rough edges on it.	DFA

III. 3″

Response	*Inquiry*	*Scoring*
1. Two figures. They're reaching arms into . . . I can't determine what sex they are. Like half male, half female.	1. (*What did you mean?*) Appeared that they had busts on top, on bottom almost phallic symbols and shoes here high heels.	DMHP
2. These look like fish, almost.	2. (*Fish?*) Way they were shaped. Had hands stuck in something, looked like the top of a fish.	DFA
3. Butterfly.	3. (*Butterfly?*) Wings. Could have been a bow tie. Actually, it looked like an upside down butterfly. (*Anything besides wings?*) No. Body was missing.	DFAP
4. Looks like someone laying on their back, kicking their leg up in the air.	4. (?) Also looked like a sea horse. (?) Way leg or tail went.	DMH DFA
5. Birds, white doves.	5. (*White doves?*) Negative space. (*What do you mean?*) The space around the inkblot itself.	SFC′A
6. Looks like a medical sign down there.	6. Had twisting lines.	drF-Sym.
7. Looks like a flower.		drFPl
8. Looks like African heads.	8. (*African heads?*) Way it was shaped. (*Anything besides shape?*) More of a prehistoric man.	DFHd

RORSCHACH SUMMARY

Response	Inquiry	Scoring

IV. 24″

1. It also looks like a leaf to me.

   1. The outline. Looked like the leaf had been dipped in ink and pressed onto card.   WFPl

2. Looks like a rosebud.

   2. It seemed that there were petals that were opening. Have to change top. Doesn't open till later on.   DF.FmPl

3. Castle in a valley.   DF Arch / SF-Ldsc.

4. People with long, flowing veils.

   4. Women. Wind blowing through them.   DF.mFH,Cl

5. A bottomless pit.

   5. (?) It was dark and center drew your eyes into it and downward.   diC′F Ldsc

6. Dogs on their hind legs.   drFM-A

7. Looks like someone's feet being tapped. You know, feet is up in the air.

   7. (*Tapped?*) Heel was up in the air, like when it's being flexed.   DMHd / *Peculiar verbalization*

8. These are all like horns coming out in the air. (*Okay*)   ddFAd

9. Kind of like a dragon. Skull here.   DF(Ad)

Second sitting (next day)

V. 2″

1. Looks like a bat. (*Giggles*)   WFA

2. Pair of tweezers.

   2. It was an opening. The way they were opened, though I wouldn't use those tweezers, because they're obviously broken because they open that wide.   DF Obj.

RORSCHACH SUMMARY

Response	*Inquiry*	*Scoring*
3. A crow.	3. Has mouth open and face. Not too accurate.	DFMAd
4. A crocodile with his mouth open.	4. (?) Reminded me of those cartoons when I was younger of a crocodile waiting in moats.	DFMAd
(Puts hand over various portions of card.)		
5. A bird in flight.		WFMA
6. Calves of legs. *(Okay)*	6. (?) Shape. No indication of foot or thigh. Looked good and muscular.	dFHd
VI. 8″		
1. Looks like a cat who's been electrocuted.	1. Head, mouth, fat body, no tail. (?) Whiskers and paws, *(What . . . electrocuted?)* Way it was flattened out and had all kinds of jagged lines and edges. *(Flattened out?)* Legs were straight out, not tucked under. Very round body. *(Anything else?)* Mainly face area. All those edges. *(Anything else?)* Stretched.	WFA
2. A leaf.	2. *(Leaf?)* Shape.	DFPl
3. Open claws.	3. *(What . . . open claws?)* Just looked that way.	diFMAd
4. Little heart.		dFAt
5. A tunnel.	5. *(Tunnel?)* A dark line going through the center, like an underground tunnel of a worm.	DC'F Tunnel

RORSCHACH SUMMARY

Response	*Inquiry*	*Scoring*
6. A starburst. (*Okay.*)	6. (*What . . . starburst?*) The gradients in tone. Had like a sunflower-type appearance.	drC′FPl

VII. 21″

1. Dancers.	1. (?) Leg being kicked in air.	DMHd
2. I get the impression of a leaf.	2. (*Leaf?*) Just shape.	SFPl
3. A bell.		SF-Obj.
4. Pig faces.	4. Snout-like, scrunched-up faces. (*Scrunched up?*) Had wrinkled. (*Wrinkled?*) Darker lines going through it.	drFcAd
5. Razor blades.	5. (*Razor?*) Flat and thin. (*Anything else?*) Square. (*Thin?*) Lightness of the ink. (*Say more?*) Just seemed very smooth. Different gradients of ink made it look like one brush stroke.	DFc Obj.
6. Elephant head.		DFAd

VIII. 10″
Pretty colors (*smiles*).

1. A fish.	1. (*Fish?*) The colors and the scales. (*Scales?*) The different shades.	WFC.FcA
2. Bird's face.	2. (*Face?*) The feathery effect and beak and shape. (*Feathery?*) Almost furry effect. Chicken's type texture, baby chicken. (*Texture?*) Way ink was stroked on paper. (*Anything else?*) Wasn't smooth outline. It was unfinished.	drFcAd

Rorschach Summary

Response	*Inquiry*	*Scoring*
3. Racoon.	3. Pair of them. Seemed perched on something. the way they were holding their heads down. And legs. (*Anything else?*) No.	DFMA
4. Flower.	4. (*Flower?*) It just kind of burst open. Colors and shape of petals.	DCF.mFPl
5. The skeletal system.	5. Seemed like bones. We used to draw bones in drawing class.	DFAt
6. Brushes. (*Okay*)	6. (*Brushes?*) Strokes and the lines. (*What do you mean?*) Lines going through the dark area that made the outline.	diC'F Obj.

IX. 12″

1. Flower.	1. (*Flower?*) Kind of exotic flower. Different colors and way it was opening up. (*Opening up?*) Top portion. It was spreading apart.	WCF.mFPl
2. Vase.	2. (?) I'd prefer it as reverse side. Makes better piece of art work. Shape. (*Anything else?*) No.	D(S)F Obj. *Peculiar verbalization*

RORSCHACH SUMMARY

Response	*Inquiry*	*Scoring*
3. Parasol.	3. Ruffled edges. (*Ruffled?*) Lines went in and out, and up and down. The edge of what looked like bottom of a parasol.	drF Obj.
4. Pool of water, puddle. Water drops, like formed on a formica table.	4. (*Water drops?*) The ink itself was mixed with water and had a transparent effect. Cluster of water that fell out on table just before it spreads out. (*Transparent effect?*) It wasn't a solid tone. Had clear, light look to it.	drcF Water
5. Blouse.	5. High collared and puffy sleeves. (?) Had chiffon look to it. (*Chiffon look?*) The way the ink is used so lightly.	DFcCl
6. Outfit. (*Okay.*)	6. Different colors.	WFCCloth

X. 0″

1. Fireworks.	1. The bursts here. (*Bursts?*) Ink was spread out. (*Anything else?*) Different colors.	DWCF Fireworks
2. Streamers.	2. Those pink. Seemed to be moving like streamers through the air. Whole card had party effect. Child's party.	DWmF.CF Obj, Party
3. Mustache.		DFHd
4. Pair of eyes.	4. (*Eyes?*) First I saw a mustache and those two dots were to complete the face.	DFHd

RORSCHACH SUMMARY

Response	*Inquiry*	*Scoring*
5. Pair of crabs.		DFA
6. Little bat in center.		DFA
7. Insect.		DFA
8. Lobsters. (*Okay.*)	8. (*Lobsters?*) Just those two areas. Had shell-like quality. Spindly claws. (*What . . . shell quality?*) Smoothness of the ink. (*Anything else?*) Shape.	DFcA

BIPOLAR DISORDER, MANIC, WITH PSYCHOTIC FEATURES

Mr. M was admitted to the hospital for the second time in the last year two days after Christmas. The Day Hospital staff had tried for most of the day to persuade him to admit himself voluntarily to the inpatient service. They had not been able to contact him for three days and he had not been seen at the halfway house where he was living. Both staffs were concerned about his deteriorating level of functioning over the last two weeks. For the last few days, he had been celebrating the holiday in the bars of a neighboring city and celebrating his decision to embark on a new career. At 29 years of age, he felt that it was time he chose a career and the day before Christmas he had decided on a career as a political lobbyist rather than entering his father's very successful restaurant supply business. Having made the decision, he felt that "the world was lifted from my shoulders." He had returned to his room to collect his personal belongings and then had come to the Day Hospital to be discharged from their care. He would not accept the Day Hospital staff's recommendation of hospitalization and instead, threatened them with legal action. He was finally hospitalized against his wishes on the recommendation of two physicians who had worked with him in the Day Hospital.

The previous Christmas, Mr. M had also been preoccupied with his career plans. At that time, he was living with his father and stepmother having given up his own apartment one year before that following a suicide attempt and brief hospitalization. He made two minor suicide attempts that previous Christmas season in the context of despair over his future and feeling guilty about his sexual attraction to his stepsister. He was admitted to the hospital, where he was given a diagnosis of major depression and responded well to a series of 10 ECT treatments. He had been discharged to the Day Hospital in June. His arrogant and disdainful attitude had kept him from making friends with the other patients in the Day Hospital. He felt he had license to treat the staff and their recommendations with contempt as his father had promised to employ him in his own company following his treatment in Day Hospital.

Mr. M's stepmother and the Day Hospital staff finally had persuaded his father of the need to withdraw this offer in order to help Mr. M develop more realistic career plans. With the offer withdrawn, the staff had grown more insistent that he adhere to the rules of the program. He became increasingly defiant and as the anniversary of his suicide attempts approached with the Christmas season, his behavior became more erratic and disorganized. When his car broke down and he could no longer come and go as he pleased, his attendance at the Day Hospital became sporadic.

Suspecting the onset of a manic episode, the Day Hospital staff began a medical workup to clear the patient for treatment with lithium and requested a psychological evaluation to help assess his present condition. Although the psychological evaluation was completed shortly before his inpatient admission, he procrastinated in gaining medical clearance for the lithium. In the face of his escalating clinical state, he was involuntarily admitted to the inpatient service.

At the time of his admission to the inpatient service, Mr. M was found to be quite distractible and overactive. His speech was pressured and his thinking was described as tangential. His affect was mildly expansive and elevated. He described his mood as "happy" as he was looking forward to his planned career as a political lobbyist and was unshakable in his conviction of boundless success. He said that in the last few days he had had a great deal of energy and hadn't needed any sleep. He apparently recognized his need for treatment, however, and requested that his legal status be changed to voluntary so that he could begin his lithium treatment. He was allowed, in fact, to convert his legal status three weeks after admission, at which time he wrote that he was requesting the change in order to pursue a "medication adjustment due to a series of hypomanic episodes."

DSM-III-R Diagnosis

Axis I: Bipolar disorder, manic, with psychotic features
Axis II: None
Axis IV: Mild—broke up with his girlfriend
Axis V: Poor—moderate impairment in both social relations and occupational functioning

Treatment and Hospital Course

Mr. M was initially treated with antipsychotic medication pending medical clearance for initiating treatment with lithium. Within a week and one-half, clearance was obtained, lithium was initiated, and adequate plasma levels were achieved. His antipsychotic medication was tapered and maintained at a lower level throughout his hospitalization. His initial response to the antipsychotic medication included diminishment of his pressured speech and grandiosity and some improvement in his concentration. His thinking remained tangential, however, and he was prone to irritable outbursts, and remained overactive. At the end of his second week on the lithium, his manic symptoms had completely remitted and he was discharged to resume his treatment at the Day Hospital and his living situation at the halfway house.

Psychological Assessment

Mr. M was assessed by the psychologist in the Day Hospital two weeks prior to his admission to the inpatient service. His referring therapist reported that he had shown a recent increase in "erratic behavior," had been talking to himself in public places, and was more irritable and uncooperative with his treatment. The psychologist was asked to assess the possibility of an emerging psychosis and the presence of an affective disorder. He was given the WAIS-R, the MMPI, Rorschach, TAT, and SCT during the course of the examination.

His behavior during testing was noteworthy. He was described as arriving promptly for his three evaluation sessions and generally was cooperative with the examination. However, he began muttering or humming to himself on several occasions and when questioned about these behaviors, would attribute them to fatigue or his interest in the flute, respectively. During a brief interview at the close of the testing, he suddenly became angry and refused to answer any further questions and would give no reason for his sudden anger.

His cognitive functioning as assessed with the WAIS-R was extremely variable. He achieved full-scale, verbal, and performance IQs of 102, 118 and 85, respectively. His subscale scores ranged from the borderline to very superior levels. His best performance was achieved in those areas where he could rely on the recall of overlearned material (*Information* and *Vocabulary*). There was no evidence of any acute disruption of either his attentional or concentration abilities. His lowest score on the verbal subtests indicated a relative impairment in his understanding of conventional social norms (*Comprehension*), although his absolute performance was within the normal range.

On the performance subtests, Mr. M demonstrated both absolute and relative deficits in discriminating essential from unessential details in pictorial representations (*Picture Completion*), a deficiency consistent with some difficulty in maintaining adequate reality testing ability. His relative deficits on the performance subtests were generated primarily by a combination of psychomotor slowing and ineffective trial and error strategies when he was unable to provide an immediate response. These difficulties appeared to be more functional than organic. Overall, his pattern of relative strengths and weaknesses suggested that he was likely to be seen by others as having more than an average intellectual endowment despite a history of little better than average educational performance and his present test performance.

Mr. M's performance on the less structured tests of the battery, the Rorschach and TAT, also indicated difficulties with reality testing. On the Rorschach, he gave a total of 44 responses and although he relied almost exclusively on the form of the inkblots to justify his percepts, his use of form was idiosyncratic or unusual in almost half of these responses (F + % = 53). His TAT stories suffered because of his fluid thinking as well. He often had trouble completing the story because he was unable to determine the details of the pictures. He would begin a story and then, as his attention became distracted by some detail of the picture, he would either revise his original story or suggest several alternative stories, depending on the interpretation of the detail. For example, his first story was told to a picture of a seated boy whose head rests on his hands. Before him is a violin and a bow resting on some papers. Mr. M began his story in a conventional way by stating that it "looks like a child who's looking over his music before he prepares to play the violin." He could not determine if the boy was preparing to play the violin or had interrupted his playing to study the music and so he turned his attention to the details of the picture, hoping to get some clue to the boy's behavior. He interpreted a shadow on the boy's face as "he has a wad of chewing tobacco in his mouth" and as he went on to inspect the face, he stated that the boy was "cross-eyed, actually. He's looking inward, both eyes are in the inside part." These details did not help him to decide between his original proposals; instead, he went on to wonder if the boy was sleeping. Finally, with no further clues to the boy's emotional state, he was unable to complete the story satisfactorily.

The distractibility and overattention to minor details found in this story were pervasive features of his Rorschach and TAT protocols and consistent with his poor discriminative judgment on the *Picture Completion* subscale of the WAIS-R. His Rorschach responses were very predominantly detail responses (39 of the 44 responses), indicating a breakdown in his organizational abilities (as noted above, also reflected in his TAT stories). For example, on *card III*, he first reported the two human figures which are frequently seen, but spoiled the response because he could neither integrate the central nor the lower details into the percept and became distracted by the ostensibly incongruous "erections" of what first seemed to him to be female figures. Mr. M was inordinately preoccupied with sexuality. On the Rorschach, he gave seven responses with "a woman's genital area" as the content of the response. Although three of these were judged to be of adequate form quality, the remainder were not and were reported because for Mr. M, a "line down the middle and two equal areas" were all that were required to form the genitalia.

The intellectualized, censored quality of his test protocol was further emphasized by the almost complete absence of either color or shading determinants in the Rorschach, evidence of his pronounced effort to contain his emotions and limit his impulsivity. The disruptive potential of allowing himself to be aroused by strong feeling nevertheless came through in the areas of the blots selected and their content. On *card II* of the Rorschach, the first and third responses were "woman's genitals" given to the central white space and the lower red detail, respectively. His second response, a popular one but somewhat idiosyncratically presented, involved the large black details which were described as "two dancing bears smooching." His final response to the card, given in what is by now a highly charged, sexual context, was of red Christmas stockings located in the upper red details. Later in the Rorschach, he saw the large pink details on *card X* as resembling Italy, but "a different kind of boot, more a work boot, to give somebody a kick."

The fusion of sexual and aggressive themes under the impact of emotional stimulation was evident on the TAT as well. His stories often had a protean quality and after beginning fairly innocuously, evolved into grim tales of sex and murder. For example, on *card 13MF*, Mr. M first noted the nude woman "with breasts exposed" and offered a story of a professor who "slept with her and got up very early, showered" and prepared to study, a story of a doctor who's been treating her and is rubbing his eyes after "a long vigil," or a murderer who "can't bear to look at what he's done."

Such disruptions as those noted on the less structured tests were also found in Mr. M's more conscious presentation of himself on the MMPI and SCT. On the MMPI, his peak elevation was on scale 8, a scale involving social and emotional alienation, lack of ego mastery, and frankly bizarre sensory experiences. He endorsed items from this scale indicating that he had "very peculiar and strange experiences" and "strange and peculiar thoughts" and agreed that there was something wrong with his mind and that he was afraid of losing his mind.

On the SCT, he served notice of the dramatic behavior that can erupt when he is emotionally stimulated. For example, he notes that *it looked impossible, so he* "dove out the window" and *when she refused him, he* "was devestated (sic)." He acknowledged having difficulty controlling his impulses (i.e. *my sexual desires* "sometimes get the better of me," *his conscience bothered him most when* "stole (sic)" and *when I think back, I am ashamed that* "I acted so selfishly at times"), but is nevertheless given to acting in ways that attract attention. He expressed wishes to be "a professional musician" or "a professional athlete," both being positions that would keep him in the public eye, and points out that his greatest fear as a child was "being ignored and overlooked by my mother"; he now fears "being abandoned." While he has difficulty with establishing adequate levels of self-control, he at the same time rails against the limits on his behavior imposed by others. On the SCT he resents "taking orders" or "conforming to rules" and regards himself as "having been held back" by his parents.

Treatment Planning and Outcome

The examining psychologist felt that Mr. M was susceptible to transient losses of reality testing, particularly when he was attempting to modulate either sexual or aggressive feelings. His present efforts to maintain an adequate level of self-esteem seemed limited to the development of somewhat grandiose ideas (he had worked in the political campaigns of several local politicians and did have some musical talent). However, in his present state, it seemed unlikely that he could marshall his resources sufficiently to actually carry out the work involved in forwarding his ideas. The psychologist felt that without swift intervention, he was likely to escalate into a florid manic state and was concerned that when he met with difficulty in putting his ideas into practice, his frustration and disappointment would again provoke suicidal ideas and attempts.

The psychologist's report was useful in helping Mr. M's treatment team in the Day Hospital adamantly pursue the need for his rehospitalization on the inpatient service and, as noted above, he responded quite well and rapidly to appropriate pharmacological intervention. Following his discharge from the inpatient service, he was readmitted to the Day Hospital. At his readmission interview, he agreed to abide by the general rules for Day Hospital patients and to improve his ability to socialize with them. He made some progress in exploring his career choices and was much more realistic in considering what would be required of him. He improved his attendance and his socialization and a referral was made to a less structured Day Hospital program where he would have more flexibility in pursuing his career goals. In the interim between programs, he decided to visit a former roommate in a nearby city and although he became mildly depressed and reported a return of some suicidal ideation during the visit, he was able to cut the visit short on the advice of his psychiatrist and successfully negotiated the transition to the new program.

EXHIBIT 1

AREA OF ASSESSMENT	CLINICAL EXAMINATION	PSYCHOLOGICAL EXAMINATION
I. Symptoms/Diagnosis		
Bipolar, manic, with psychotic features		
Elevated and expansive mood	Has had world lifted from his shoulders	Strained efforts to control affect and impulses; underlying depression
Increased activity	Spent last three days in bars "making friends"	Pressured flow of associations without adequate controls
Pressured speech	Pressured speech	Speaks rapidly
Flight of ideas	None	At times has more ideas than he is able to convey. Sexually preoccupied
Delusional grandiosity	Complete confidence in becoming a political lobbyist	Expresses wishes for public adulation; impaired reality testing
Decreased need for sleep	Hasn't slept in 3–4 days but feels fine	None
Distractibility	Very distractible	Easily distracted and derailed by minor details
Overinvolvement in activities with potentially painful consequences	Cannot recognize three day absence caused problems at residence and Day Hospital	None
II. Personality Factors	None	Inability to persist in achievement of long-term goals
		Easily feels rejected and "overlooked"

AREA OF ASSESSMENT	CLINICAL EXAMINATION	PSYCHOLOGICAL EXAMINATION
III. Cognitive Abilities	None	Probably average intelligence although appears brighter leading to expectations in excess of ability. Uses intellectualization extensively.
IV. Psychodynamics	None	Grandiose ideas used to shore up impaired self-esteem
		Evidence of psychosexual confusion and defenses against experienced psychosexual inadequacy
V. Therapeutic Enabling Factors	Prior response to somatic treatment	None
	Vocational goals somewhat consistent with past accomplishments	Still functioning on an overall average intellectual level
VI. Environmental Demand and Social Adjustment	Contemptuous of efforts to set helpful limits	Feels dominated when expected to conform to external demands
	Able to make friends but unable to keep them	Limited empathic ability; self-centered

EXHIBIT 2

WAIS-R SUMMARY

Verbal Subtests	*Scaled Score*
Information	13
Digit Span	15
Vocabulary	14
Arithmetic	14
Comprehension	10
Similarities	12

Performance Subtests	
Picture Completion	6
Picture Arrangement	10
Block Design	7
Object Assembly	8
Digit Symbol	8

Verbal IQ	118
Performance IQ	85
Full Scale IQ	102

MMPI SUMMARY

F'KL: 8"597'46-230/1:

RORSCHACH SUMMARY

Number of Responses	45
Rejections	0
Populars	8
Originals	3
Average R/T Chromatic	26"
Average R/T Achromatic	13"(2RT's missing)
F%	84
F+%	53
A%	29
H%	11
Sex%	17

RORSCHACH SUMMARY

Geog%		27
W:M		5:5
M:Sum C		5:0.5
m:c		2.0
VIII-X%		29
FK + F + Fc%		84
(H + A):(Hd + Ad)		15:3
Apperception	W	11%
	D	60%
	d	13%
	Dd + S	16%

EXHIBIT 3

RORSCHACH SUMMARY

Response	*Inquiry*	*Scoring*

I. 1″

All these images are coming to my mind.

1. It kind of looks like a head of a wolf, here and here.	1. The way it stuck out, the long snout that the coyote has.	DFA
2. The whole thing looks like a woman's genital area, anyway.	2. The way it's formed, shaped. (*What in particular?*) The line down the middle and two equal halves.	WF-Sex
3. This looks like a woman's breast.	3. The shape.	dFSexO
This looks like a coyote's nose, from Road Runner.	(*Separate response?*) It's the snout, Part of the one I said before.	
4. These look like hands or claws, here.	4. (*Hands or claws?*) Hands, I guess. (?) Shape.	dFHd
5. If these two things were tilted, they'd look like the Matterhorn in Switzerland which I've been to.	5. It's formed that way. That's the shape. Here's the peak.	dFGeo.
That's about it.		
6. This sort of looks like the bottom of a spine, like somebody's coccyx.	6. I don't know, down the bottom, the long straight line looks like a spine, and the thing sticking out at the bottom.	dF-At

II. 18″

1. Again, it looks like a woman's genital area, here's openings.	1. Same. Up and down slit. Just the openings.	SF-Sex

RORSCHACH SUMMARY

Response	*Inquiry*	*Scoring*
2. It looks like two dancing bears, smooching here in the middle, touching noses.	2. Right here. See. (*Bears smooching?*) That's how I see it. They're shaped that way and they're touching.	WMAP
3. This also looks like a woman's genital area down here.	3. Just shaped like it. Another slit down the middle.	DFSex
4. I don't know what these two red things are supposed to be. Almost looks like Christmas stockings.	4. Whatever. They look like stockings, curve to the left or right, except they were backwards or upside down (shifts uncomfortably). Stockings could look like red stocking of Boston Red Sox.	DFCCloth
5. Actually, this side sort of looks like a map of New England (*names states*), no not New England, it's like when you see a map of Connecticut and Northern Westchester (*names places*). Also, you can half see New England, the top part, New Hampshire and Vermont.	5. That's just how it's shaped—like a map of those places.	DF-Geo

III. 25″

Hmm, this, boy that's a strange picture.

RORSCHACH SUMMARY

Response	Inquiry	Scoring
1. This looks like two women with high heels are balancing some kind of wide, long, large wide cushion in front of them, this looks like some kind of globe. But it doesn't make any sense that it's women because they both have penises. They look like women with heels but it's very strange because they both have erections.	1. They were leaning on some kind of large foot cushion, or looks like a globe, stationery thing, revolves around. (?) You know how in a house or library there's a globe sitting in a framework. You spin the globe around. (?) Yeah. The only thing I can think is that some men are fooling around from behind, and their erections are sticking out between the women's legs. I don't know how to make sense of that one.	WM.FmH, Obj,Sex P
2. This part looks like butterfly.	2. I don't know, looks like a butterfly, wing spread, I don't know.	DFAP
3. These two things look like a map of Cyprus, each of them.	3. It's shaped like a map. Looks to me like Greece or Cyprus—a country in the Mediterranean. That's all.	DF-Geo
This looks like Greece, I can't really tell.		
4. They also kind of look like electric guitars, crazy electric guitars.	4. I don't know. That's what it looks like to me. The neck, the body. See it.	DF-ObjO
5. Also, if I'm looking at it upside down it looks like two horses, like the old Denver Broncos helmet, way back . . . with one leg kicking back.	5. It has the same kind of shape. The leg sticking back here.	DFM(A)
6. Did I say this looks like somebody's pelvic area?	6. (*Pelvic area?*) Kind of side (*gestures*) sweeping, kind of looks like a pelvis.	DFAt *Peculiar verbalization*

RORSCHACH SUMMARY

Response	*Inquiry*	*Scoring*
7. The pelvic area also looks like a Long Island area, with strips of land sticking into the bay.	7. See the strips of land. It looks like they're jutting out into the water or something, the way it is in Long Island with the bay.	DF-Geo

IV. 14″

1. Well, this again looks like a woman's genital area.	1. It's shaped that way. The whole thing sort of looks like a woman's private area.	drF-Sex
2. I don't know, this looks like a, something, I don't know what the hell it is, some kind of a, if you take the whole thing, it looks like the head of a turkey down there.	2. It's strange, like the head of a turkey. It's got that shape.	DFA
	1. It also could be some kind of long branch hanging down. The same shape. (*Hanging down?*) The position of it. The direction it's pointing in.	Add: DFPl
	2. You know, this up here sort of looks like an anus. (*Anus?*) Same shape. Could be a hole here.	Add: dF-AtO
3. This looks like the Metropolitan area, Long Island, Bronx, Brooklyn, Queens, Westchester, Connecticut, Rhode Island, Massachusetts	3. I looked at it and thought of the locations of all those places.	DF-Geo

V. 13″

1. This *entire* thing looks like a butterfly. Either a butterfly or, yeah, butterfly.	1. The shape.	WFAP

RORSCHACH SUMMARY

Response	Inquiry	Scoring
2. This area here looks like the Eastern end of Long Island. This is north, south fork. Hamptons, Montauk.	2. Like the others. It's shaped that way.	DF-Geo
3. This kind of looks like a wishbone down here.	3. Just the shape.	DFAto
4. This again looks like a woman's genital area, the lips here, maybe the clitoris here.	4. It's the shape. The two lips.	DF-Sex

VI. 13"

Hmm (*Looks at me*).

Response	Inquiry	Scoring
1. The entire thing looks like a bear skin rug.	1. The shape. That's all.	WFAdP

Hmm (*Sighs, looks at me*).

Response	Inquiry	Scoring
2. This whole left area looks like a map of France (*names parts*), if it didn't stick out so much it would look like a map of France.	2. The same as the others. It has the form of country.	DF-Geo
3. This kind of looks like a mouth and some kind of trapping device of a beetle or insect. Here, except this part.	3. The shape.	dF-Ad
4. This kind of looks like the Eastern seaboard, Florida.	4. Another one where I looked at it and that's what it reminded me of, the East coast down to Florida.	drF-Geo

RORSCHACH SUMMARY

Response	*Inquiry*	*Scoring*

VII. 11″

(Shifts, hums)

1. This part *really* looks like a woman's genital area. This is sort of the crack of her back side.

   1. I don't know. Just did. With the crack of her back side down there.

   dFSex

2. What else is there? Oh, hmm. These look like two young people, here, children, yeah. Looks like two young children, looking at each other. Wearing Indian feathers, and they're either carrying children in some back pack, or something else. Maybe these *are* back packs and these are the looking at each other, to get a better look.

   2. Shape of children's faces. They are looking at each other.

   DMH,ObjP

3. This looks like a map of Queens and Brooklyn (*names parts*).

   3. I just see it as a map and the shape is like Queens and Brooklyn.

   DF-Geo.

VIII. 8″

1. Oh, um, these two things look like two, I don't know, wolverines or badgers, they look like a lion, not beaver, legs are too long, same thing on either side.

   1. The shape.

   DFAP

2. Hmm, it looks like there's two outlines of bats over here. These two look like bats.

   2. That's what they look like. Cause they had the wings. (*Shrug*).

   DF-A

RORSCHACH SUMMARY

Response	*Inquiry*	*Scoring*
3. This whole thing kind of looks like a mountain.	3. The shape. That's all. The peak is here.	DFGeo
(*Anything else?*) Mmmm.		
4. This looks like France a little bit. This is probably Netherlands, then Germany.	4. It just does. I just see it as a map of those countries.	drF-Geo

IX. 45″

1. They kind of look like dogs over here, a little dog with short tail, legs here, sticking out there, and paws.	1. Just the shape.	DF-A
2. This kind of looks like a thermometer, up the middle, the head is kind of round.	2. Shape.	drFObj
3. This also kind of looks like the Howard Johnson's symbol, the baker leaning forward to give the little boy something, this is the back of the apron, maybe, doesn't quite make sense, this is the cook's hat, baker's hat.	3. The form of the whole thing. It looks like he's leaning forward.	DM(H)

X. 33″

(*Mutters, hums, whistles*)

1. This very small area here looks like heads of horses.	1. I don't know. I just looked and that's what I saw, the shape of a horse's head.	ddF-Ad
2. The entire blue thing kind of looks like a crab.	2. The shape.	DFAP

RORSCHACH SUMMARY

Response	*Inquiry*	*Scoring*
3. This looks like the pelvic area of somebody again, down here.	3. The spine and, then, the pelvic bone. The picture just has that form. That's all.	DF-At
4. Yeah, this kind of looks like Italy, but it's a different kind of boot, more a work boot, to give somebody a kick. That's why there's no heel, unlike Italy, with sharp point. To give somebody a kick.	4. It was kind of swung back, and swings forward, to give somebody a boot.	drMHd,Cloth
5. These kind of look like crabs, also. These look more like crabs, actually.	5. Same shape.	DFA
6. This one yellow area kind of looks like Alaska.	6. Shape of Alaska.	DF-Geo.

EXHIBIT 4

THEMATIC APPERCEPTION TEST

CARD 1 (*Takes off glasses, inspects*) Looks like a child who's, um, looking over his music before he prepares to play the violin. (*Pause*) Either he's preparing or he's played a little and he's kind of dumbfounded by the music and he's looking over the music before he plays again. Kind of a strange looking kid. He looks like he has a wad of chewing tobacco in his mouth and this eye looks kind of . . . (?) Looks kind of drowsy. (*Eye?*) Kind of cross-eyed, actually, looking inward. Both eyes are in the inside part. (*Done?*) Well, perhaps he's played the beginning, now he's looking over the rest, first page, or could be second page. He actually could be sleeping, but I don't think he is. (*Ruminates a bit further*)

CARD 5 Hmm. This looks like a woman who's looking into a room and is disturbed by what she sees. Or surprised. It looks like she's surprised. Anyway, she's looking into the room, not at the table, it looks like there's a couch. (*Wait*) Past the table, like she's looking in on somebody. Actually, it doesn't look like she's surprised or shocked, she's just looking in on somebody, like a child or an old person . . . (*more description of room*) (*What led up and how turn out?*) Doesn't look like it's anything really eventful. It looks like she's going to look in, close door, and go back to where she was.

CARD 6BM This looks like a mother and her son. It's probably during the winter because he has a top coat on. She's looking out the window, seems like watching for something. (*What?*) Like a taxi, or maybe somebody's coming to pick him up. He's going somewhere. (*Pause*) Now it could be the police that are coming, and he's going to jail. (*For what?*) I don't know, it looks like he's well-mannered, so maybe a white collar crime, embezzlement. Looks like a young guy. Maybe he's a bank teller who's stolen money or a junior accountant who's juggled the books. (*Let's stop*)

CARD 10 Hmmm. Well. This looks like a priest consoling one of his parishioners. This is definitely an adult. This doesn't look like a child because the nose is too long. Maybe it's an adolescent. He's kind of consoling this person. He looks very tearful and unhappy. (*More?*) No. I think it definitely looks like a priest. Consoling person. It might be an old woman, mourning the death of someone. Looks like somebody's grandmother. This one's definitely a priest. My first thought was that it was two homosexual men. But it really doesn't look like that.

CARD 12M This looks like someone has either just died or is very sick.

Probably very sick. This person looks like they're trying to heal them. (*Pause*) Either that or they're being given their Last Rites. (*OK*).

CARD 13MF Hmm (*Takes off glasses, inspects*). This can be one of two things. Obviously there's a woman lying on the bed, nude, with breasts exposed. This man either slept with her and got up very early, showered, or at least got dressed very early. (*Wait*) Either to leave early, or there's books here, so maybe he's a professor, or else he's going to study here, but probably not, because he has his tie on. There's a few other things it could be. He could be a doctor, he's been treating her, it's been a long vigil, he's rubbing his eyes, maybe he's never been to bed with her. He's probably not a doctor, though. (*Wait*) The other alternative is that she's just died, and he has his hand over his face because he can't bear to look anymore. He might be a doctor but I doubt it, because she's unclothed. (*Wait*) And the last thing it could be is that he's just murdered her, and he can't bear to look at what he's done, and he's looking away and hiding his eyes.

CARD 14 Hmm. Oh. It looks like a man looking out a window. Like at the moon. Either the moon or the sun has just come up. Not a young man, 35–45, a nice head of hair. Looking out window. Maybe he's star gazing at night. But it looks like the sun has just come up, because it's dark in here and bright out there. (*Thinking and feeling*) I think he's thinking about the day to come, and he's just thinking about the day to come. Maybe thinking of a woman, I don't know, he might be an alcoholic, he's just woken up, he's trying to clear his head, or maybe a drug addict, or maybe a musician. I don't know. Because you can't see anything of the room.

CARD 15 (*Looking at me often, staring when I look up.*) Hmm! This looks like someone who's standing in the middle of a graveyard, with crosses, headstone. Looks like he's looking at this cross, in very deep thought, thinking of the person who's buried here. (*p*) Looks like a woman, because it looks like a woman's hands. Her hair is pushed up on one side. Plus it looks like a woman's coat. (*Wait*) (*Huge yawn*) Like I say, kind of looks like in deep thought or mourning. Looks like the woman's lost a good deal of weight, drawn in cheekbones. (*Mutters*) (*Did you say something?*) I'm tired today . . . I got up at 5:30 to come here! (*Lost weight?*) Yes. (*Describes picture*) (*Why?*) Cause she's in mourning. This is her husband who died. Or her child.

EXHIBIT 5

SENTENCE COMPLETION TEST

2. *He often wished he could* be a professional musician.

3. *It looked impossible, so he* dove out the window.

5. *When she refused him,* he was devastated.

6. *I used to feel I was being held back* by actions taken by my parents.

8. *As a child my greatest fear was* being ignored and overlooked by my mother.

17. *Sometimes he wished* he was a professional athlete.

19. *I could hate a person who* forced his will upon others.

23. *When I met my boss,* I was wary of him.

24. *When I think back, I am ashamed* that I acted so selfishly at times.

36. *Taking orders* is a necessary evil.

37. *I dislike* to conform to stupid rules.

53. *My sexual desires* sometimes get the better of me.

54. *His conscience bothered him most when* he stole.

68. *When they put me in charge,* I feel good.

72. *When he was punished by his mother,* he felt resentful.

77. *When they told him what to do,* he felt angry.

83. *More than anything else,* he needed structure.

87. *I am afraid* of being abandoned.

DISCUSSION

Mr. M, a 29-year-old, single male was tested during an escalating manic episode for which he was hospitalized. Thus, his test results provide a picture of classic manic behavior in the testing situation. He had symptoms of pressured speech, expansive and elevated affect, boundless energy, exaggerated self-confidence, and grandiose career plans. In unstructured situations, his thinking was idiosyncratic and unusual. He was quite distractible, and often energetically embellished his responses to small and insignificant stimulus details. The content of many of these responses is evidence of his sexual preoccupations. The testing confirmed the clinical impression that he was beginning to escalate into a full-blown manic episode.

The manic symptoms were brought under control with the stucture of the hospitalization and medication. At that point, the issue of life goal expectations surfaced, as the wealthy father expected his son to take over the family business and had difficulty recognizing his son's illness and disability. Family sessions with psychoeducational material were used to assist the family in readjusting their expectations of the son. With the assistance of some freedom from the family expectations and of the medication that dampened his own grandiosity, Mr. M was able to recognize his need for a day hospital which could help him develop some career goals of his own and related work skills. He was discharged to a relatively unstructured day hospital where these goals were successfully pursued.

The case of Ms. G, a 23-year-old, single female, was much less prototypic in regard to manic symptoms and behavior. Prior to her first hospitalization, she was gaining weight and becoming lethargic, but began to function in a job with the encouragement of her family. During her eighth week of hospitalization, she was referred for testing due to continued uncertainty regarding her diagnosis. The brevity of her acute symptoms and the atypical nature of her presentation made it difficult for the hospital staff to settle on a confirmed diagnosis. She was given a discharge diagnosis of schizotypal personality disorder.

While she presented few typical symptoms of mania prior to the hospitalization, her next admission shortly after her discharge clearly seemed to be precipitated by a manic episode. Thus, the test results from her first hospitalization are those of a young woman in a very disturbed, but non-psychotic, episode that predated by several months a clear-cut manic episode. Irritability was manifest in her flip, hostile comments, some of which she immediately retracted. Her cognitive organization and controls broke down in the unstructured parts of the testing. Her expansive and overinclusive thinking was dramatically demonstrated in the object sorting task.

Likewise, her 74 responses on the Rorschach evidenced verbal expansiveness and idiosyncratic use of small details, color, and shading combined into non-popular responses. While she doesn't present with clear affective polarities, her thinking was expansive and flighty rather than unusual or weird. Also, she engaged people rather than putting them off.

Like the previous case of Mr. M, the hospitalization was successful in reducing manic symptoms and preparing the patient for discharge. The family had high aspirations and was relatively successful, and their expectations of the patient had to be lowered through psychoeducational means. This patient had more thinking disturbances outside of manic episodes than did Mr. M (note her diagnosis of Schizotypal at first admission), and thus she was discharged to a more structured day hospital. Here she received very direct and structured help in the development of vocational skills.

It is a common clinical myth that bipolar patients need lithium treatment and little else. This is often not the actual situation, and these two cases are illustrative of the multiple vocational and family/social issues bipolar patients face between illness episodes. Thus, treatment planning for bipolar patients must always include, but not be limited to, medication treatment.

CHAPTER 5

Anxiety Disorders

A. OBSESSIVE COMPULSIVE DISORDER WITH AND WITHOUT PERSONALITY DISORDER

Obsessive compulsive disorder is classified as one of a number of anxiety disorders on Axis I. The essential features are recurrent obsessions or compulsions of such severity as to involve marked distress, consume great amounts of time, and/or significantly interfere with normal routine. The most common obsessions, that is, persistent ideas, thoughts, impulses or images, experienced as intrusive, are repetitive thoughts of violence, contamination and doubt. Compulsions such as handwashing, counting, checking, and touching are the repetitive intentional behaviors that are the stereotypic responses to obsessional thoughts. This disorder is often associated with depression, anxiety, and phobic avoidance.

The Axis I disorder is distinct from, but may be related to, Axis II Obsessive Compulsive Disorder, one of the Cluster C (including avoidant, dependent, and passive/aggressive) personality disorders characterized by anxiety and fearfulness. The essential feature of obsessive compulsive personality disorder is a pervasive and longstanding pattern of perfectionism and inflexibility.

OBSESSIVE COMPULSIVE DISORDER

Ms. H arrived at the hospital at the exact time she had been given for an intake evaluation. She presented as a petite, meticulously groomed young woman of 25 years of age who smiled shyly when first introduced to the interviewer. She stated that "my present condition is of a compulsive nature and it is making it uncomfortable to lead a normal life." As the interview continued, it became apparent that she had led a progressively more restricted life, with much of her time and energy being devoted recently to rituals of cleanliness and unrelenting preoccupations with the possibility of contamination by "grease." She feared contamination of her person, her clothes, and her home.

Her concerns had grown to the point that her cleaning rituals, which she herself recognized as out of proportion to the realistic possibilities of contamination, required many hours of her time each day. The time she devoted to these rituals had expanded as more and more personal items required her attention. Her routines had become more and more rigid so that if interrupted in her endeavors, she would have to begin all over again to insure the cleanliness of her articles of clothing, various personal effects, and her own body. One month prior to her admission, she had left her job in order to be able to devote sufficient time to maintaining the immaculateness of her person and her wardrobe.

Ms. H was a devoutly religious Catholic and her obsessions and compulsions had first developed five years previously after terminating a pregnancy by abortion. No one in her family knew of either her sexual indiscretion or her abortion; in fact, until her present admission and despite three brief attempts at outpatient treatment and one brief psychiatric hospitalization, she had kept the events concealed from everyone.

Her social and sexual life revolved around her boyfriend. She had broken off her relationship with him a year and one-half ago while he was on an extended business trip. Shortly after, she had noticed "small bugs" in her bedroom. She had thoroughly cleaned the room, her clothing, and her personal effects, but remained preoccupied with the possible reinvasion of her room and had finally called the exterminator. Feeling that the apartment was indelibly contaminated, she had moved into another apartment.

More recently, fearing that these quarters had also become contaminated, she had returned home to live with her parents in her childhood bedroom. Her mother became involved in helping the patient clean and did several loads of wash for her each day, often washing the same articles several times a day. Her wash had to be done separately from the rest of the family's wash, particularly her father's soiled clothes, as his work often brought him into contact with greasy and oily machinery and she feared that her clothing and, ultimately, her person also would become contaminated.

Apart from her preoccupations with contamination, there were no other disturbances in her cognitive functioning noted on mental status examination. She did describe her mood as "sad," but was otherwise unable to clearly describe her emotional state and, clinically, her affect was judged to be constricted and dysphoric. She also reported a decrease in appetite and difficulties in sleeping of two to four weeks duration. She recognized that her fears regarding contamination were unrealistic and that her cleanliness was overdone. She felt that her overconcern perhaps was related in some way to the humiliation she had experienced at eight or nine years of age when she had been sent home by the school nurse because of head lice which she and several other children had contracted. She stated that she had profited somewhat from her previous brief hospitalization. Her treatment at that time had included pharmacotherapy, which she had discontinued after being discharged. She agreed to be admitted for evaluation and treatment of her obsessive and compulsive difficulties.

DSM-III-R Diagnosis

Axis I: Obsessive compulsive disorder, rule out major depressive disorder
Axis II: Deferred
Axis III: None
Axis IV: Moderate—recent death of her grandfather to whom she had felt close
Axis V: Fair—moderate impairment in both social and occupational functioning

Treatment and Hospital Course

Ms. H's initial evaluation focused principally on the severity of her depressive symptomatology and, shortly after admission, a diagnosis of major depressive disorder was confirmed. She was begun on an antidepressant and after she had achieved and maintained adequate serum concentrations for one month, there were noticeable improvements in her sleep, appetite, and mood. The treatment staff wished to begin to address her cleaning rituals, but were uncertain how to proceed. Strict limits were placed on the amount of time she was allowed to engage in these activities and the amount of time was gradually decreased over the weeks following admission.

In the face of significant symptomatic improvement, Ms. H was offered the opportunity for a long-term hospitalization in order to resolve her long-standing difficulties with dependency on her family and her inability to express herself emotionally. Attention was also to be directed at helping her to increase her capacities for vocational functioning through a structured vocational plan. Although she seemed willing to go along with the treatment staff's recommendation, she was actually quite ambivalent about staying in the hospital.

Psychological Assessment

Ms. H was referred for psychological testing at the start of her second month of hospitalization. At that time, although there had been some improvement in her depressive symptomatology, her psychiatrist had begun to feel that she would need continued treatment with antidepressants to realize further gains. Questions regarding the extent and severity of her depressive symptoms and, in light of her primary diagnosis of obsessive compulsive disorder, a recommendation as to whether a supportive or exploratory psychotherapy would be more appropriate at the present time was requested. Finally, in light of her possible willingness to work on other interpersonal issues while remaining in the hospital, the referring psychiatrist also wished help in considering how to approach these issues with her.

Ms. H was given a WAIS-R, Rorschach, TAT, and DAP by the examining psychologist. She cooperated with the evaluation but, throughout, seemed disconnected from the examination and approached the tests with a detached air of intellectual curiosity. Her manner was ponderously deliberate and, at times, when unsure of her response, she would flatly reject any attempt by the examiner to engage her in an exploration of her uncertainty.

Ms. H's WAIS-R results revealed a full-scale IQ of 83, a verbal IQ of 92, and a performance IQ of 76. These scores were seen as inconsistent with her premorbid level of functioning and were found to be lowered in part by her overly cautious response style which denied her the benefit of additional points for prompt completion of the task. For those subtests without time constraint, occasionally successful efforts at encouraging her to guess when she was unsure of the correct response revealed both adequate knowledge and startling gaps in her general fund of information. For example, after she replied "I don't know" when asked to identify Louis Armstrong, the examiner requested that she guess. She then revealed that she had thought he had "something to do with music" and was "a saxophone player." When the examiner asked her to identify the continent on which Brazil is located, she first claimed she did not know and, when encouraged, she refused to guess. In response to a second request at the end of the examination, she answered correctly. Alternatively, she thought Labor Day was in May and that Robert E. Lee had once been President of the United States.

Her relative strengths were in the areas of rote memorization of digits, understanding of social norms, and capacity for abstract thought. Graphically reflective of her indecisive and deliberate manner, she noted on the Picture Arrangement subtest, "I can't figure this one out. It doesn't make sense to me. It would take me too long, but if I had enough time, I would come to some sort of decision." In short, the WAIS-R gave abundant evidence of the procrastination, ruminativeness, and ambivalence characteristic of obsessive compulsive disorders.

On the projective tests, particularly the TAT, there was considerable evidence of depression. Death and separation, fear of intimacy and ultimate rejection were perseverative themes and typically occurred in the context of longing for sustained emotional contact, which somehow did not occur during life. For example, *card 15* prompted her to tell a story concerning "a very old man standing in a cemetery late on a winter night . . . depressed about being alone since his wife died." He has come to the cemetery to talk to his wife "to get as close to her as he could" and talking to her, he feels "comforted." In the same vein, she told a story to *card 12M* involving a grandfather taking his leave from his grandson, who feigns sleep in order to avoid saying goodbye. A few days afterwards, the grandson calls the grandfather "and lets him know he was awake but felt too sad to actually say goodbye and the grandfather understood."

These themes of sadness and longing typically arise because life's events move too swiftly and she is perennially surprised at what happens next. It would be "wonderful" if she "could do the same thing every day" (*card 14*), but is frequently left trying to "understand what she had just seen as being a normal part of life" (*card 3GF*). However, even the total routinization of life fails to prevent emotional upheaval, as she recognized in her story to *card 13MF*. Her story revolved around a man who goes into the den at the same time every evening to consult his law manuals and, on this occasion, finds his wife dead. She had "slit her wrists because she felt that she was losing control of her life and he wouldn't acknowledge that. He wouldn't acknowledge she was ill in any way and refused her to see a doctor." Such stories help to forge a link between her obsessive concerns with isolating the contamination, the "disease" of emotions, by adherence to orderliness. Unfortunately, an inner emptiness and impoverishment are her chief rewards.

Her Rorschach provided additional examples of her impoverishment and despair. *Card V* produced "a dead chicken" because the legs look "lifeless . . . like if a person relaxed their legs and they were just hanging there." *Card VI* led her to tentatively suggest "possibly the inside of a pit, like from the inside of a piece of fruit." Inquiring into the reason for its resemblance to a pit, she was able to say that "you can just tell that you're down to rock bottom . . . if you were to tear a pit open, you'd see its deep center, its core." Finally, *card X* revealed "a baby without arms" because of the "head and legs and they were small." Her figure drawings were of tiny persons with asymmetric, shrunken bodies and enlarged heads. The house was represented only by a roof out of which a chimney extended and above which was a large, unconnected billow of smoke. Leading from the front door was a path which broadens out as it extends upwards above the peak of the roof and terminates in the air.

Treatment Planning and Outcome

The psychological report was useful to Ms. H's treatment team in helping them to confirm their suspicions of a concurrent depressive disorder for which she continued to receive pharmacological treatment and to which she responded. Her indecisiveness, her attempts to keep herself unmoved by emotion, and her pedantic tone all were seen as consistent with her admission diagnosis of an obsessive compulsive disorder. Her general lack of interest in what motivated either her own or others' behavior, her limited psychological resources, and her need for a high degree of structure and task focus argued against a reliance on an interpersonal therapy as the treatment of choice. A recommendation of a behavior modification approach to her compulsive cleaning difficulties was accepted and implemented with some success.

Also described in the examining psychologist's report was a suspicion that Ms. H's compulsivity was in part an effort on her part to stave off a more pervasive regression and decompensation. There were concerns that unless her treatment were to continue in a structured setting, such as an inpatient unit, attempts to address her fears of intimacy and her long-standing anger at her family would prove too much for her to manage. Her treatment team therefore moved quickly to help her accept their recommendation of continued inpatient treatment and were able to enlist her parents' support for continuing the hospitalization.

Although some headway was made in helping Ms. H to become more emotionally expressive and more emotionally involved with others, she was not felt to be ready to return to work and to an independent living situation at the conclusion of her hospital stay. She was referred to a day hospital where she could continue to receive help with these issues and to a halfway house. Her individual psychotherapy was carried out by the psychiatrist who had referred her for inpatient treatment.

She disliked the halfway house and attempted on several occasions to persuade her parents to let her return to live with them, but they refused to give permission. She was ultimately unable to utilize the day hospital program and after repeated attempts to engage her in working towards increased socialization and improved vocational functioning, she was discharged after four months. She continued in her individual psychotherapy and at the time of her discharge from the day hospital, was preparing to return to work.

E X H I B I T 1

AREA OF ASSESSMENT	CLINICAL EXAMINATION	PSYCHOLOGICAL EXAMINATION
I. Symptoms and Diagnosis		
Obsessive compulsive disorder		
Obsessions	Contamination by dirt, especially grease	Perseverative thinking
Compulsions	Ritualized grooming and cleaning in excess of hygenic requirements	Compulsively deliberate
Distress and interference with role functioning	Quit job to devote time to cleaning	Aware of inefficiencies in functioning due to present distress
II. Personality Factors	Procrastination and indecisiveness	Becomes indecisive in the face of uncertainty to avoid confrontation
III. Cognitive Abilities	Average intelligence	Below average intelligence with cognitive inefficiencies due to rigidity and other personality factors
IV. Psychodynamics	Dependency gives rise to hostility to ward off the expected rejection	Avoids intimacy for fear of becoming too dependent and being rejected
V. Therepeutic Enabling Factors	Aware that her fears and her response to them are out of proportion to realistic circumstances	Reality appreciation is largely intact.
	Prior treatment response to medication	None
VI. Environmental Demand and Social Adjustment	Excellent premorbid functioning in highly structured and routinized work setting	Functions best in structured situations
	Extremely limited social life; no enduring close relationships	Difficulties in establishing and allowing close relationships

EXHIBIT 2

WAIS-R Summary

Verbal Subtests	*Scaled Score*
Information	5
Digit Span	11
Vocabulary	9
Arithmetic	6
Comprehension	10
Similarities	10

Performance Subtests

Picture Completion	7
Picture Arrangement	7
Block Design	6
Object Assembly	5
Digit Symbol	8

Verbal IQ	91
Performance IQ	76
Full Scale IQ	83

Rorschach Summary

Number of Responses	17
Rejections	0
Populars	6
Originals	0
Average R/T chromatic	58″
Average R/T achromatic	95″
F%	53
F + %	65
A%	41
H%	12
W:M	3:1
M:Sum C	1:0
m:c	3:4
VIII-X%	29
FK + F + Fc%	71
(H + A):(Hd + Ad)	7:2

RORSCHACH SUMMARY

Apperception   W   18%

D   59%

d   0%

Dd + S 23%

E X H I B I T   3

Rorschach Summary

Response	*Inquiry*	*Scoring*

I. 3″

1. Looks like a butterfly to me. Can I change that? It looks like a bat to me.

    1. In here reminds me of a bat's head or something. (*Bat?*) The whole shape of the ink on the card. (*Anything else?*) Not really. Just looked more like a butterfly. I guess it was the pointy sides. A butterfly has wider, floppier sides, and butterflies are pretty. To me, it looked a little more scary to me. Just that it really looked like a bat to me and I'm really scared by bats. The little head bothered me. It looked leathery like a bat. It seemed creepy to me. (*Creepy?*) Just was.

    WFcAP

2. Looks kind of like a leaf.

    2. The parts that jutted out and came to a point and the fact that it was irregular. Leaves are like that. Sometimes they're missing their tops and sides. (*Anything else?*) No. It's like a crusty old leaf. No, now that I say that I'm embarrassed because it doesn't look that much like a leaf.

    drFc-Pl

3. Looks like a woman's body without a head. That's it.

    3. This looks like her hands reaching upward. It doesn't make sense that it doesn't have a head but I could really clearly see a woman's outline.

    DMHd

RORSCHACH SUMMARY

Response	Inquiry	Scoring

II. 32″

1. It looks like a . . . uh . . . crab. | 1. Just the shape and those pointy things that came out, like antennas from the front of it. (*Anything else?*) No. | DFA

2. And it looks like a heart. I don't mean, maybe I do mean both. The actual heart organ. And that's it. | 2. I guess just the shape of it. (*Anything else?*) No. | drFAt

3. This part in here looks like something but I'm not sure if I'm supposed to respond to this part. (*Whatever you like*). This part looks like a hurricane lamp to me. | 3. Just the shape of the top of it reminded me of a hurricane lamp, and also had the stem-like bottom. (*Anything else?*) No. | SF Obj

III. 15″

1. Looks like a bowtie. Part of it looks like a bowtie. That's it. That's all I see. | 1. Shape | DFClothP

2. I guess the same part resembles a butterfly. | 2. Again the shape. | DFAP

IV. 72″

I don't know. Doesn't look like anything to me.

1. Maybe down here this and this remind me maybe of rabbit's feet. That's it. | 1. The part of the blot sort of went out like that (*motions*) and the rabbit's feet look big and fluffy, and they go out like that. (*Fluffy?*) It looks soft and furry. | DFcAd

---

RORSCHACH SUMMARY

Response	Inquiry	Scoring

V. 45″

1. (*Drops card*). It reminds me of a dead chicken. That's it.	1. All things that jut out are like a dead chicken. It's so lifeless. Like the rest of the body's hanging up here and the legs down here look lifeless. Doesn't look so much like chicken legs up here. (*Else?*) No. Just those things that I call legs. (*Other parts of body?*) No. (*Dead rather than alive?*) Yeah. Lifeless legs. They weren't straight lines, like if a person relaxed their legs. It's like a chicken that's just hanging down dead.	WFm-(A) *Confab*

VI. 1′15″

It doesn't really look like anything to me.

1. Possibly the inside of a pit, like from the inside of a piece of fruit.	1. Especially in here where it gets darker. (*Anything else?*) I guess it must have looked like . . . you can just tell that you're down to rock bottom. I don't know, it's hard to explain. (*Rock bottom?*) If you were to saw a tree in half, you'd see the grain. It's just like if you were to tear a pit open you'd see its deep dark center, its core. (*Certain piece of fruit in mind?*) No.	diFC′-Pl *Confab*

RORSCHACH SUMMARY

Response	*Inquiry*	*Scoring*

VII. 2′45″

Are you only supposed to look at these one way, the way you hand them to me? (*Whatever you like*).

I really don't see anything at all.

1. One side of it looks like a little dog with its one paw up. That's it.	1. The way that a dog sits and the little thing that I called the paw. (*Anything else?*) No.	DFMA

VIII. 50″

1. I see a frog.	1. Just the shape of it, and it just looked like frog's legs, the way they were spread apart like that. (*Else?*) No.	DFM-A
2. Two animals. I don't know what they're called . . . possums . . . you know, they even look a little like rats to me. It would really surprise me if someone else would look at this inkblot and not see the rats or possums. It's almost like they were painted on there. It's so clear. That's it. That's all I see.	2. The more I looked at it they looked like rats to me. They really did! (*Rats?*) Just the shape. (*Else?*) I could just very clearly see the outline of rats! (*Reaction?*) I don't know why. Don't know if I've ever seen a rat. (*Feel affected by these?*) I just keep thinking that if I ever saw one of those in a room with me alone, I don't know what I'd do. I remember hearing that there was a rat who lived in the wall of an apartment I used to live in.	DFAP *Confab*

RORSCHACH SUMMARY

Response	*Inquiry*	*Scoring*

IX. 1′40″

Nothing. I don't see anything.

1. I think all of them kind of remind me of bugs. Like if you were to take a bug and look at it under a microscope, this is what you'd see. They all seem to have little feelers or arms to them. That's really it. Feelers or arms to them.

1. I'm thinking of one bug, probably just from looking through books and seeing a picture of a bug and then seeing it up close and, oh! (*Holds head*). It looks much scarier when it gets magnified. (*Many or one?*) I think all of the cards I've seen so far have reminded me of bugs. (*Bugs?*) Guess I saw little feelers on them all. (*Feelers?*) Like where I traced on the last card, antennae-like things. They just remind me of little arms or feelers or antennae.

WF-A
Confab

X. 2′15″

1. The only thing I see is needle-nose pliers.

1. The part that looked like the baby's legs to me, that made it look like needle-nose pliers, the way they come together at the top.

DF Obj.

(*Holds card up to face, back down, back up, back down*).

2. I suppose I see a baby without arms. That's it.

2. It just looked like a baby to me. I could see a head and legs and they were small. (*Baby rather than person?*) I guess just the size of it. (*Without arms?*) I couldn't see any arms on it. I probably shouldn't have said it unless I saw the whole thing.

DF-Hd

E X H I B I T   4

THEMATIC APPERCEPTION TEST

CARD 1 1'5″ There's a little boy sitting at the table with a violin in front of him. I forgot the questions. He, the little boy, is sad because he wanted his father to play the violin with him, his father also has a violin. His father said they, he didn't have the time, he was working on a sales presentation. And the little boy is feeling very sad and shut out because he had asked his father several times to play with him but he was always too busy, it seems. (*End?*) Later on that evening the little boy was reading and his father walked in playing his violin and suggested that they play together for a while. And the little boy ran out of the room to get his violin.

CARD 2 1'25″ In the picture is a man and a woman and their niece who was visiting from New York. And she had come out to the field to see what her aunt and uncle were doing before she went off to the library. (*Thinking or feeling?*) Well, the niece is, feels amazed at how hard her uncle is working and she feels sad . . . that he has to work so hard to maintain what he has. And the story ends . . . uhm . . . I don't know . . . And the story ends by the niece promising that she will visit every summer because she knows that that would mean more to them than anything money could buy.

CARD 3GF 30″ Okay. In the picture is a young girl about 24 who's coming out of her father's chicken coop. She had gone down there to ask her father if he would mind giving her a ride to her grandmother's and she opened the chicken coop door and she saw that he was just killing a chicken and she turned away in disgust . . . and she was feeling hate. (?) Toward her father. (*End?*) It will end by the girl deciding . . . not even to ask for the ride and walking instead to try and understand what she had just seen as being a normal part of life.

CARD 5 35″ In the picture there's a lady who's looking into her living room from her bedroom. She was looking out the door because she thought she'd heard a noise and she's feeling scared and her heart is beating very fast. And the story ends by the lady hearing the milkman's truck pulling away from the curb and she realizes that the noise she heard was her milk being dropped in her metal box and she feels very relieved.

CARD 10 35″ In the picture is a man and a woman. The man is holding the woman and the woman is upset because she came home to find . . . that the delivery truck had left off her couch and chair and they had been recovered in the wrong fabric. And the woman is feeling very disappointed and

THEMATIC APPERCEPTION TEST

a little angry. (*What's the man thinking or feeling?*) He's feeling understanding and angry. (?) That the store could do such a stupid thing. (*End?*) The story will end by the man making a deal with Macy's that they would not only fix what they had done but would also do an additional love seat for the same price.

CARD 12M 1′45″ I see an old man looking at his grandson and the grandfather had come really to say goodbye but found his grandson sleeping. At first he thought he'd wake him but decided just to look instead. And the grandfather was feeling a great deal of pride just seeing how beautiful his grandson was. (*Grandson feeling?*) The grandson was asleep. I take that back. The way I was going to end it was the grandson was awake so he could have been feeling something. The grandson sensed the grandfather's presence in the room and felt upset because he knew he had come to say goodbye and the way the story ends is that the grandson calls the grandfather several days later and lets him know he was awake but felt too sad to actually say goodbye and the grandfather understood.

CARD 13MF (*Turns card over, then back.*) 1′25″ I would say a man and a woman . . . (2′25″) . . . and they're in a den . . . in a house, in their house, and the man had come into the den to consult some law manuals as he did every evening at the same time and found his wife . . . dead . . . And he felt . . . well, he was shocked. (*How did she die?*) She slit her wrists. (*Why'd she do that?*) Because she felt that she was losing control of her life and he wouldn't acknowledge that. (?) He wouldn't acknowledge she was ill in any way and refused her to see a doctor. (*End?*) . . . The story will end by the man going back to work and resuming his normal . . . lifestyle.

CARD 14 These are hard. (1′45″) In the picture, there's a . . . young man looking out of a window on the top of a high tower overlooking the ocean. And he had come up to the tower to sit and think as he often did in the early morning hours. (*Thinking or feeling?*) He was thinking how wonderful it would be if he could do the same thing every day. (?) Come to this same spot everyday because after only a few hours there his mind seemed somewhat clearer. And the story ends . . . by him hearing a fire whistle and he knew it was time to get back to the grind. (*What was grind?*) Just like everyday stuff. (*Like?*) Work, family, friends.

CARD 15 1′10″ In the picture, there's a very old man standing in a cemetery late on a winter night. And he came to the cemetery because he couldn't sleep. And he was feeling very gloomy and depressed about being

THEMATIC APPERCEPTION TEST

alone since his wife died. And when she was alive, they had some of their best talks late at night, so he felt it appropriate to get as close to her as he could and the story ends by the man having had a conversation just as though his wife had been standing there, and he felt . . . comforted. (*Could he talk with his wife?*) No. She didn't answer back.

OBSESSIVE COMPULSIVE DISORDER WITH MIXED
PERSONALITY DISORDER

Mr. J is 22-years-old, presently unemployed, and living with his mother. He was first hospitalized at age 18 following his high school graduation and in the context of his father's sudden death in an automobile accident. He became overwhelmed with anxiety, leading to frequent, acute attacks of panic. He had failed to respond to two brief hospitalizations and subsequently spent almost a year at a long-term, private psychiatric hospital where his anxiety and panic attacks remitted without pharmacological treatment. He was able to live alone and attend college with the help of individual psychotherapy and attendance at a structured day hospital program, but his anxiety and panic returned. He was given trials of several anxiolytic and antidepressant medications without any apparent benefit. He moved in with his younger sister and finally with his mother, but for the last six months, his increasing fears of contamination by other people's bodily substances and an ensuing host of hygienic rituals and rigid avoidance of contact with objects touched by others have made it extremely difficult for him to be managed outside the hospital.

Mr. J agreed with his mother's recommendation that he seek hospitalization and he was readmitted to the private hospital where he had been treated previously. His functioning deteriorated further and, dissatisfied with his progress, he requested transfer to a different hospital. His mother supported the transfer, feeling that he needed a greater amount of structure in his daily living which was not being provided by the hospital staff. He had been "very depressed" for the last two months. He slept as much as 12 hours a day in order to avoid becoming preoccupied with his fears of contamination. He lost weight since his fears of contamination required him to limit his food intake. Unable to ward off his intrusive thoughts, he had become suicidal.

At the time of his transfer, he stated he was requesting admission because "I've had paranoid episodes since I was 17. Beginning this February, I started to be afraid to touch anything." He began the interview by placing a handkerchief on the seat of the chair, explaining that he did not want to become contaminated by the chair. He said this fear was irrational, yet he could not sit down until allowed to use the handkerchief. Throughout the examination he kept his hands in his pockets. He touched nothing for fear that he would contaminate any object with which he came into contact. He reported he was very tense and he looked anxious and was restless. His speech was digressive, but there was no evidence of a formal thought disorder noted during the examination. He reported persistent, intrusive thoughts having to do with contaminating or being contaminated by bodily substances. He washed his hands frequently in order to protect himself from these contaminating substances.

DSM-III-R Diagnosis

Axis I: Obsessive Compulsive Disorder
Axis II: Mixed personality disorder
Axis III: None
Axis IV: Severe—recent hospitalization; dropped out of school
Axis V: Fair—moderate impairment in both occupational and social functioning

Treatment and Hospital Course

Following his admission, the hospital staff developed a highly structured, milieu treatment plan that included a daily diary of his thoughts, feelings and activities. He was confronted by the staff around his compulsive rituals and was allowed to spend progressively less time engaged in them as treatment progressed. He developed some insight into the relationship between his anger and his intrusive thoughts and compulsions and, as he became better able to express and tolerate his anger, his intrusive thoughts and compulsions diminished. As he began to evidence some moderate degree of improvement, his depressive feelings and hypersomnia remitted. He continued to have difficulties in his social relationships and spent little time with others.

Psychological Assessment

Mr. J made a good adjustment to the structured treatment plan implemented by the hospital staff. He was referred for testing during the first week of hospitalization to help with his differential diagnosis, to determine the nature of a previously reported learning disability, and to assess his potential for psychotherapy. The primary issue in the diagnostic differential was his capacity to adequately test reality, given the dramatic effect of his obsessions and compulsions on his behavior. He was given an MMPI, Rorschach, TAT, SCT, and DAP to help with the diagnostic differential and psychotherapy assessment. He received a battery of neuropsychological screening tasks, including the WAIS-R, Wide Range Achievement Test

(WRAT), Raven's Progressive Matrices, and Spreen-Benton Battery to help assess his neuropsychological difficulties.

His behavior during testing was largely unremarkable with the exception of a great deal of restless motor activity such as jiggling his leg. He had no difficulty following the examiner's instructions when they involved handling test materials, but otherwise kept his hands in the pockets of his shorts.

On the WAIS-R, he obtained full-scale, verbal, and performance IQs of 96, 97 and 94, respectively. Compared to the results reported three and four years previously, there was some lowering of his verbal IQ. The pattern of his various subscale scores suggested relative weaknesses in concentration, attention, and visual-motor coordination and speed. His DAP also suggested difficulties with visual-spatial integration.

His visual-motor deficits were partly neuropsychological in origin. He evidenced a moderate graphaesthesia in both the right and left hands and a mild finger agnosia on the left side. Fine motor coordination was impaired to a moderate degree. In addition to these sensorimotor deficits, he also gave evidence of some mild articulation problems and intermittent word-finding difficulty. His WRAT performance placed him at sixth grade levels in both spelling and math and at only the ninth grade level in reading. His accounts of his school difficulties, both behavioral and academic, and his strategies to circumvent his reading difficulties in particular were suggestive of long-standing neuropsychological impairments. These impairments may have been related to a specific learning disability for which he had learned to compensate partially or perhaps to a more diffuse pattern of atypical cognitive development. In either case, these neuropsychological deficits had compromised his integrative cognitive abilities and continued to make it difficult for him to use these abilities, particularly when psychologically distressed. His distress was evident in his MMPI where seven of the 10 clinical scales (*scales 1, 2, 3, 6, 7, 8 and 0*) and his F scale all had pathologically high T scores of 70 or greater. The remainder, with the exception of *scale 9*, were scored at 65 or above.

Mr. J's relatively higher WAIS-R subscale scores showed a preference for factual material and a heightened sensitivity to environmental cues. Mr. J relied on his hyperalertness to preserve his reality testing abilities which, on the whole, were found to be reasonably intact. On the Rorschach, for example, he gave seven popular responses in an expansive record with a total of 42 responses, but managed only a borderline adequate consensual appreciation of the form of the inkblots ($F+ = 79\%$). However, there was a striking total absence of responses which incorporated color, reflecting an extremely guarded emotional reactivity. Instead, he was overly ideational and ruminative ($M = 6$) and was captured by the shading of the inkblots and the black and white contrast, features of his Rorschach record which indicated the presence of a great deal of anxiety and internal tension. His sense of this anxiety was that it was potentially explosive. For example, on *card 1*, this was clearly projected in his report of two tiny details which reminded him of "a nuclear bomb cloud."

The sense of total annihilation which developed from a single, small detail was perhaps clarified by his TAT stories. He was obviously preoccupied with death and the disruption and loneliness that resulted for those who had survived the death. On the TAT, the majority of the stories involved very negative themes. The causes of death included a heart attack (*card 5*), suicide (*cards 14* and *15*), acts of war (*card 10*), terminal cancer (*card 13MF*), madness (*card 3BM*), and a deadly childhood disease (*card 12M*). In each case, the survivors failed to make a successful adjustment to the loss and, in each case, the catastrophe resulted from someone's attempt to establish a life outside the parental home.

In these stories, he made it clear that growing up and establishing a life that was independent of his childhood home was to invite certain disaster. Any such attempt would be punished by death. It is little wonder that such a pervasive fear would give rise to an intolerable amount of anxiety and episodes of acute panic in the context of efforts directed at independence and maturation. The solution to this dilemma appeared to lie in the rigid maintenance of a compliant and submissive posture and a complementary avoidance of situations and people who might stimulate forbidden aggressive or sexual wishes. In addition, protective devices such as the "boxing gloves" and "goalie mask" reported on *card IX* of the Rorschach must be employed to effectively survive.

Mr. J's TAT and SCT responses made it clear that he felt unable to negotiate the adult world of work and relationships. On the SCT, he reported that he felt happiest when "I daydream" and that when with his mother, he felt "protected." Since childhood, his greatest fear was that "my parents would die" and he felt to blame when "his father died." His father was described as the ideal man and always "was nice to me." His lost relationship with his father was clearly quite important to him. On the TAT, the only story with a positive outcome (*card 7BM*) concerned a father and a son. The father encourages the son to accept a scholarship to college rather than a high paying job and, following the father's advice which "turned out eventually to be a good decision in the long run," the son "turned out to be a successful businessman."

He continued the theme on the next card (*6BM*) where a mother and son were separated by the son's decision to take a better paying job out of town. The mother and son were described as "really, really close, especially since her husband died, his father, and he lives right near her now that he's grown up and takes care of her." Although the son moved away, leaving the mother "shocked and depressed and confused," he "doesn't like being away from his home and he really misses his mother" and he eventually "quits his job and moves back home" where he is "a lot happier."

Mr. J appeared to yearn for a restoration of his earlier family situation and seemed willing to renounce independent strivings. However, such a renunciation would require him to accept a view of himself as a resourceless and hopelessly ill child. This view was graphically portrayed in his male figure drawing. He drew a tiny, empty, smiling figure on bended knee with outstretched arms whom he described as 24 years old or so and "happy . . . reaching out to grab something." Surprisingly, his female figure was drawn in exactly the same posture but was described as "confident, happy, strong and aggressive." These two desexualized figures were interchangeable except for their hairstyles and a small halo which was drawn over the head of the male. The great similarity of the figures, but certainly not of their descriptions, suggests the conflict he feels in adopting a helpless, dependent, child-like role. This conflict and the trap it posed for him also surface in the Rorschach. In one response to *card II*, he used the internal red details to identify "a man screaming, he's trapped in something." On inquiry, the eyes are "eyes in a frowning face enclosed in here, in the black, like a cell."

Treatment Planning and Outcome

Mr. J had made substantial progress in reducing the amount of time he spent engaged in washing rituals and in allowing himself to physically contact his environment under the structure of his nursing supervised, behavioral care plan. However, his success was itself a source of anxiety for him for he felt it implied a rapid discharge from the hospital and an ensuing loss of support. This theme of abandonment in the face of success, which was consciously recognized by him in the context of his hospital treatment, provided the psychologist and his treatment team with a focus for their treatment recommendations.

His neuropsychological deficits were acknowledged by the treatment team and were explained to him as setting real limits on what he could accomplish. His need for consistent support to develop compensatory strategies was accepted as valid and he was able to work productively with the therapeutic activities department to develop compensatory skills. He was also helped to see that outside of these real deficits and his realistic fears for his own ability to maintain an independent existence there were irrational elements to his fear which were a source of conflict for him.

He was offered an opportunity to explore these fears in greater depth in his individual psychotherapy. He gradually came to understand that his obsessional thoughts and compulsive behaviors served primarily to defend him against his feelings of anger, guilt, and frustration which had crystallized around his father's death and were perpetuated by his real concerns over his mother's health and his fear of losing her as well. In his group psychotherapy, he was able to recognize that anger and tension held less destructive potential than he had imagined and he became increasingly able to express his own feelings in this context.

Equally important to his further progress was his family therapy. The psychological assessment was first utilized to help Mr. J's mother understand his real neuropsychological problems. She had worked in medical settings and found these results easy to accept. Initially, she felt they confirmed the need for Mr. J to remain dependent on her. She later became aware of and able to express her own limitations and conflicts with regard to how much she could do for him. Over the next several months, he learned that his mother did not need for him to be dependent and his mother learned that he was able to lead a happy life away from her.

Mr. J's hospitalization lasted almost a year. At the end of that time, the hospital staff recommended to him that he live in a halfway house, attend a day hospital, and continue with his individual and family psychotherapy. These plans were accepted by him and he made a good adjustment after leaving the hospital.

EXHIBIT 1

AREA OF ASSESSMENT	CLINICAL EXAMINATION	PSYCHOLOGICAL EXAMINATION
I. Symptoms/Diagnosis		
Obsessive compulsive disorder		
Obsessions	Will contaminate or be contaminated by others	Obsessive preoccupation with catastrophe and death
Compulsions	Excessive hand-washing, keeps hands in pockets	None
II. Personality Factors	Mixed personality disorder with dependent and schizotypal features	Marked immaturity and very limited insight, but reality testing not grossly disturbed
		Odd speech; paranoid ideation; marked social anxiety and isolation
III. Cognitive Abilities	Possible history of learning disabilities	Sensorimotor and spatial orientation impairment; academic performance much below college grade level
IV. Psychodynamics	Dependent on mother	Unwarranted guilt over father's death; fears his independence will be difficult for his mother
		Infantile yearnings for a protective environment
V. Therapeutic Enabling Factors	Functioning improves in a structured environment	Adept at using external cues and direction to organize his behavior
		Is capable of compliance when safety is guaranteed
VI. Environmental Demand and Social Adjustment	Unable to maintain independent living	Poor planning and organization without external structure; expects to fail

Area of Assessment	Clinical Examination	Psychological Examination
	No close friends; no leisure pursuits	Limited empathic skills and uncertain psychosexual identification

EXHIBIT 2

WAIS-R Summary

Verbal Subtests	Scaled Score
Information	11
Digit Span	8
Vocabulary	10
Arithmetic	8
Comprehension	9
Similarities	11

Performance Subtests

Picture Completion	14
Picture Arrangement	11
Block Design	7
Object Assembly	8
Digit Symbol	8
Verbal IQ	97
Performance IQ	94
Full-scale IQ	96

MMPI Summary

F*LK: 8!2**7"610'345-9/

Rorschach Summary

Number of Responses	43
Rejections	0
Populars	8
Originals	1
Average R/T Chromatic:	7"
Average R/T Achromatic:	12"
F%	56
F+%	79
A%	44
H%	16
W:M	6:7
M:Sum C	7:0
m:c	6:6
VIII-X%	21

RORSCHACH SUMMARY

FK + F + Fc%		63
(H + A):(Hd + Ad)		21:5
Apperception	W	14%
	D	63%
	d	9%
	Dd + S	14%

EXHIBIT 3

RORSCHACH SUMMARY

Response	*Inquiry*	*Scoring*

I. 4″

1. It's a wolf. Do I describe the picture or something? (*Just tell me what it looks like. Some people see more than one thing.*)	1. Whole thing. (*Wolf?*) The ears and the triangular-type face.	WFA
2. And I see two birds-like statues of two birds.	2. Here. The top part. (*Bird-like?*) Like the ear part of the wolf looked like it had a feathery tail and beak. Just the general shape. (*Feathery?*) The shape and the way the ink is light and dark in places. Reminds me of something light and feathery. (*Statues?*) It looks still.	DFcA
3. And I see, um, I see like little paws of a clam—no not a clam—a, a lobster. Little legs (*gestures*).	3. The shape.	dFAd
4. Looks like two—two mushrooms of a nuclear bomb cloud. A mushroom cloud.	4. They were, like, foaming on top, and they shot up like a mushroom. (*Foamy?*) Um, they just, uh, the top of them looked like, like gaseous-like.	dKF.cF Expl
5. And it looks like little—like, like . . . like amoebas, or small animals, floating around.	5. They seemed to be very small and swimming very fast and erratically. (*Seems that way?*) The way they seemed to be bumping into one another, and the way the ink went—like they were in motion.	ddFMA

RORSCHACH SUMMARY

Response	*Inquiry*	*Scoring*
6. And it looks like a top of a teapot—a percolator, you know, that type of thing. That's about all.	6. This here. (*Percolator?*) Just the shape sort of reminded me of one.	drF-Obj

II. 14″

1. The pelvis . . . area. Like an x-ray of the hip. Pelvis.	1. Here—it's everything but the red. Here's the sacrum—what do you call it-the Xray bottom of the backbone. (*X-ray?*) That's the only way you could see the different parts. I guess—the color. (*Color?*) Just the black versus white.	WFk.FC'-At
2. There's, uh . . . two . . . dogs that are rubbing noses.	2. This half here and this half here. (*Including this?*) No, none of the red; just the black split in half. (*Dogs rubbing noses?*) Shaped that way. The way they're touching.	WFMAP
3. There are fighting munchkins-like, little, fighting . . .	3. Heres, these two red things. (*Fighting?*) The way the red dots came off them. (*How was that?*) It seemed—just seemed to make 'em seem to be more in turmoil. (*Munchkins?*) I don't know—they just seemed like small people.	DM(H)
4. And there's like, I think it'd be like a type of a crab or a shellfish with sort of antennas.	4. Here. (*Shellfish?*) The overall shape. Antennas.	DFA
5. There's uh, like a lamp you see in the park, to light the walkway.	5. The white. (*Lamp?*) Just the shape.	SF Obj

Rorschach Summary

Response	Inquiry	Scoring
6. There seems to be a man screaming—he's trapped in something—trapped in a cell or something. (*Cell?*) Yeah, a room of some type.	6. Just—well it's not as good on both sides, but you can see in this red in here, like eyes on a frowning face. Like enclosed in here, in the black, like a cell. (*Cell?*) He just seemed trapped in it. (*Trapped?*) His face— that he was sad and stuff.	DM-Hd, Arch.
7. I see an outline of a dog's head. That's all I can see.	7. Here. Just the shape.	dFA

III. 6″

Response	Inquiry	Scoring
1. There's a bowtie.	1. The red thing in the middle. (*Bowtie?*) Just the shape.	DFClothP
2. Another picture of the hip.	2. Right in here. (*Picture of a hip?*) Just looked like it . . . in this one, well, it's mostly in both of them-the part that looks like the coccyx. The part of the spine that sticks down there in the middle. (*Show me*) Yeah, there, it's that line there. Not so much in this one, but you can see it here. And also, the shape of the sides.	DFkAt
3. Two women fighting over something.	3. This here and here. And they seem to be in a tug-of-war type thing. Pulling this here.	WMHP

RORSCHACH SUMMARY

Response	*Inquiry*	*Scoring*
4. Two, like, uh, I don't know what you'd call them—like cartoon characters, something you'd see in a cartoon. And they seem, like, screaming back and forth to each other.	4. Yeah, here and here. And what makes them look like they're arguing is the way the ink comes off them there. Arguing verbally. (*Show me*) There. (*The dots?*) Yeah. (*Cartoon characters?*) Yes, the head, the arms, tail. Has to be a tail.	DM(H)
5. And, like, two mushroom clouds again.	5. Here and here. (*Clouds?*) The shape. (*Anything else?*) No.	drFCloud
6. And then, uh, two men with, with, who are very stern and have big noses. (*Hums to self, puts foot on chair and jiggles it.*)	6. Right here, this is the neck, their head, the eyes, the lips, the nose. (*Stern?*) The, the, the way their lips were, and their chin. (*Mean?*) Drooped, like. The chin drooped.	DMHd
7. And uh, two guns. That's all I can see.	7. Right here, here's the trigger and the barrel. The same over here. (*Gun?*) Just the shape.	DF-Obj

IV. 45″

1. Uh, the, the spinal column.	1. Uh, here. And that looked like the bottom. (*Spinal column?*) Um, the shape. And like, on each of the bones, they have a spine or something that comes off them, like condiles. (?) Yeah, protuberances, and those looked like that.	DF-At
2. There's two, there's a boot.	2. The shape. The points here.	DFClothP

RORSCHACH SUMMARY

Response	*Inquiry*	*Scoring*
3. There's a shadow of a bird—like the ones you make with your fingers, that you shine in front of a light (*gestures with hand*).	3. Here and here. (*Shadow?*) Uh, just like the beak and stuff. (*Show me?*) Uh, here. Doesn't look like a real birds' head. It could be like the shadow. (*So not looking real made it seem like a shadow?*) Yeah, not looking real. (*Anything else?*) No. I don't think so.	DF(Ad)
4. Looks like a bear rug.	4. The whole thing. This is the head, these are the arms, and that's the tail. (*Bear rug?*) The shape. The head was there, and the tail.	WFAdP
5. It's, looks like kind of like where they light the flame for the Olympics, or a torch, like in a temple. Like in a Buddhist temple.	5. I meant like a torch stand. This part here, and this part going up. The flame would go in there. (*Torch stand?*) The shape.	DFObj

V. 5″

1. A butterfly.	1. Uh, this way. (*Butterfly?*) Wings. Shaped like one.	WFAP
2. Ah, a dolphin.	2. Here, this, this is its body, this is its head and mouth. And it looked like it's in motion. (*Dolphin in motion?*) I don't know—just looked that way.	DFM-A
3. A back view of a rabbit. Uh . . . (*long pause*) That's all I can see.	3. Here, here's its ears and its tail. A back view.	dFA

VI. 4″

1. Um, it looked like a wolf's head.	1. Here. (*Wolf's head?*) Shape.	DFAd

RORSCHACH SUMMARY

Response	*Inquiry*	*Scoring*
2. A, a guitar. (*Sighs, puffs*)	2. Well here's where the strings go and then here— you notice how the color changes?—it goes out and down here and then back.	drFC'-Obj
That's about all I can see.		

VII. 4″

1. Two girls, Indian girls, staring at each other.	1. Outlines. (*Indian girls?*) They had a feather, kind of, on their heads.	DMH,ObjP
2. Two elephants. And then (*Hold on*) . . .	2. Well, well, the elephants go kind of the way you're looking at it. Here's the eyes, and the head and the trunk.	DFA
3. Two pigs.	3. Just upside down. Here's the eyes and the nose. This is a little thing off the head.	DFA
4. And then, uh, a domed arena. That's all I can see.	4. This thing here, this whole thing. (*Domed arena?*) Just the shape. (*Show me parts of it?*) Here's like, the roof. And these are the sides. I sort of filled in here so it would be like level.	DF-Arch

VIII. 3″

1. Looks like two water rats.	1. Here. (*Rats?*) The shape.	DFAP

RORSCHACH SUMMARY

Response	*Inquiry*	*Scoring*
2. Looks like a ghost.	2. Here are its eyes, these are its arms. This is the rest. It looks all swervy-like, that's why I saw that. (*Swervy?*) It looked like, uh, just like there were creases. Like he was very inanimate . . . just creases. (*How did creases make it seem inanimate?*) It made it seem like light and spooky . . .	DFc(H) *Peculiar verbalization*
I can't see nothing else.		

IX. 8″

Response	*Inquiry*	*Scoring*
1. Two witches facing each other.	1. Just the shape. (*Whole figures?*) Yeah, whole figures.	DM(H)
2. A rabbit's face.	2. Here are the eyes. OK, it ends about here, and it goes up here into the bright—here are the ears—and down around here. (*Rabbit's face?*) The eyes and the ears, the shape. (*What about eyes?*) I don't know, just reminded me of a rabbit.	D(S)F-Ad
3. Two boxing gloves.	3. Looking this way at them, you can see it. This is like the thumb in here. It's just the shape.	DF-Obj
4. Um, a goalie's mask, like in hockey.	4. OK, here's the eyes. It goes down here and up, up here. For some reason, it looks very thick. I guess it's the shading. So anyhow, it goes down to here and around here.	dr(S)FcObj
That's all I see.		

RORSCHACH SUMMARY

Response	*Inquiry*	*Scoring*

X. 6″

Response	Inquiry	Scoring
1. Bugs crawling up a pole.	1. Here's the bugs here and these are the antennas. And this is the pole.	DFMA,Obj
2. Two seahorses (*Inspects card carefully, taps card*).	2. Right here. The shape of seahorses.	DFA
3. Two wolves looking at each other nose to nose.	3. Right here-here's the heads and here's the nose. (*Wolves?*) Just reminded me of wolves. That kind of shape.	DFMA
That's all I can see.		

E X H I B I T 4

THEMATIC APPERCEPTION TEST

CARD 1 Uh . . . hmm . . . um. The kid got in trouble in school for getting bad marks. And he was sent—his parents sent him to his room to study, and he's uninterested and he's moaning about it. (*Hold on*) And uh, he—he decides to try and, and learn the work he has to learn. And he goes into school and he fails anyway. And it seems that no matter how hard he tries, nobody believes he tries, and he still seems to fail anyway. And—that's it. (*He doing?*) Studying for a test—or studying for school in general.

CARD 3BM A lady becomes, uh, really depressed, and uh, because she becomes so depressed and everything, she starts to lose her family and her job and everything. So—one day she eventually loses everything—her family, her friends and her job —and she can't function and she becomes hysterical. She starts crying and becomes so hysterical, she loses it. (?) Like she's gone crazy. She eventually just dies from not eating and the elements—she just walks around in the city and nobody knows her. She just dies because of her, you know, her life situation. (*How does she lose everything from being depressed?*) She just becomes so hysterical that she doesn't care anymore—she doesn't care about anybody or anything—she just pushes them away. (*What led up to depression?*) The pressures of home, and uh, her job, and just— the—pressures of those things. (*Dies from not eating and the elements?*) Yeah— she just wanders in the streets.

CARD 4 Uh, a man and wife go on vacation and uh, the, the, and they go into a hotel and the guy at the desk is—extremely rude to the guy's wife. And he's really angry and wants to hit 'im, and his wife is scared and is holdin' him back and tryin' to calm him down. And what happens is, uh, they—they—the guy at the desk and the woman's husband—they just argue and no violence breaks out and they just go on and have their vacation and nobody says anything about it and it's forgotten. (*How does guy keep from hitting him?*) His wife talks him out of it. (*How was guy rude?*) He was verbally abusive—rude and snide—and used foul language. (*Any reason?*) Just had a bad day.

CARD 5 Ok. This, this lady is sitting on the—sitting in the first floor of a house, and, uh, all of a sudden she hears a large bang or a loud noise in a bedroom. So, uh, she runs up-upstairs and, uh, opens the door, and she looks really ah—she looks very shocked and petrified. What she sees is that, um, her husband had, uh, had a heart attack and had fallen to the ground. (*Hold on*) While he was painting the ceiling of the room. And, uh,

THEMATIC APPERCEPTION TEST

she, uh—whatchamacallit—she, uh, it turns out that her husband died. And she's—she survives—but it turns out that her life is depressing and her—her children aren't around anymore, and she's just really alone. That's—that's it.

CARD 6BM   A, a mother and son are really, really close, especially since her husband died. His father. And he lives right near her now that he's grown up, and takes care of her. And one day he finds out that because of his job he has to move away. He decides—and when he tells her here, he's really saddened, and she's shocked and depressed and confused, and doesn't know what she's gonna do. He finally moves away and she seems to adjust, but he doesn't like being away from his home and he really misses his mother. So eventually he moves back to—home—quits his job, and moves back home. And even tho' he can't make as much money and things like that, he's a lot happier being home. (*What does he miss?*) Family and friends.

CARD 7BM   OK, uh, a kid around 20 years old gets, uh, an offer for a good-paying job, and at the same time he gets a scholarship to college. Now he doesn't know exactly what to do. In the picture here he's talking it over with his father. He's confused and scared, because this decision will affect him for the rest of his life, so (*hold on*) so he decides, uh, to—his—him and his father—with the help of his father he decides to go to school. At first the decision didn't seem to be a good one, because he had to give up a job, but it turned out eventually to be a good decision in the long run. He turned out to be a successful businessman. (*Father thinking and feeling?*) He's feeling sympathetic towards the son, that he has to make a difficult decision. (*Why decide school?*) He feels it would be—him and his father think it would be better for him in the long run—he'll have better opportunity.

CARD 10   Uh, a couple in their early 60s have just found out that their—their youngest son had died. He was, uh—he was, um, in—at war and he got shot and killed. And they're very sad and depressed and they, they try to comfort each other. But they decide to stay and uh, stay alive and try to get over that because they have two other children and they have grand-children. But in—in time, they really don't—miss this—miss the son that much. And they—they live with their oldest child and their grandchildren, they live very happily, considering what happened to their youngest son. That's about what happened. (*They think of not staying alive at first?*) No.

CARD 12M   A young orphan contracts, uh, a deadly childhood disease. he—he suffers for a while and eventually dies. The priest who ran the orphanage that he was staying at administers the Last Rites. The child contracted what he had because he didn't have the right food or medicine. And the priest was more upset and more despondent about that, because the death was needless. So—after the child dies, the father works and works and works to try to improve the conditions for the children. But no matter—even though he works hard, no matter how hard he works, children still die and he feels very angry and upset that children die. But no matter how hard he tries, he can't help everybody. (*When did child get sick?*) At the orphanage. (*Why can't priest improve things?*) Because prices go up and he has to take care of more children and more children each day and support for him goes down.

CARD 13MF Uh, uh, a guy's, um, wife, she's, uh, do I have to start at the beginning? (*How do you mean?*) Do I start at the beginning, or should I think it all through first like I did last time. (*Do it the way that's most comfortable for you.*) A young couple get married and uh, soon after they get married, uh, the—the wife becomes very ill. And—uh—uh, the—the couple goes to a doctor, they go to a doctor, and they find out that the wife's gonna die—she's got terminal cancer. (*Hold on*) So they decide to spend—she has about two or three months to live—so they decide to spend all their time together. And what happens—this is when she dies. She's dead, she don't know what's going on. But he's really upset and bereaved and confused. And, uh, so he—he eventually leaves where they're living and moves away and gets a new job. He never remarries or anything, but he does okay, I guess. (*She died at home?*) Yeah.

CARD 14 A young—a guy about 24 is, uh, is, is married and uh, he's—he's cut 'em—he cut himself off from everybody—his family, his brothers and sisters, his cousins and everything. (*Hold on*) And what happens is, is his wife leaves him. She—she goes—she went crazy and she—she killed herself. And, uh, this—this guy is just sitting on a windowsill wondering what to do with his life now. He wouldn't—he doesn't kill himself or anything, but what he decides to do (*hold on*) is to go back and try to be close to his family again. He tries and tries, but he keeps thinking about his wife. And even though the family gets close again, he's never as close as it was before he met his wife. (*Why cut self off?*) Cause all he cared about was his wife. And—and nothin' else. (*Why she leave him?*) Cause she went crazy—she didn't know what she was doin'. (*How he feeling?*) Depressed.

CARD 15 An old man is—is—is all alone and his friends have all died,

THEMATIC APPERCEPTION TEST

so what he decides is to go to the cemetary and visit 'em. And—and he goes early in the morning to visit 'em, and, uh, he stays there all day—uh, looking and going through the tombstones of each of his friends. He—he stays there until about midnight—and, he puts his hands together and starts crying because he's so alone. And what happens is, uh (*hold on*) so what happens is, at about 12 midnight he decides to leave, and he feels so alone that he doesn't think life is worth living. So he killed himself, and nobody knew about it, or cared, or missed him.

EXHIBIT 5

SENTENCE COMPLETION TEST

4. *He felt to blame when* "his father died."
8. *As a child my greatest fear was* "my parents would die."
9. *My father always* "was nice to me."
10. *The ideal man* "is my dad."
13. *My first reason to him was* "fear."
16. *Most fathers* "are caring."
35. *When he thought of hismother, he* "wished he could be near her."
41. *If I can't get what I want, I* "pretend I do not care."
42. *When I am criticized, I* "pretend not to care."
46. *When they didn't invite me, I* "pretended not to care."
47. *He felt very tense when* "he has to compete."
70. *When my father came home, I* "always got something."
74. *I feel happiest when* "I daydream."
87. *I am afraid of* "everything."
94. *When he was with his mother, he felt* "protected."

DISCUSSION

Obsessive compulsive disorder is equally prevalent in males and females. Our male case, Mr. J, reported compulsive symptomatology which arose in a two-year context of anxiety and panic following the death of his father. By the time of hospitalization, the core conflictual theme was an intense fear of contamination, leading to multiple restrictive rituals and behaviors. This notion, in fact, may have had something to do with the referral for psychological testing. The central questions in this referral concerned the extent to which his reality testing was intact, a referral question which is quite common with obsessive compulsive individuals who require hospitalization. The issue of his ability to test reality is also related to the referring therapist's question about the ability of the patient to profit from psychotherapy.

The test results seemed quite congruent with the clinical picture and were quite helpful in addressing the referral questions and furthering the treatment plan. He was extremely ruminative and overideational, with a lack of emotional reactivity. His projective test findings revealed the depth of his preoccupation with loneliness and catastrophic death. On the other hand, there was some evidence that he could reach out to parental figures for help and guidance. In addition, while reality testing was at times borderline, he was able to produce a number of popular responses and the plan of a supportive but gradually more exploratory therapy seemed feasible.

The case of Ms. H, a 23-year-old woman with rituals of cleanliness and fear of contamination, provides some similarities and contrasts. Like Mr. J, her obsessive compulsive behavior seems related to a significant life event. While Mr. J's preoccupations with death are related to the sudden death of his father, Ms. H, a devout Catholic, first developed her symptoms after terminating a pregnancy by abortion, a fact which she hid from her family and a behavior which conflicted with her deeply held religious beliefs. Prior to the onset of Axis I obsessive compulsive symptoms, she possessed many traits of the obsessive compulsive personality disorder, traits that seemed less prominent in Mr. J.

The testing referral came after some progress in treatment involving symptomatic relief with antidepressant medication, but future therapeutic efforts hinged on the depth of depression and whether or not the patient could respond to an expressive or a supportive psychotherapy. Her full-scale IQ of 83 and her cognitive style emphasizing rote memory and the understanding and adherence to social norms suggested that a more supportive approach to treatment might be more congruent with her cognitive and personality styles. Her Rorschach responses revealed a profound sense of despair and emotional impoverishment and suggested that expressive psychotherapy would be too ambitious an undertaking.

The psychological test material also suggests that her depression is of an anaclitic type, with a profound sense of inner impoverishment and a hunger for contacts with others. She appears to have mixed personality disorder traits, including dependent, obsessive compulsive, and passive aggressive characteristics. She seems chronically dysthymic, with little energy, and chronically at the borders of despair. Her self-concept of a small child seen in her figure drawings might suggest that she would approach a therapist as a distant authority figure and proceed to engage in passive/aggressive maneuvers.

It is interesting to note how the Axis I obsessive compulsive behaviors resolved in these two individuals. Mr. J, through treatment, experienced relief in the exploration of his father's death and what it meant to him. His obsessive compulsive symptoms disappeared and he returned to his prior level of functioning. He was discharged to a day hospital and halfway house because he had been unable to function independently since his adolescence. In some contrast, Ms. H found little symptom relief in her exploration of her dynamics in therapy and returned to an anxious and dependent mode of operation. She seemed the more likely of the two to reexperience Axis I obsessive compulsive features in the future.

B. POST-TRAUMATIC STRESS DISORDERS CHRONIC AND DELAYED

This is an Axis I disorder in which symptoms follow a seriously stressful event which is typically beyond the realm of usual human stressors. The traumatic stressors under consideration are typically those of military combat or civilian experiences such as earthquakes, floods, rape, assault, airplane crashes, large fires, etc. The symptoms that follow the traumatic event include disorder-specific symptoms such as recurrent and intrusive images of the traumatic event, an experience or feeling that the event is reoccurring and/or intense distress at exposure to stimuli that symbolize or resemble the traumatic event, and efforts to avoid thoughts or feelings associated with this trauma. They also include nondisorder-specific symptoms such as difficulty falling asleep, irritability, difficulty concentrating, and hypervigilance.

Since military combat and its deleterious effects are the most obvious and occur to so many individuals, especially after an occasion such as the Vietnam conflict, the diagnosis is probably mostly utilized in these situations and underutilized in the civilian population. It is also among combat veterans that the disorder has been most often investigated. Psychological testing of combat veterans with and without PTSD has revealed that the former are more seriously disturbed, with higher scores on symptom scales measuring depression, fatigue, confusion, anger, and anxiety (Fairbank, Keane & Malloy, 1983; Hyer, O'Leary, Saucer, Blount, Harrison & Boudewyns, 1986). We have chosen two quite different cases of PTSD, one involving a male combat veteran and the other a female who was a victim of domestic combat involving sexual and physical abuse.

POST-TRAUMATIC STRESS DISORDER, CHRONIC

Ms. B is a 39-year-old teacher who has been unable to work for the last few months because of back problems. She has been supporting herself on social security disability. In the last few weeks, she has become increasingly depressed and preoccupied with events of her early childhood. She was admitted to a psychiatric evaluation unit on the advice of her physician for a period of observation and evaluation.

This was her first psychiatric hospitalization, although she was seen as an outpatient on several occasions since age 19. She had been bulimic in the past, but had recovered in treatment several years ago. However, she had continual difficulty functioning on her job and in her social life because of her problems in early life which constantly preoccupied her. At age seven, she had been blamed by her family for an injury sustained by her younger brother. Since that time, she remembered being repeatedly beaten by her mother and made to stay in the dark in an upstairs linen closet for hours at a time by her older brothers, who repeatedly abused her sexually from the age of 10 until her late adolescence.

Over the years, she had not been able to keep herself from thinking about these events. When confronted with external cues such as television shows or other women with similar histories she encountered during her work, she would vividly recall these events and suffer nightmares. These nightmares would continue for many nights and she would then be afraid to sleep and become severely depressed. At these times especially, she became wrapped up in her guilty feelings and once again she would attempt to unravel the circumstances of her younger brother's injury and her own motivations at the time of his injury.

Although she could vividly recall the immediate circumstances of her brother's injury, she could never see beyond the brief moment of his having been injured. She did not know if her guilt was brought on by having survived the accident unscathed or because in some way, as her family believed, she had been responsible for its occurrence. She wondered if she were in some way responsible for her brothers' sexual abuse of her as well. In any event, she no longer trusted her memory and complained of having trouble concentrating.

At the time of the admission, Ms. B was dressed casually and presented as a thin, middle-aged woman whose physical appearance was consistent with her chronological age. She cried intermittently throughout the evaluation, especially when recounting the events of her early life. She was clearly preoccupied with these events and the guilty feelings she had about them. At times, she became so physically tense that she would shake. She described her mood as "sad" and her affect was depressed and somewhat constricted. On gross clinical examination, no abnormalities of consciousness or higher intellectual functioning were found.

DSM-III-R Diagnosis

Axis I: Post-traumatic stress disorder, chronic. Major depression, recurrent, without psychotic features
Axis II: None
Axis III: Idiopathic lumbar pain
Axis IV: Severe—serious illness leading to disability
Axis V: Fair—moderate impairment in social relations and mild impairment in occupational functioning

Treatment and Hospital Course

Ms. B was treated with an antidepressant which began to alleviate her depressive symptoms. However, she still continued to be preoccupied with the events of her early life. Her psychiatrist attempted to address these in an exploratory psychotherapy; however, she experienced no relief from this brief course of treatment.

Psychological Assessment

Ms. B was referred for psychological testing two weeks after her admission. Her psychiatrist was chiefly interested in an assessment of her personality functioning to help place her present difficulties in a broader context and to rule out the possibility of a psychotic disorder. She was evaluated over three testing sessions and her examination included the WAIS-R, Rorschach, TAT, MMPI, SCT, Bender Gestalt, and DAP.

Her full-scale and verbal IQs were 119 and 114, respectively, placing her in the high average range of intellectual functioning. Her performance IQ was somewhat lower (105) and in the average range. There was relatively little intertest scatter in her subtest performance. Her relative strengths were in the areas of abstract reasoning, general range of information, and knowledge of words; in all of these her intellectual functioning was superior. Her relative weakness was in the area of psychomotor speed where her performance was most likely compromised by her depressive disturbance.

The remainder of her performance gave some evidence of mild impairments in concentration and attention (*Arithmetic* and *Digit Span*) and reflected the degree to which anxiety was able to encroach on her otherwise quite adequate performance as, for example, on the Bender Gestalt. These test results also lent some psychometric credence to her complaint of difficulties in concentration. Among the performance subtests, her relatively high score on the *Picture Completion* subscale indicated a tendency for hyperalertness and vigilance.

Her MMPI profile also contained evidence of her vigilance combined with her mistrust of others (*scale 6*) occurring in the context of significant depressive disturbance (*scale 2* > 80), including multiple somatic concerns. She also reported a history of episodes of depersonalization and derealization, but denied any other psychotic symptomatology. There was no evidence from the Rorschach of more serious difficulties in reality appraisal. However, of the 25 responses given to the Rorschach, the occurrence of five hard anatomy responses (e.g. "pelvic bone") and the use of black/white contrast or shading as determinants for eight of the responses were consistent with a depressive disorder and her preoccupation with unexplained back pain.

The interplay of these various factors revealed significant information about her personal style of dealing with emotionally evocative material. For example, on *card VIII* of the Rorschach, the first fully chromatic card in the series of 10 cards, she initiated her first response quickly. She described the whole card as looking like "the insides of the shell of a dead horseshoe crab, the skeletal structure with a lot of gaps. This would be the bony part." Her second response continued with the same sense of hard and durable substances which are preserved from insult. She reported the whole card as giving the impression of the "inside of a skull with the sinuses. An X-ray of the inside of the skull and sinuses. Bone structure and sockets for eye orbits and spaces for the sinuses." In describing the outer, protective surfaces she saw, she is careful to note that they appear in contrast to the "gaps" and "spaces."

Comfortable now with the colorful aspects of the card, she reported her last response. Again, using the whole card, she saw "water with rocks or grass and a lion . . . lurching from one side to the other [and] his reflection in the water." Now the durable substances (rocks and grass) are stepping stones for a powerful animal (lion) who is none too surefooted in his traverse. The sequence, content, and determinants of her responses readily evidenced the inner emotional tumult and vulnerability she experiences. This gives rise to her need to maintain a protective outer shell against further hurt, which she experiences as a highly precarious and effortful endeavor.

In the interpersonal arena, the same tension appeared in the context of "frustration" and "confusion," as well as in conflict over goals and outcomes. On *card 1* of the TAT, the young boy "stays frustrated and confused" because "he's torn between trying to please his parents and playing with his friends." Her story to *card 6GF* involved a young woman who is "surprised" and "startled" at "a dirty old man propositioning her" and in the end, "she just moves away from him and keeps it to herself." Although avoidance appeared to be her primary response to conflicting feelings, in one instance she was able to propose a more hopeful solution. *Card 4* depicts a man in silhouette against an open window with an arm and a leg raised above the lower sill. Ms. B described the card as "this guy is in a dark room and there's a window that's the only source of light. I don't know if he wants to be there. Maybe he's lonely and he's isolated himself. He looks like he's reaching out of the window trying to join in with the rest of life and people, but he's afraid to." She went on to describe him as "curious" and felt "he wants to give up the way he feels . . . he looks eager." When asked to complete the story, she concludes that "I guess he goes out and gets over his feelings."

Her hope that feelings could be confronted and worked through was a positive finding in her protocol. She reported a restricted social life (scale 0 from the MMPI > 75) but, while avoidant, was not disinterested in people; nor was she without some understanding of positively supportive and altruistic motives in others. For her, these motives were best captured in those with scientific or academic interests. Her first figure drawing was of a man wearing the traditional white coat of a scientist. He was drawn with glasses and was described as someone who "dislikes suffering" and who wished that "he could make everybody healthy and make the world a happier place." Her second drawing was of a woman, her sister-in-law. She again expressed a positive sense of the figure, noting that she "dislikes my mother" and wishes that "I would be happy; that people wouldn't get sick; that my brother would be more open with her." Although presumably smiling and wishing to be helpful, the figure was nevertheless drawn with her hands behind her back and appears more frightening than warm. The eyes of the figure are wide open and slightly malevolent; her smile paradoxically reveals a mouth filled with sharp, pointed teeth.

Treatment Planning and Outcome

The examining psychologist reported that the test findings gave abundant evidence of a major depressive disorder and that there was no evidence of significant difficulties in reality appraisal that would suggest a psychotic disorder. Additionally, the psychologist felt that her reported intrusive recollections of and recurrent dreams about past traumatic events, the test findings supporting her estrangement from others, difficulty concentrating, mild hyperalertness and vigilance, and somewhat constricted affect were all supportive of a diagnosis of a chronic post-traumatic stress disorder.

Ms. B's psychiatrist recommended that she continue her inpatient treatment at a hospital specializing in the treatment of post-traumatic stress disorders. She accepted the recommendation and made arrangements for an admission in two weeks when they had an opening available. She was subsequently admitted and treated with narcotherapy and psychotherapy, with some minimal symptom relief. Following this course of inpatient treatment, she was able to return to work and continued in an outpatient psychotherapy.

EXHIBIT 1

Area of Assessment	Clinical Examination	Psychological Examination
I. Symptoms/Diagnosis		
Post-traumatic stress disorder, chronic		
A. Recognizable stressor	Chronic, severe physical and sexual abuse	Perseverative thinking emphasizing her own vulnerability
B. Evidence of re-experience of trauma		
—recurrent and intrusive recollections	Repeatedly plagued by recollections for many years	Offers reports of child-hood trauma and recurring dreams without solicitation
—recurrent dreams	Recurrent dreams	
C. Numbing or reduced involvement		
—markedly dimin-ished interest	Socially withdrawn	Social withdrawal
—feeling of detach-ment or estrangement	None	Reports transient feelings of depersonalization and derealization
—constricted affect	Affect depressed and constricted	Depressed and con-stricted affect
D. Two symptoms		
—hyperalert	None	Hyperalert and vigilant
—sleep disturbance	Chronic difficulty	None
—survivor guilt	Related to brother's accident	None
—trouble concentrating	None	Mildly impaired concentration
—exposure intensi-fies symptoms	Television shows and clin-ical histories of others exacerbate intrusive recollections	

Area of Assessment	Clinical Examination	Psychological Examination
II. Personality Factors	Possible psychosis influencing personality fuctioning	Intact reality appraisal; no evidence of psychotic symptomatology
	Possible histrionic personality disorder	No significant hysterical features but may overreact to minor events symbolizing earlier traumatic events
III. Cognitive Abilities	None	Average to superior intellectual abilities with present functioning compromised by depression and anxiety
IV. Psychodynamics	Performance anxiety and strong wish to please lead to avoidance and impairment of personal relationships	Strong wish to please but mistrustful of others; unresolved passive-dependent feelings
V. Therapeutic Enabling Factors	Successfully resolved past history of bulimia	Reports past success in resolving bulimia
		Eager for greater involvement with others and hopeful about successful resolution of present difficulties
		Adequate range of internal coping abilities but these are presently underutilized
VI. Environmental Demand and Social Adjustment	Limited history of intimate personal relationships	Self-protectively avoids close personal relationships for fear of hurt

EXHIBIT 2

WAIS-R SUMMARY

Verbal Subtests	*Scaled Score*
Information	14
Digit Span	12
Vocabulary	14
Arithmetic	11
Comprehension	13
Similarities	15

Performance Subtests	
Picture Completion	12
Picture Arrangement	11
Block Design	11
Object Assembly	11
Digit Symbol	9

Verbal IQ	119
Performance IQ	105
Full Scale IQ	114

MMPI SUMMARY

F'L/K: 82"06'3491-7/5#

RORSCHACH SUMMARY

Number of Responses	25
Rejections	0
Populars	9
Originals	0
Average R/T Chromatic	9"
Average R/T Achromatic	11"
F%	56
F + %	92
A%	48
H%	20
At%	16
W:M	10:3

Rorschach Summary

M:Sum C		3:0
m:c		3:3
VIII-X%		32
FK + F + Fc%		68
(H + A):(Hd + Ad)		13:4
Apperception	W	40%
	D	48%
	d	8%
	Dd + S	4%

EXHIBIT 3

RORSCHACH SUMMARY

Response	*Inquiry*	*Scoring*
I. 18″		
1. Looks like a pelvic bone.	1. The shape of it and the spaces in between. Possibly an X-ray of bones—black and white . . . dark greyish color.	W(s)Fk.FC′At
2. Looks like a bat with the wings.	2. Wings here. Body here. Basically looks like a bat. Eyes here and little hands here.	WFAP
3. This part looks like a crab with little pincers or claws.	3. The shape—the bulgy eyes and the little claws.	DFA
II. 2″		
1. Looks like wings of a butterfly with the long tail and the antenna on top.	1. Wings here. Long tail here. Antenna here. The shape. Swallow tail.	DFAP
2. Looks like two dogs with their noses touching. Looks like ears.	2. Ear . . . snout . . . profile.	DFMAP
3. Pelvic bone, hollow middle.	3. The shape of it and the holes.	W(s)FAt
III. 10″		
1. Looks like a butterfly.	1. The wing shape and the little body in the middle. The shape.	DFAP
2. Looks like the head of a fly with those huge bulging eyes.	2. Like a National Geographic. A close-up photo of enormous compound eyes.	DFAt
3. There could be two women carrying jugs or two dancers and they're dancing around this thing in the middle.	3. Head, neck, back. Looks like a woman because of the bust.	WMHP

RORSCHACH SUMMARY

Response	Inquiry	Scoring

IV. 26″

1. These look like wings to me, of some kind of manta ray or something.

1. Big flat—almost like a flounder. The shape basically.

WFA

2. Back of the head of a dog. These would be the ears. Look furry.

2. (*Top half*) The ears and the fur. (?) The shading looks like it's furry.

drFcAd

V. 1″

1 Looks like a bat or a butter-fly. Feet, wings, antenna, little head. Great big wing spread.

1. The wings and the rest.

WFAP

VI. 6″

1. Looks like something from marine bioogy.

1. Like in Jacques Cousteau. An odd creature at the bot-tom of the ocean. The odd shape. Head here—flippers or appendages here. Lying.

WFMA

2. This looks like the snout of a lion. This looks like the mark that often comes down the face. This the eyes, and this the nose.

2. Not a live lion—but a pic-ture. The coloration. These would be the eyes (?) The dark, the light and the shape.

dFcAd

VII. 4″

1. Looks like two cupids or angels. Looks like they're facing each other and this is the profile of the face. Could be women with this the ponytail or Indians with this the feather.

1. Not real definite shape—like cherubs. With fluffy nondescript outline, looks like a profile of a face—neck, hair, nose, top of head.

DMHP

2. Clouds.

2. (*Bottom half*) Looks like light and dark. (?) The shading. And no sharp outlines.

D(S)KF
Clouds

RORSCHACH SUMMARY

Response	*Inquiry*	*Scoring*
3. Looks like a picture of a lampshade. This the middle of the lamp and this the base.	3. The shape.	SF Obj.

VIII. 2″

1. Looks like the shell of a horseshoe crab . . . cavities.	1. Looks like inside of the shell of a dead horseshoe crab. Skeletal structure with a lot of gaps. This would be the bony part.	D(S)FAt
2. Inside of skull with the sinuses.	2. X-ray of inside of skull and sinuses. Bone structure and sockets for eye orbits and spaces and sinuses.	WFlk-At
3. Water with rocks or grass and a lion or a 4-footed animal and he's lurching over from one side to the other. And this would be the reflection in the water.	3. This would be the water here. This the shape of a cougar or panther or something. Looks like he's trying to get from here to here.	WFM.FKAP

IX. 20″

1. Looks like a pelvis. Hip bones (*green*) acetabulum here. This is the illiac crest. This would be the bladder (*white*) ovaries and fallopian tubes. Uterus here.	1. Reminds me of the shape of it. Shape of the fundus of the uterus.	WF-At

X. 12″

1. Two crabs. Fiddler crabs with one claw bigger than the other.	1. The shape.	DFAP
2. Part of a face—eyes (*yellow*), nose, and this would be a moustache—the green thing.	2. Here and here and here. The shape.	D(S)FHd

RORSCHACH SUMMARY

Response	Inquiry	Scoring
3. Eyes (*yellow*) and furrows in the forehead (*green*) and chin here (*gray*).	3. The shape. Like a caricature of a face.	D(S)F(Hd)
4. Someone parachuting.	4. Here. The shape. Man and the parachute here.	DMH

E X H I B I T   4

THEMATIC APPERCEPTION TEST

CARD 1   This is a little kid and he's looking at his violin and he's supposed to be practicing. But he doesn't feel like it. He's torn between trying to please his parents and playing with his friends. He's frustrated and doesn't know what to do. Wishing the violin would go away I guess. (?) The end he stays frustrated and confused.

CARD 4   A man and a woman and she's very much in love with him but he seems unable to commit himself to one woman. He doesn't seem capable of a lasting relationship because there's a picture of a woman in the background. He just has casual affairs with a lot of women. She loves him a lot. She's trying to hold onto him and reach him, but she really can't. (?) She cares for him but part of her is hurting. She wants him but she's frustrated. (?) I don't think it'll work out.

CARD 6GF   A man and a lady in a living room in a party or alone. I don't know. He's either suggesting something to her or telling her something that she finds unpleasant or disturbing. She has a surprised look on her face. Maybe he's a dirty old man propositioning her and she's surprised. She doesn't know what to respond to him . . . or to tell someone what he was telling her. She's just kind of startled. (?) She doesn't say anything about what happened. She just moves away from him and keeps it to herself.

CARD 7GF   I can't make it up. A mother and a daughter and the mother seems to be interested in the daughter and the daughter is not interested. She seems distracted and looks like she wishes she were somewhere else. She seems like she feels more grown up than the way she's treated. She'd rather be out doing more adult things than playing like a kid. She doesn't seem very happy.

CARD 12   Two men. I guess one is the father or the grandfather and the one lying down is the son or the grandson. He's sleeping or just lounging around. He doesn't look like it's bed time. He's just sloppy and unkempt. He has kind of a funny look on his face like . . . I don't know. The old man is approaching him and trying to wake him up—but he's afraid of what reaction the guy will have. He seems intimidated by the younger guy—like maybe he's snotty or abusive. I don't think he (*younger*) treats him very well. In the end I think he probably backs off and walks away.

CARD 13MF   A man and a woman and the woman is in bed partly exposed. I don't know if she's dead or alive. I think maybe she's dead or

---

---

something. He feels . . . apparently he's done something to her. He raped and then murdered her and then he feels guilty or ashamed. Like he's done something and not realized what he did. The reality hits him and he doesn't know what to do. I think he runs away out of fear.

CARD 14 This guy is in a dark room and there's a window that's the only source of light. I don't know if he wants to be there. Maybe he's lonely and he's isolated himself. He looks like he's reaching out of the window trying to join in with the rest of life and people—but he's afraid to. Only half of him wants to be out in the sunshine. (?) He's afraid and confused. Kind of curious though. He wants to give up the way he feels. But he's afraid to make that step. He looks eager though. (?) I guess he goes out and gets over his feelings.

E X H I B I T 5

SENTENCE COMPLETION TEST

3. *I want to know if my family* "really loves me or not."
6. *At bedtime sometimes I'm* "afraid to go to sleep because of bad dreams."
7. *Men are* "attractive to me but I'm afraid of them sometimes."
12. *I feel* "mixed up a lot of times."
23. *My mind is* "pretty good, but sometimes it gets mixed up."
28. *Sometimes I wish* "I could disappear."

POST-TRAUMATIC STRESS DISORDER, DELAYED WITH ALCOHOL ABUSE, EPISODIC

Mr. W was a 34-year-old veteran who was married, had five children, and had worked for the last 14 years for the city parks department as a grounds keeper. After graduating from high school, he was stationed in Vietnam in the mid-1960s and served as a rifleman in an infantry platoon near the demilitarized zone. Shortly after he returned from Vietnam, his uncle had helped him to get his job with the parks department, where he was known as a steady and reliable worker.

Over the last few years, he became interested in the history of the war in Vietnam. He began to withdraw from his family and spent more and more of his time in the bedroom thinking and reading about Vietnam. As he became immersed in his studies of the war, he became increasingly angry at the situation of many of the Vietnam war veterans and also began to recall more vividly some of his own war experiences which he had not remembered in years. He remembered and relived his disgust at the dead and mutilated bodies of American soldiers he had seen. He also began to realize that he and his outfit must have killed many civilians and perhaps American servicemen in battles in the "free fire" zones where his platoon typically patrolled.

His recollections alternately moved him to anger and sadness and he began to drink more heavily to ease these feelings. As his drinking became heavier, he began to reenact his war experiences. A few months before his admission, he had set a fire in the woods late one night, claiming that he was "burning out the Vietcong." His wife began to find him crawling through the yard at night with his gun as if he were back in actual combat. A few weeks before his admission, his reliving of his war experiences began to encroach on him even when he was not intoxicated. While out hunting with his friends, he had felt that another hunter was firing at him and had started to fire back but was stopped by a companion.

He became increasingly frightened that he would do something to hurt his family and was particularly concerned about hurting his wife. During one of his reliving experiences, he had pointed a gun at her and spoken to her in a sexually degrading manner. Recently, he had taken to calling her "mama san" during sex and had begun to remember his physical abuse of Vietnamese prostitutes. He finally agreed to enter the hospital after he had gotten drunk at his uncle's house and injured him in a fight. He had fled in panic and wrecked his car, finally running out into a nearby field to escape the pursuing Vietcong.

At the time of admission, Mr. W was tense and anxious. He spoke movingly about his fear that he would "maybe do something to hurt my wife and kids" and realized that his behavior had changed over the last few years as he had begun to study the war. He would give only vague accounts of his war experiences, however, claiming that he did not remember the specific details, only how he had felt during that time. He described his mood as "concerned"; his affect was anxious. There was no evidence of hallucinations, delusions or other alterations in his sense of reality that could be elicited, with the exception of those related to his reliving of his traumatic war experiences. His concentration, attention, memory, abstracting ability, and general fund of information were judged to be adequate. He acknowledged that there were impairments in his judgment around his reliving experiences, but otherwise his judgment seemed intact.

DSM-III-R Diagnosis

Axis I: Post-traumatic stress disorder, delayed. Alcohol abuse, episodic
Axis II: None
Axis IV: Severe—multiple exposures to dead and mutilated servicemen during his military service
Axis V: Fair—moderate impairment in his social and marital relationships

Treatment and Hospital Course

Mr. W made a good initial adjustment to the hospital unit. He presented no difficulties in his management and readily complied with the psychiatrist's recommendation that he begin Alcoholics Anonymous meetings for education about and treatment of his difficulties with alcohol. In his individual psychotherapy, he was able to recount his combat experiences with a good deal of affect. He was alternately, and always appropriately, angry and tearful, but continued to claim that he remembered few details of these experiences. Unless specifically asked about his war experiences, he avoided talking about them altogether. He acknowledged that talking about them caused him a great deal of emotional upset which he preferred to avoid.

Although his treatment was progressing satisfactorily in some respects, he continued to be reluctant to fully address the relationship between his war experiences and his reliving experiences which had led him to seek hospitalization. Because of the emotional turmoil induced by his discussing these experiences and his obvious need to avoid discussing them in any detail, his psychiatrist asked for a full psychological evaluation to help determine if Mr. W could tolerate the affective arousal likely to be induced by a more exploratory stance on the part of the psychiatrist.

Psychological Assessment

Mr. W was referred for psychological testing in order to help determine his capacity to utilize a more exploratory psychotherapy. Consequently, his reality testing abilities, style of affective management, and capacity for establishing a working alliance in treatment were all in need of assessment. He received a battery of tests, including the WAIS-R, Rorschach, and DAP.

Mr. W's WAIS-R examination yielded scores which placed his full-scale, verbal and performance IQs in the Average range. His scores were 99, 98 and 100, respectively. The apparent evenness of intellectual ability implied by his IQs was belied by a closer examination of his subscale scores. These ranged from the Borderline to Very Superior levels. His most conspicuous weaknesses (Borderline level) were on the *Comprehension, Object Assembly* and *Digit Span* subscales; his relative strengths were found on the *Arithmetic* and *Picture Arrangement* subscales, the latter a test of anticipatory planning (*Very Superior* and *Superior levels, respectively*). This pattern of strengths and weaknesses suggested that while he had inherently adequate powers of concentration and showed better than average abilities to plan and anticipate, his performance was susceptible to disruption by anxiety and he was prone to lapses in practical judgment.

On the WAIS-R, there was no evidence of serious defects in reality appreciation. His Rorschach protocol further substantiated this finding (F + % = 87). He was generally able to maintain adequate reality testing, but did produce a significant number of unusual responses reflecting his preoccupation with his combat experiences even within a somewhat constricted record (19 responses). For example, on the first card, his last response was "something a gook would put on its head, a helmet" which was offered with the card in its inverted position. During inquiry, the helmet is described as having horns, "like a Viking helmet." Additional responses related to his military preoccupations, included a "flack vest" to *card IV* (again in the inverted position), "a good place to have an ambush" to *card VI*, and references to a 50-caliber machine gun and "tops of trees" seen from the vantage point of a helicopter (*card X*).

Mr. W's style of affective reactivity was vividly portrayed in his Rorschach protocol. He made relatively frequent use of shading (reflecting anxiety) and of color (6 of 19 responses); in four of these instances, either the shading or the color was the dominant determinant. His color responses were almost invariably incendiary and dramatic and included "fire" (*card II*), "an explosion" (*card IX*), "a volcano" (*card IX*), and "blood" (*card X*). On balance, his Rorschach protocol gave evidence of difficulties in the modulation and adaptive expression of affect. He generally experienced affect as disruptive and potentially explosive and was frightened that he had inadequate means of containing and integrating his emotional life. However, his generally adequate reality testing and availability of adaptive cognitive controls held out the promise of helping him to effectively integrate and regulate his emotional turbulence.

Mr. W gave several human percepts (two—*cards III* and *VII*) and these made up almost one-half of his popular percepts. He also produced fairly adequate human figure drawings. The latter were presented in a somewhat stiff and rigid fashion, with frozen smiles and disproportionately short arms, casual clothing, and a steady, straightforward gaze, but still acceptable in terms of concept. These features lent support to the notion that he could be engaged in meeting the challenges of a more exploratory psychotherapeutic approach in a straightforward fashion without undue distortion or regression. On a negative note, he exhibited a paranoid component to his thinking and the use of projection as a possible defense (e.g. the "evil face" on Rorschach *card I*). Furthermore, he was currently uncertain over and preoccupied with his sexual identification. This was mirrored in his response to Rorschach *card III* of figures with both male and female sexual characteristics and his drawing of a woman who appeared to be wearing both a skirt and pants.

Treatment Planning and Outcome

Based on the results of his psychological evaluation, Mr. W's psychiatrist was encouraged to proceed with his plans to assist him in integrating the emotional impact and intrusive nature of his war experiences and to encourage him to explore his feelings in more depth than he had heretofore allowed. In anticipation of this work, Mr. W was reassured that he had the resources to engage in this exploration. After hearing what he could be expected to experience during this phase of his treatment, he agreed to proceed. He worked with the psychiatrist to develop a plan that would allow him sufficient opportunity to express and explore his feelings at a slow but steady pace. Over the next few weeks, he was gradually able to discuss his combat experiences in more detail and to analyze his reactions to them despite the anger and anxiety they frequently aroused in him. He was able to see how virtually all of his reliving experiences had been elaborations of those aspects of his combat experiences about which he was most troubled. Over the course of his treatment, he stopped having reliving experiences and he began to incorporate his Vietnam experiences into his life in a way that left him feeling he now had some control over them.

EXHIBIT 1

AREA OF ASSESSMENT	CLINICAL EXAMINATION	PSYCHOLOGICAL EXAMINATION
I. Symptoms/Diagnosis		
Post-traumatic stress disorder, delayed		
Recognizable stressor	Vietnam war combat experiences	None
Evidence of reexperience of trauma		
—sudden acting as if the traumatic event were reoccurring	Sets fire in woods "to burn out Vietcong" Shoots at hunters and other imagined enemies Stalks enemies in his own house	Is preoccupied with his combat experiences
Numbing or reduced involvement		
—markedly diminished interest	Spends most of his time alone reading about the war	None
—constricted affect	Avoids feelings related to his war experiences	Attempts to minimize affective expression without much success
Two symptoms		
—sleep disturbance	Difficulty sleeping	None
—exposure intensifies symptoms	Symptoms activated by his study of the war	None
II. Personality Factors	Avoidance of strong feelings	Strong feelings give rise to fears of loss of self-control Some paranoid elements to his thinking

AREA OF ASSESSMENT	CLINICAL EXAMINATION	PSYCHOLOGICAL EXAMINATION
		Adequate cognitive controls given time for anticipation and planning
III. Cognitive Abilities	Average intelligence	Average intelligence but current performance impaired by anxiety
IV. Psychodynamics	Attempts to repress and deny feelings associated with his combat experiences result in his "reliving" these experiences	Susceptible to explosive emotional reactions when confronted with aggressive or catastrophic feelings
		Uses projection as a defense
		Preoccupied with his masculinity
V. Therapeutic Enabling Factors	Good premorbid adjustment and initial post-combat adjustment	Internal resources are presently underutilized
	Accepts the need for treatment	None
VI. Environmental Demand and Social Adjustment	Good work history	None
	Has maintained a social network and is concerned about his family	Some capacity to identify with others

EXHIBIT 2

WAIS-R Summary

Verbal Subtests	*Scaled Score*
Information	11
Digit Span	7
Vocabulary	9
Arithmetic	15
Comprehension	6
Similarities	10

Performance Subtests	
Picture Completion	10
Picture Arrangement	13
Block Design	10
Object Assembly	6
Digit Symbol	8

Verbal IQ	98
Performance IQ	100
Full Scale IQ	99

Rorschach Summary

Number of Responses	19
Rejections	0
Populars	5
Originals	0
Average R/T Chromatic	12″
Average R/T Achromatic	9″
F%	47
F + %	87
A%	13
H%	32
Explosion%	11
W:M	11:3
M:Sum C	3:4
m:c	3:2
VIII-X%	37

RORSCHACH SUMMARY

FK + F + Fc		68
(H + A):(Hd + Ad)		5:2
Apperception	W%	58
	D%	43
	d%	0
	Dd + S%	0

EXHIBIT 3

RORSCHACH SUMMARY

Response	*Inquiry*	*Scoring*
I. 3″		
1. Looks like a jet at first	1. Got wings on its front here. Big wings like an F104. Body of plane is here. Wings here—fins for the back. Looks like a jet looking down. Back guns here.	WF-Obj
2. Looks like an evil face if you look in the middle of it.	2. Big eyes, mouth, eyes like a jack-'o-lantern, mouth across here. (*Evil?*) Looks like a Brothers Heidelberg album cover. A mythical picture of a creature. I've associated it with their paintings.	W(S)FHd
3. Could look like a bat.	3. Mouth here. Little yicky teeth on its wings. Tail here.	WFAP
4. Could be something a gook would put on its head—a helmet.	4. Head would go here. Peak here. Protection over the ears. Horns look like a Viking helmet. (?) No.	WF Obj
II. 12″		
1. Looks like a space ship or rocket taking off.	1. Rocket inside it. Has the stuff shooting out of the rocket. (?) Dust rolling up around it. (?) It's dark. (?) It's red . . . it's fire.	D(S)Fm.CF Obj
III. 2″		
1. I've seen this already. Two women.	1. Boobs sticking out. They're lifting something together. Carrying some old basket of clothes or something here. High heels on—how does that grab you.	WMHP

Rorschach Summary

Response	Inquiry	Scoring
2. Two men with their cocks sticking out.	2. Cocks sticking out here. Can call them fairies 'cause they have boobs sticking out (?) I don't know. I'd never see it.	WMHP

IV. 10″

Response	Inquiry	Scoring
1. Looks like a creature out of the Trilogy.	1. Big feet here. Tail here. Big, big, big. Here's the top. Here's the dinky head. Looks like he's got hooks for arms. (?) He's ugly. (?) Look at the face (?) Small.	WF(A)P
2. Looks like someone with a flack vest. Looks like the outline of a guy's shoulders.	2. Here. Here's the outline of ammo pockets (*all but Central D*). Zipper here. (?) The shape of it. The dark spots look like where the pockets would be.	WFcH

V. 12″

Response	Inquiry	Scoring
1. Looks like a kite.	1. Looks like a kite in a movie. Wings here. Looks like a kite of a flying dragon (?) On TV or a movie. In Japan they have all them dragon kites. (?) Mouth and tail like a dragon kite.	WF Obj

RORSCHACH SUMMARY

Response	*Inquiry*	*Scoring*

VI. 10″

1. Looks like a good place to have an ambush. Looks like two mountains with a road through the middle of it. Looks like a river.

   1. River is dark where the vegetation might be. As it comes up along a hill, vegetation wouldn't be so dark. The center could be a road. (mountains?) the banks. Came up on both sides (?) The shading. An ambush—wouldn't go nowhere if you got caught in there. Would be a cross fire down there.

   WFK.FcLdsc

2. Here's a delta or something.

   2. Comes down and washes out. Spreads out. Water and dirt all built up here (?) Water is light and dirt is dark.

VII. 20″

1. Looks like two people looking at each other, but I don't know what's on top of their heads. Looks like just half of them up there.

   1. Faces here. Look like twins looking at each other. Body would be here and hands may be back at the sides here. (?) Only half of them.

   DMHP

VIII. 15″

1. Looks like someone's backbone with ribs on it. Here are his shoulders here.

   1. Backbone here, ribs here. I don't know what's coming down over the top of him. Looks like he's got his shoulders shrugged saying what the hell am I doing here?

   DF-At

RORSCHACH SUMMARY

Response	Inquiry	Scoring

IX. 10″

1. Looks like an explosion or something.

    1. Flames shooting up at top. Dust again. Dust again. Looks like a bomb going off. (?) Orange color looks like flames. The dark part (*green*) in the middle is dust. I don't know what the pink is doing here (?) Not part of the explosion.

    DCF.mF Expl

2. Looks like a volcano—like Mt. St. Helens.

    2. Top of the volcano here with dust on top, dirt, fire shooting out of it. (?) The red part. But really isn't red enough to look like fire (*Dust?*) dark.

    WCF.mF Expl

X. 20″

1. This looks like a gun sticking out here.

    1. Looks like a hand with a 50 millimeter gun sticking out (?) A kind of gun.

    DFHd aggr

2. This looks like blood here. Looks like the color of blood here.

    2. The color of it looks like blood. Maybe a drop of water hit it. (?) It's light on top and gets dark toward the bottom.

    DCF.FK Blood

3. Tops of trees or something.

    3. (*Blue*) These here and here look like looking out of a helicopter at trees from on top (?) Shape.

    DFK Ldsc

4. Looks like a wishbone.

    4. Looks like a wishbone or maple seed. It's exactly the shape of it.

    DFAt

DISCUSSION

Like most veterans with PTSD (Hyer et al., 1986), Mr. W had minimal problems before combat and, in fact, initially made a good adjustment upon return. He was hospitalized for preoccupation with and reenactment of combat experiences in the context of alcohol abuse. Psychological testing was requested not to assist in the diagnosis of PTSD, as this evaluation was based upon objective and clear behaviors, but rather to assist in the overall evaluation of Mr. W's relative strengths and his capacity for utilizing exploratory psychotherapy in an attempt to help him integrate the horrifying experiences during combat. The results of psychological testing were quite consistent concerning this question. He had an average IQ and his reality testing seemed adequate in both structured and unstructured testing situations. The ability to hold onto and appreciate conventional reality seemed like a real strength for this man. In contrast, it was his affective lability and his difficulty in modulating and integrating emotion that emerged prominently in his testing. Thus, the testing was quite helpful in recommending an exploratory treatment with the aim of helping an emotionally reactive man integrate his appalling past experiences, a therapy which subsequently succeeded.

In contrast to Mr. W, Ms. B, a 34-year-old, single female, was admitted with depression and a preoccupation with traumatic events that had occurred in her youth. She had been repeatedly beaten by her mother and forced to stay in a dark closet for hours at a time. She was sexually abused by her brothers from age 10 until late adolescence. She experienced the stigmata of traumatic stress disorder involving nightmares and intrusive daytime thoughts about these events.

Psychological assessment was not required to make the diagnosis of posttraumatic stress disorder, but the patient was referred for assessment after treatment was begun to evaluate the possibility of psychotic thinking and to place the stress disorder into the overall context of her strengths and weaknesses. This is a recurrent theme in this book: DSM-III diagnoses, from a symptomatic point of view, are most typically made through clinical interview and history. Initial treatment planning can begin with this. However, as the treatment begins and initial symptomatology is alleviated somewhat, the evaluation of the more enduring strengths and weaknesses of the patient become a necessity for more finely tuned treatment planning.

The test findings were helpful in clarifying the question about the patient's reality testing. While her test results showed mildly impaired concentration and suggestions of some depersonalization and derealization and a cognitive style of hyperalertness and vigilance, there was every indication that there was adequate reality appraisal with no current or anticipated psychotic thinking. There was strong evidence from the testing, therefore, that her symptomatology was indeed consistent with a post-traumatic stress disorder. The patient showed important therapeutic enabling factors such as an average to superior intellectual ability and qualities that suggested the possibility of a positive treatment alliance, including a wish to please others, past success in resolving bulimia, and an eagerness for involvement with others.

CHAPTER 6

Adjustment Disorders

As implied by the name, an adjustment disorder is a maladaptive and symptomatic response to specific and identifiable stressors in an individual's life. There must be some indication that the maladaptive pattern is related temporally to the onset of the stressors. This is concretely defined in DSM-III-R as the onset of symptoms (of up to six-months duration) within three months after the stressor. Typical stressors of serious moment to individuals in our culture include divorce or other marital difficulty, occupational difficulties, health problems, and stress brought on by developmental events such as becoming a parent or retirement. Symptoms which are typical in reaction to such stressors include anxiety, depression, physical complaints, and inappropriate behavior which violates the rights of others.

ADJUSTMENT DISORDER WITH MIXED DISTURBANCE OF EMOTIONS AND CONDUCT

Ms. K, a 16-year-old high school sophomore, was accompanied to the hospital by her mother who had arranged to have her admitted without her knowledge. She had been caught by her mother sneaking in from a date with someone her mother disapproved of and she and her mother had a loud and angry argument. She had packed a suitcase and threatened to run away from home. Ms. K and her mother had been arguing often and her mother had sent Ms. K to a therapist to get help with her "rebellious" attitude. On the advice of Ms. K's therapist, the mother had called the police on the evening of the threat. After the acute crisis had passed, she had again consulted Ms. K's therapist who had recommended a psychiatric admission for evaluation and recommendation of subsequent treatment. Ms. K was not told of the impending admission until the morning of the intake evaluation. Although she had finally agreed to accompany her mother to the hospital, she had done so under protest.

The intake evaluation was conducted in a highly charged emotional atmosphere. Ms. K was by turns loudly angry and tearful. She and her mother argued about almost everything, agreeing only that things between them had become more conflictual in the last few weeks. She found her mother's attempts to enforce rules regarding telephone use, whom she was allowed to have in the home, what she could wear, and how she could decorate her room, among other things, impossible to accommodate. She felt decisions about these things rightfully belonged to her and did not understand her mother's recent insistence on monitoring her activities more closely.

Her mother was by turns demanding and placating. She felt she had a right to insist on these things and claimed that her daughter's recent school probation for failing work, along with what seemed to her to have become a morbid preoccupation with sinister and anarchic elements of Ms. K's teenage subculture, justified her increasing adamancy. Her mother acknowledged that these things had been left to Ms. K's discretion in the past and that in some respects Ms. K's deviance had been a source of pride. Not long ago, her mother had been contacted by a family friend who asked to interview Ms. K and her "punk" friends and had featured them in a local TV news program on teenage lifestyles and values. However, since separating from her husband a few weeks previously, she had become alarmed by these very same elements and now wished to see her daughter adopt a style of dress and manner more consistent with her own middle class values and attitudes. Ms. K's mother held up Ms. K's younger brother as a model worthy of emulation in these matters. Ms. K disparaged her younger brother as "an air-headed preppy" and was disgusted at the very idea of transforming herself into someone so "superficial."

A formal mental status examination revealed a young, white female who was slightly overweight and quite unusually groomed and attired. She sported a "punk" hairstyle with her hair gathered into a short-cropped topknot dyed a bright green on top. She wore a metal-studded, leather jacket and steel-tipped, leather boots, a t-shirt tie-dyed in several colors, and a pair of faded and torn jeans. These clothes were her usual attire. Her affect and mood were alternately angry and tearful, but always appropriate to circumstances. Her general manner was somewhat defiant and challenging, but not unreasonably hostile, and she cooperated with the examination. She agreed that her parents' recent separation had saddened her and was surprised to find herself feeling this way as she had hoped for a separation between her parents for quite some time out of an awareness that her mother and her father shared little with one another.

She admitted to threatening her mother with running away, but saw this as representing no grave danger to herself since she had intended to stay with friends. She denied any suicidal or homicidal ideation. She gave neither a history of nor evidence of any significant cognitive or perceptual abnormalities. She stated that her own reasons for entering the hospital were "to get away from home for evaluation" and agreed that a period of separation would help everyone to "chill out." However, referring to her mother's past history of depression and her mother's sister's suicide attempt, she argumentatively suggested that her mother, rather than she, be offered the services of a psychiatric hospital.

DSM-III-R Diagnosis

Axis I: Adjustment Disorder with Mixed Disturbance of Emotions and Conduct

Axis II: Rule out Borderline personality disorder

Axis III: None

Axis IV: Severe—Divorce of parents; chronic marital conflict prior to divorce

Axis V: Fair—Fails to work up to potential in school; limited circle of friends

Treatment and Hospital Course

Following her admission to the unit, Ms. K quickly calmed down. She made a rapid and satisfactory adjustment to the unit. She was able to admit to being more depressed since her parents' separation. She initially placed most of the blame for her difficulties on her mother, but was soon able to acknowledge that "about one-half" of the difficulties were of her own making. Her initial treatment plan involved individual psychotherapy sessions and additional family sessions between Ms. K and her mother as she became less angry at her mother and expressed an interest in having her therapist help effect a reconciliation.

Her mother supplied a report of a previous psychological testing, done when the patient was nine years old, giving evidence of an earlier depressive episode and emotional turmoil. This examination had taken place shortly after Ms. K's aunt, who was closely involved with her at the time, had been hospitalized for a suicide attempt and accompanying depression. Because of Ms. K's renewed depressive concerns in the context of her parents' recent divorce, her hospital psychotherapist requested that she be given a psychological evaluation to assess the extent of her depression and its relation to her personality functioning.

Psychological Assessment

Ms. K began her psychological evaluation at the end of her second week of hospitalization. She was given the WISC-R, Rorschach, TAT, Sentence Completion Test, and a Bender Gestalt by the examining psychologist. During the testing sessions, she was described as cooperative, although somewhat withdrawn and lethargic. The examining psychologist also commented on her unusual style of dress and personal appearance.

She achieved a verbal IQ of 115 and a performance IQ of 131, yielding a full-scale IQ of 126 on the WISC-R. This placed her in the superior range of intellectual functioning, with subtest scores ranging from the average to very superior levels. Her visual-spatial skills and her ability to attend to detail were instrumental in helping her to achieve her best performances on the *Block Design, Object Assembly* and *Picture Completion* subscales. These abilities were consistent with her acknowledged interest in visual art, an area of talent she had been cultivating for quite some time. She did poorest, but nevertheless gave an average performance, on a visual-motor test of new learning ability. Among her verbal subtests, her scaled scores ranged from 11 to 14, with her best performance given on the *Vocabulary* subscale and her worst performance given on the *Information* subscale. These subscale scores and her Bender performance, which showed good organizational abilities and good recall, supported her better-than-average intellectual abilities.

Given Ms. K's obvious intellectual abilities, perhaps the most striking feature of her Rorschach, SCT, and TAT results is their general poverty. On the Rorschach, she gives little better than one response to each card and the majority of these responses are fairly global and only loosely determined by their form. She seems little interested in exploring the blots unless something happens to catch her attention. The majority of her responses are banal—the cat's face on *card I*, the monster on *card IV*, the bat on *card V*—and show little of her creative talents. This general sense of impoverishment is also in evidence on the TAT. Here, she had great difficulty in deciding on a context for the story, in ascribing motivations or feelings to her characters, or in imagining the outcome of the scenes she describes. People are described as "waiting" (*cards 2, 5 and 12 F*), perhaps for the "bad news" mentioned in her story to *card 3GF*.

When she developed any interaction between the characters, it was sometimes consistent with the typical theme for the particular card, as for example *cards 1* and *10*. To *card 1*, Ms. K told a conventional story of a boy receiving a violin for a gift who was allowed to return it after the person who gives him the gift "sees that he's not happy with it." Her story to *card*

10, which usually prompts a story concerning peer interactions, concerned a reunion between a mother and a son who are glad to see one another again. However, in stories told to *card 12M*, where she was unable to decide between the possibilities of aggression and assistance, and *card 13MF*, where the sexual connotations of the semi-nude female figure were completely ignored, she seemed to be unable to rely on any sense of the conventional in deciphering human actions and motivations. At times, she was not reluctant to use her imagination to supply perceived, missing aspects of her environment (e.g. *card IX* of the Rorschach). She seemed, however, to be largely in the position of the character in her story for *card 14*, simply mildly curious about the state of the world's affairs so as to know whether or not "warm clothes" and a "raincoat" would be best.

The possibilities of being abused and misunderstood seemed to be behind many of her SCT responses. As she noted in describing her fears, it is "powerful idiots" of which one must be most afraid. She wishes she could "be truly free to express herself," but finds that she "wasn't being listened to" and so had developed a resistive, distrustful orientation towards others and is wary of their demands. She adopts a pretense of not caring (e.g. items 22, 42, 46, 49, 60, 71, 72, 81, 82 and 93) and when pressured, resorts to deceit in order to avoid beind held back by "restriction." Despite some tacit compliance with external demands, her general view is that others make unreasonable requests of her, a trait she finds prominent in her mother (item 99). However, she is aware that she needs relationships with other people (e.g. items 74 and 83) and recognizes that lying to them and losing her temper are problems she must solve.

When looking to solve these, or any other problems, for that matter, her basic motivation is to look outside herself, to change her surroundings or her situation. There seems little evidence that any clear sense of internal motivation for self-change is likely to spontaneously carry her through these difficulties. Her attitude is perhaps best described by her basic view that many people are "unhappy" and her own gratification comes from finding "an expression that she felt comfortable with." As she also indicated on the SCT (#97), she experiences a sense of inferiority because she is not from a happy family.

Ms. K's wary attitude towards others, her resistive and usually oppositional stance towards authority, and, by clinical history, her occasional outbursts are suggestive of borderline personality disorder features. In contrast to these features were her general lack of impulsivity, her self-definition, although by opposition in part, and her emotional warmth when not feeling put upon. These latter findings, when taken together with her presentation when she was feeling under pressure, suggested her difficulties were more reactive than enduring in nature.

Treatment Planning and Outcome

In the report made to the referring therapist, the examining psychologist summarized the test results as reflecting experience of depressive moods, but found this to be largely in reaction to recent events. Other aspects of her personality style were also reported as more consistent with a reactive disturbance than indicative of abnormal personality development. The chief concern expressed by the examining psychologist was Ms. K's self-reliance and preference for focusing on problems of external reality, so much so that there seemed to be little insight into her own or others' motivations and little interest in self-change. The examining psychologist thought these personality traits would likely make it difficult for her to generate sufficient motivation for change.

These impressions were very much in keeping with those formed by her treatment team. As a consequence, Ms. K and her mother were encouraged to work out a contractual solution to their difficulties in living together. Various responsibilities were discussed and arranged to be contingent on Ms. K fulfilling certain obligations which her mother felt she could meet. In return, her mother agreed to allow Ms. K a certain measure of freedom to decide things for herself. In order to facilitate this process and insure that it continue successfully once Ms. K was discharged, she and her mother and younger brother began to meet regularly with someone who would continue to work with her family following her discharge.

With the intercession of an intermediary able to reflect both Ms. K and her mother's realistic concerns and unreasonable demands, she and her mother were able to make rapid progress on outlining the parameters of their relationship together following discharge and Ms. K was discharged two weeks later. They continued to see the outpatient therapist for a few weeks and then terminated the work when things seemed to have resumed a more stable course. Subsequently, sporadic difficulties in their relationship arose, but they were able to make use of periods of brief intervention by Ms. K's former therapist and a family therapist to quickly set these aright. Over the next few months, Ms. K changed schools and made a more successful adjustment to her new academic setting. Her mother was able to find many things about her daughter's new life and interests that she could genuinely support.

EXHIBIT 1

AREA OF ASSESSMENT	CLINICAL EXAMINATION	PSYCHOLOGICAL EXAMINATION
I. Symptoms/Diagnosis		
Adjustment disorder with mixed disturbance of emotions and conduct		
Reaction to identifiable stressor within three months of onset	Parents have recently separated	None
Maladaptive reaction indicated by		
—impairment in school functioning	Failing in school	None
—symptoms in excess of normal reaction	Overreacts with anger and suicidal threats to mother's attempts to set limits	Avoids emotional reactions by pretending to not care while wary of others
Not just one instance and not an exacerbation of another disorder	Fights with mother are more frequent and increasingly antagonistic	No evidence of more serious psychopathology
Less than six months duration	Less than six months duration	None
II. Personality Factors	Can be headstrong and quick to defend her personal values	Oppositional when confronted by others, especially authority
III. Cognitive Abilities	Above average intelligence	Above average intelligence
	Academic performance is below her ability	Preference for activity and concrete experience may result in poor academic performance
IV. Psychodynamics	Conflicts over autonomy and interdependence	Empathic experience of others is avoided out of fear of entrapment

AREA OF ASSESSMENT	CLINICAL EXAMINATION	PSYCHOLOGICAL EXAMINATION
V. Therapeutic Enabling Factors	A willingness to share some responsibility for her actions	Recognizes her own problems but looks to external environmental change for a solution
	Recognizes a need for professional intercession to establish a better relationship with her mother	Cooperation with treatment is likely to be conditional on a *quid pro quo* negotiation
VI. Environmental Demand and Social Adjustment	Passively resists demands for appropriate school performance	Resistance to others demands is seen as serving autonomy
	Has friends who are chosen for their social deviance	Friendships based on acceptance and nonintrusive support

EXHIBIT 2

WAIS-R SUMMARY

Verbal Subtests	Scaled Score
Information	11
Similarities	13
Arithmetic	13
Vocabulary	14
Comprehension	14

Performance Subtests	
Picture Completion	16
Picture Arrangement	13
Block Design	14
Object Assembly	19
Coding	10

Verbal IQ	115
Performance IQ	131
Full Scale IQ	126

RORSCHACH SUMMARY

Number of Responses	13
Rejections	0
Populars	4
Originals	0
Average R/T Chromatic	22″
Average R/T Achromatic	17″
F%	38
F + %	73
A%	38
H%	23
W:M	7:3
M:Sum C	3:3
m:c	3:1
VIII-X%	23
FK + F + Fc%	46
(H + A):(Hd + Ad)	6:2

RORSCHACH SUMMARY

Apperception	W	54%
	D	31%
	d	0%
	Dd + S	15%

E X H I B I T 3

RORSCHACH SUMMARY

Response	*Inquiry*	*Scoring*

I. 48″

I'm supposed to tell you what I see or something. I don't know.

1. Looks like a face or something like a cat—like a cat kind of a . . . some kind of animal.	1. The eyes, the teeth, nose, ears. I don't know what these things are, didn't use them. (*Cat?*) The fact that it was shaped like one and looked like one.	W(S)FAd

(Sometimes people see more than one thing.)

I don't see anything else.

RORSCHACH SUMMARY

Response	Inquiry	Scoring

II. 18″
It's hard.

1. Uhmm . . . well one thing I know this is weird—Can I say several things? (*Entirely up to you*) This looks like a horseshoe crab. (*Laughs*) I don't know why.

2. This looks like two things dancing, the black part, like bear skin rugs or something,

And I don't know what that is on the bottom.

1. This red blotch. Strange, but it looked like it a lot. (*Horseshoe crab?*) The shape. (*Anything else?*) No.

   DFA

2. And the black things were the two things dancing, and the other ones, didn't see anything. (*Can you tell me more about the idea of two bearskins dancing?*) Well, at first I thought it was two bears, but they're too disfigured to be bears. I was thinking of something that could be large. (*Were the bear skins dancing?*) Yeah, they look that way. That's the way I saw it. (*Bearskin rug?*) The shape, I used to have a lambskin rug like that and it reminded me of it. (*Anything else?*) No.

   DFMA *Confab*

RORSCHACH SUMMARY

Response	*Inquiry*	*Scoring*

III. 3″

1. Looks like two people, two women kind of, leaning forward or something and kind of—no, it looks like a woman looking in a mirror, posing or something.

    1. (*Woman looking in the mirror?*) Because the black figures are shaped like a woman and the fact that there are two of them made it look that way. (*Posing?*) The position was the way her head was up made it look like she's not looking down at what she's picking up but it's kind of a pose.

    WMHP

2. This too. A bow.

    2. (*Bow?*) Something in the background in the room she's in. I used it in the picture. I didn't ignore it. (*Bow?*) The shape.

    DFObjP

3. And the things on the top here are some kind of lamp or something.

    3. (*Lamp?*) The shape. They're in the background too.

    DF-Obj

Rorschach Summary

Response	Inquiry	Scoring

IV. 37″

1. I think it looks like some kind of animal, just the face and fur. It looks like it's leaning down against something. Just the head, kind of photography or something that uses black and white only, no gray areas and that's what it reminds me of, the face of an animal like that.

1. The whole. These are the eyes and the nose and mouth area—and this is kind of shaggy and it kind of looks like fur in that kind of photography. When something's in between it either decides to be black or white. The ears would be up here and there would be more of the face around—but I'm just talking about the general face area. (*So you're saying there should be more?*) I'm saying there would be more. I'm just talking about the face. There would be ears and more of the body. I'm just concentrating on the face part. (*So in the blot you don't see some of the parts?*) Right. Looks like a tiger skin rug that just kind of sits on the floor and the head is the part you see. (*What do you mean by shaggy?*) I mean the lines going off in different directions. (*Head?*) Just what I saw—the shape and the way the rugs always have sad or stunned faces and the eyes look sad the way they go down—mostly the shape.

W(S)Fc-A

RORSCHACH SUMMARY

Response	*Inquiry*	*Scoring*

V. 12″

1. Looks like a bat or something like that cause the wings are small.

1. (*Bat?*) It's almost exactly shaped like one—I guess other people might have said butterfly but the wings aren't like a butterfly, more like a bat. (*Yawns*)

WFAP

VI. 18″

1. Well um, the only thing I can see is in this part—it looks like a cat. They must think I have a cat obsession. (*Who's they?*) Whoever's going to be reading this—shaped like a caricature of a cat—looks a lot like a cat caricature. I don't know what this is in the background, I was only using this.

1. Mouth. It's like it's howling or something. You know how cats have, on either side of their nose, brushed back, that's what this is. He's looking up or something. (*Nose?*) Like a caricature, looking up, hair falling down. My brother has a book, Bloom County, and that's what it looks like, sort of, Bill the cat. Two faded lines. Looks like his arms, going down straight in front of him. (*Cat?*) Looks like the cartoon cat, it's shape.

drFM-(A)Fab

Rorschach Summary

Response	Inquiry	Scoring

VII. 15″

I have no idea.

1. I mean it looks like two bobby-sox type girls looking back at each other, with their ponytails flying up (*Laughs*). I don't know why, it looks like cartoon girls looking back at each other. Looking over their shoulder, walking away from each other. (*Their ponytails flying up?*) (*Laughs*) It's so ridiculous, but you . . . (*Flying up?*) Like the, swinging their heads really fast.

1. The bottom, kind of their skirt or something. (*Their bottom?*) I don't know what it is—just kind of when I looked at it, that's what I saw, I didn't think about it very much so I guess you take this thing over here. (*Take out?*) I'm not using this part here. Umm, the faces look so detailed, nose, mouth, sticking out tongues at each other, these are eyelashes coming out.

WM(H)P

VIII. 12″

1. Um, looks like some animal walking across a river bank, by a river bank. Like on a short cliff over water. That's it.

1. This is the animal, the pink. This is the bank, kind of, and the reflection, the water. (*Animal?*) Exactly what I saw, first thing. (*Blot?*) The legs, face, even has a dot for an eye, the back. (*River bank?*) Whenever there's a river, there's a darker part where the rock has broken away and that's what this looks like. (*Reflection?*) Because it's the same on both sides.

W(S)FM.CFA, LdscP

IX. 15″

1. I don't see anything. Just looks like a mess of colors sort of. (*Turns*)

WCdesAbs

RORSCHACH SUMMARY

Response	*Inquiry*	*Scoring*
(*Can you try?*) Doesn't look like any figure or anything. I really don't see anything.		

X. 25″

1. Upside down it looks like some kind of "Dungeons and Dragons" kind of thing like a face like an evil type person. (*Yawns*) That's it.	1. These are the eyes and they're kind of angry and yellowish and that looks like a nose or something. And that's the evil smile and (*Laughs*) and has a pointed head like all the villains do in the old movies.	drF/C.M-(Hd)

EXHIBIT 4

THEMATIC APPERCEPTION TEST

CARD 1   Well, you mean a story like an essay? Lots of questions. Looks like since the violin is lying on some kind of paper someone gave him a violin for his birthday or maybe some other reason and he doesn't really want it. He wanted something else. He doesn't look too happy at all. (*What happens?*) What do you mean? The person who gave it to him looks at him and sees that he's not happy with it and offers to let him return it and the little boy gets something that he likes.

CARD 10   Umm, uh, looks like a little boy or a girl, you can't even tell. I guess a little boy who's saying goodbye to his mother. No, he came back from somewhere and he missed her and he's giving her a hug. The reason he's not leaving is cause he looks relieved or kind of happy so I was thinking he'd be coming back. Umm and it looks like the mother—her eyes—she's smiling cause there's a dimple on her chin—and she has smiling eyes or whatever they say—I don't know where the boy's coming back from—I can't think—I don't know what happens next—the mother made a big dinner for him and they're coming back and the whole family will be there. He looks like Marlon Brando, you don't have to write that. (?) The guy, the little boy or girl, who it was meant to be.

CARD 5   Umm, (*Yawns*) this woman is uh, is waiting for her husband to get home because she has some bad news to tell him or something. You can tell by the expression on her face that she's not exactly looking forward to it and that's all I can relly tell. Oh, should I say what happens after? Her husband gets home early and she tells him her news and he (*Thinks*) and for some reason he wasn't upset.

CARD 12M   Umm, looks like this person is sick or something and this guy is going to feel his head or is just checking on him or else he's going to try to suffocate him with his hand or something but it looks more like he's sick from the position he's lying in, can't tell what the man with his hand up is thinking because you can't see his face (*Puts card down*).

CARD 18GF   Mmm, Looks like this person just strangled this other person by the way the hands are grabbing and the expression on her face. (*Whose face?*) The person who's doing the strangling—and this person's dying—looks like there was some kind of fight before it because her hair's all messed up.

CARD 3GF   Umm, This person is umm, wants to be alone or something

---

THEMATIC APPERCEPTION TEST

---

and wants to shut the door cause she just found out some bad news. Something she didn't want to hear and she wants to lie down or be alone. (*Anything else?*) Nope.

CARD 2   I don't know, it looks like this farm girl, or whatever it is, is going off to school. She's waiting for someone to pick her up or something. That's all I see. (*What's she thinking or feeling?*) She doesn't look like she's too happy about going to school but she looks like she's waiting for a while and just kind of bored.

CARD 12F   Umm, I don't know, it looks like the woman in front is umm, waiting to do something she looks kind of nervous and the woman behind her is a nun or something. (*Yawns*) And she's there to be reassuring for comfort or something and she looks kind of worried herself. I don't know what the woman is waiting for. Umm, she looks kind of happy actually and I don't know. (*What happens?*) I don't know, the woman looks kind of proud or something like she's going to go up and get an award or something and the woman behind looks happy but nervous and suspicious so I don't know what happens. (*What's she suspicious of?*) No, it looks like she knows something that the girl doesn't.

CARD 13MF   Umm, it looks like these are husband and wife or whatever, a couple, and he's just getting up in the morning and the light. He's stretching or something and the light is bothering him and he has to go to work so he got dressed quickly and he didn't want to wake his wife. (*That's it?*) Yes.

E X H I B I T   5

Sentence Completion Test

2. *She often wished she could* "be truly free to express herself."
7. *She felt proud that* "she had found an expression that she felt comfortable with."
12. *I was most depressed when* "I felt I wasn't being listened to."
22. *When people made fun of her, she* "ignored them."
42. *When I am criticized, I* "ignore the criticism."
46. *When they didn't invite me, I* "did something else."
49. *People seem to think that I* "don't care."
60. *My mother always* "thinks she's doing what is best for me."
71. *Her reaction to me* "didn't matter."
72. *When she was punished by her mother, she* "didn't care because it was unfair."
74. *I feel happiest when* "I'm with my friends."
81. *Most women act as though* "they don't care."
82. *When I feel others don't like me* "I avoid them."
83. *More than anything else, she needed* "company."
84. *Most people are* "happy."
87. *I am afraid of* "powerful idiots."
93. *When introduced to people, she* "appeared happy."
97. *She felt inferior when* "with happy families."
99. *I wish that my mother* "were more reasonable."

ADJUSTMENT DISORDER WITH DEPRESSED MOOD

Mr. T, a 38-year-old, separated, corrections officer, was brought to the hospital by his department's psychologist. He hadn't reported for duty and when his landlord had gone to his apartment to check on him at the request of the duty sergeant, Mr. T was sitting with his service revolver in his lap looking dejected. Spread out on the bed before him were pictures of his four children (aged 4 through 10), his wedding ring, a card, and a ribbon from a school athletic competition his son had recently given him. Mr. T had the hammer cocked and pointed the gun at his head several times, finger shaking, before his landlord was able to talk him into giving it up. The department psychologist was called and by the time he arrived, Mr. T was feeling embarrassed and apologetic.

Mr. T had been separated from his wife and family for nearly three years. Recently, his wife had initiated efforts to extend the legal separation for another year. Perhaps adding insult to injury, his girlfriend of the last few months had also decided to break off her relationship with him. Feeling hopeless about a resolution of his difficulties with his wife and girlfriend, and financially burdened by supporting both his own and his wife's household, Mr. T had filed for divorce. On the morning of his hospitalization, he and his lawyer were scheduled to meet with his wife and her attorney to negotiate the terms of the divorce settlement.

Mr. T acknowledged that he had been in a low mood the last month or two and had at times been overwhelmed with feelings of futility and despair. He would feel a little better on the two or three nights a week he had a few drinks with his friends in the evening after work. Although he hadn't missed any work, he had been distracted at work and recently his preoccupation with his personal troubles had resulted in difficulties with his duty sergeant. His chief and fellow officers, however, played down these troubles. Everyone knew the sergeant had a "difficult personality." Despite their reassurances, Mr. T remained concerned about his sergeant's evaluations.

His first separation from his wife had come after she had filed a series of complaints against him for intoxication and abusive behavior. News of these complaints had gotten back to Mr. T's coworkers, a fact that was a source of great embarrassment for him. Moreover, the whole situation had strongly reminded him of his own father's difficulties. Mr. T's father had been allowed to resign his commission in the military some years earlier as his drinking began to compromise his job performance.

Mr. T had agreed to seek counselling when these difficulties began and he and his wife had attended a number of conjoint sessions where he acknowledged his occasional difficulties with alcohol and seemed prepared to address other problems in the relationship as well. His wife, on the other hand, felt that all their difficulties stemmed from his drinking and stopped attending sessions and filed for a separation when it became apparent that neither the first nor the second counsellor they visited was prepared to adopt her view that all their problems could be traced to her husband's drinking.

At the time of his admission to the hospital, Mr. T was embarrassed by his behavior of that morning and stated that "I don't feel I can handle it anymore," a reference to his situation with his wife. This was his first psychiatric hospitalization and he stated that "severe depression" was his reason for seeking admission at this time. He was noticeably despondent, with a persistent, sad affect, and described his own mood as "discouraged." He was oriented in all three spheres, gave no indications of or history of delusions or hallucinations, and showed no evidence of either short-term or long-term memory impairment on examination. His insight and judgment were described as fair. His counsellor considered him a reliable informant and found no reason to contradict his description of his own behavior or mental status.

DSM-III-R Diagnosis

Axis I: Adjustment disorder with depressed mood
            Alcohol abuse, episodic
Axis II: Mixed personality disorder with dependent and depressive
            features
Axis III: None
Axis IV: Severe—Impending divorce; prolonged separation from
            family
Axis V: Serious Symptoms—suicidal ideation, increased alcohol
            abuse

Treatment and Hospital Course

For the first few days after arriving at the hospital, Mr. T appeared rather subdued and isolated. He was carefully observed for signs of alcohol withdrawal and none were noted. Shortly, he settled into the unit routine and gradually became less isolated and better able to interact with the hospital staff and the other patients. He felt "relieved" to be in the hospital and was glad to have the opportunity to "talk with someone about all the things on my mind." He focused specifically on problems with his marriage. After he and his wife were seen together, it became clear that no possibility for reconciliation remained. The marital relationship had been chronically unsatisfactory for both.

Although Mr. T was clearly experiencing difficulty around the situation with his wife and children, in all other respects he appeared to be able to function at quite a high level. He quickly assumed a leadership role on the unit, enjoyed his activities, and began to participate in the hospital's Alcoholics Anonymous program. Psychological testing was requested to help in assessing his impulsivity and level of depression and to identify any characterological issues which Mr. T might begin to address while in the hospital.

Psychological Assessment

Mr. T received a WAIS, Rorschach, TAT, and Bender Gestalt during the third week of his hospital stay, as well as an MMPI within a week of his admission. He was cooperative with the testing procedures but seemed to resent being examined.

His MMPI profile indicated a moderate level of denial and efforts to make a good impression (L 6; F-K = -15). His *scale 4* elevation is not unusual for law enforcement personnel and indicated his inclination for activity and perhaps some impulsiveness. A history of alcohol abuse is common in individuals with this profile feature. His elevation on *scale 8* revealed, on closer inspection, to consist of feelings of social alienation and mistrustfulness. Overall, the profile was seen as consistent with a history of alcohol abuse, poor interpersonal relationships, and difficulty in dealing with emotionally-charged situations in an adaptive way.

Mr. T's WAIS performance yielded a full-scale IQ of 103 with verbal and performance IQs of 108 and 99, respectively. His best performance was given on the *Similarities* subtest where he achieved a superior score of 15 and his worst performance, which was somewhat below average, was given on the *Block Design* subtest where he achieved a scaled score of 8. Apart from these subscale scores, his WAIS profile gave evidence of relatively little scatter (scaled scores of 9-12).

Perhaps the most noticeable feature of his WAIS performance was his relative inefficiency on the performance subtests. His interchanging of two fingers on one *Object Assembly* item, his successful completion of two block designs only in overtime, and his slow and methodical performance on the *Digit Symbol* subtest all suggested he was having some difficulty in readily mobilizing skills which appeared easily in his grasp. His Bender performance demonstrated that he was aware of his difficulty and made some perfunctory efforts to compensate for them.

On the Rorschach, Mr. T's performance was characterized by the same sense of struggle and inefficiency. He often struggled to make something out of the blots. Where he could find evidence for it, he preferred scenes of gaiety and liveliness (e.g. *cards II* and *III*). Even here, however, people need something to hold on to such as the champagne glass in *card III*. His frequent use of shading (*cards II, IV, VI*) indicated his underlying anxiety and tension and lent an air of defeat and despair to his responses. He sought refuge in the conventional, for when faced with life's problems, he seldom feels up to the task and is "cornered" (*card VI*) by his own inability to act. Alcohol, because of its association with happier times (*card III*) and tenderer feelings (*card X*), offers itself as a temporary escape from the rigors of adult life.

As with his Rorschach performance, Mr. T's performance on the TAT was infused with his hope for a stable, conventional world. He made no apology for his strong desire for "happy endings" and almost invariably attempted to find one. Despite this desire, there seemed to be little sense of how one might proceed from the present tragedy to the happy ending: "hopefully" things will turn out for the best (*cards 3BM and 12M*), or the wisdom of age (*7BM*) or divine providence (*12M*) will prevail. Somehow, when things don't seem as if they will work out well, the characters simply must learn to "deal with that" in their lives (*card 15*), but nowhere does he specify how this task is to be accomplished.

Treatment Planning and Outcome

In the psychologist's report, Mr. T's struggles with his depressive feelings and his need for nurturance and support were emphasized. The psychologist noted that Mr. T might wish for an older, paternal figure who could function as a source of support and guidance, but that his own guilt and angry sense of loss would probably impair his ability to make use of such a figure. The psychologist's recommendation was for a continuation of a supportive psychotherapy which would help Mr. T to build up his own defenses. Finally, although there were some indications of a poorly contained impulsivity, he was not seen as presently suicidal.

Mr. T continued to work in individual psychotherapy and gradually came to accept the need for him and his wife to follow through on their divorce. With the help of his therapist and his social worker, he and his wife were able to work out an arrangement for him to maintain contact with his children and she brought them to visit him in the hospital on several occasions.

He felt supported and aided by the hospital staff and, for the first time, began to talk about his experiences while serving with the Navy in Vietnam. He began to recognize that his experiences there had taught him to divorce himself from his feelings and had contributed to his sense of futility and despair about making changes in himself or his life. This insight helped him to begin to look at his own attitudes towards his present situation and to begin to confront his own feelings more directly.

At the end of his one-month hospitalization, Mr. T had made arrangements to continue with the divorce and to live with a fellow officer until he and his wife could come to a more acceptable financial arrangement. He was able to refrain from drinking while on passes from the hospital and agreed to continue with the AA program on discharge. He appeared grateful for the help the hospital had given him and has not required any additional hospital treatment since his discharge.

EXHIBIT 1

Area of Assessment	Clinical Examination	Psychological Examination
I. Symptoms/Diagnosis		
Adjustment disorder with depressed mood		
Reaction to identifiable stressor within three months of onset	Meeting with attorneys for initiation of divorce proceedings	None
Maladaptive reaction indicated by		
—symptoms in excess of normal reaction	Suicidal ideation with aborted attempt	Coping strategies seem inadequate in light of assessed ability
Not just one instance and not an exacerbation of another disorder	Only suicidal episode but drinking has increased	Persistent feelings of inadequacy and depression concerning intimacy
Less than six months duration	Less than six months duration	Present difficulties are at odds with demonstrated abilities suggesting a recent onset
II. Personality Factors	None	Underlying feelings of immobilization and resultant dependency which he denies
III. Cognitive Abilities	Average intelligence	Average intelligence with evidence of some impairment in performance abilities due to current depression
IV. Psychodynamics	Guilt and anger combined impair adaptive problem solving	Feels defeated and self-derogatory and at the mercy of a primitive view of benevolent fate
V. Therapeutic Enabling Factors	Readily responds to a supportive environment	Hopefulness may assist in developing a therapeutic relationship

AREA OF ASSESSMENT	CLINICAL EXAMINATION	PSYCHOLOGICAL EXAMINATION
	Functions best when supported in taking appropriate action	Feels more comfortable and makes better use of his resources when in a structured setting
	Has successfully utilized psychotherapy in the past	None
VI. Environmental Demand and Social Adjustment	Good work history despite interpersonal troubles	After initial anger and resentment, cooperative if not fully engaged
	Has made and kept several friends	None

EXHIBIT 2

WAIS-R SUMMARY

Verbal Subtests	*Scaled Score*
Information	12
Digit Span	11
Vocabulary	11
Arithmetic	10
Comprehension	10
Similarities	15

Performance Subtests	
Picture Completion	12
Picture Arrangement	12
Block Design	8
Object Assembly	9
Digit Symbol	9
Verbal IQ	108
Performance IQ	99
Full Scale IQ	103

MMPI SUMMARY

K-FL/4"892-371/0:

RORSCHACH SUMMARY

Number of Responses	18
Rejections	0
Populars	8
Originals	2(-1)
Average R/T Chromatic	15"
Average R/T Achromatic	11"
F%	56
F+%	75
A%	44
H%	28
W:M	10:3
M:Sum C	3:1
m:c	1:3
VIII-X%	33

RORSCHACH SUMMARY

FK + F + Fc%		56
(H + A):(Hd + Ad)		9:4
Apperception	W	56%
	D	39%
	d	0%
	Dd + S	5%

E X H I B I T   3

Rorschach Summary

Response	*Inquiry*	*Scoring*
I. 20″		
1. A butterfly. Or a bumble bee.	1. It reminds me of a butterfly because of a central body, wings on either side of it. At the furthest part from the center there appears to be a pointed part.	WFAP
2. Some kind of flying type insect. That's what it reminds me of. It has to be viewed upright. (*No*).	2. The whole, the same thing almost like a shadow effect because of dark color.	WFM.FC′A
II. 15″		
1. Two people dancing and touching hands and knees.	1. Here are their heads, and here's where they are touching at the hands and knees.	WMHP
2. A facial expression, nose, moustache, mouth.	2. A large moustache, mouth, nose, eyes. (*Moustache?*) A big, thick moustache, bushy, coming from the center of the nose. (*Bushy?*) A bushy effect—little lines, like painted, shapes.	W(S)cF-HdO
III. 8″		
1. Two people, holding onto something in the center. And a champagne glass in the center.	1. With arms stretched out. Arm here and here, leg here and here, holding onto champagne glass in middle.	D(S)MH,ObjP
2. A bow, or whatever red piece represents.	2. A bowtie in center. (?) Just shape.	DFCP

Rorschach Summary

Response	Inquiry	Scoring

IV. 25″

1. Something laying down, some kind of animal laying down.

1. Legs, arms, head gives me general impression of bearskin rug lying down, laying on the back as opposed to the front. (*Back of a bearskin?*) Dark coloration.

WFC′AP

V. 4″

1. Back to the butterfly again.

1. Two little antennae and two little legs in back.

WFAP

VI. 5″

(*Laughs*) I don't know. No recognizable shape to it. I'm not sure it represents anything to me.

1. I was thinking starfish but it doesn't even have that complete shape.

1. The general outline.

WF-A

2. Only thing that comes to mind is that two portions meet and might be a corner of a room.

2. An inside corner like a wall that comes together, see that came there. The coloration, gets darker in corner. Darker and gets lighter going away.

WFC′-ObjO

VII. 25″

1. Like Tinker Bell looking at one another.

1. A girlish type face looking at one another. Chin, head, hair, profile.

DM(Hd)P

2. Almost looks like these are also faces. Nose, eye, mouth.

2. (*Eye?*) Oval—with little dot. Over here, but not as pronounced.

DFHd

VIII. 12″

1. Two animals, the pink portion on either side. Have four legs.

1. Two of them looked like it's got legs, several, out on either side.

DFAP

RORSCHACH SUMMARY

Response	*Inquiry*	*Scoring*
2. The blue and grey. I don't know why fish comes to mind but some kind of crustacean or crab, something like that.	2. Pincers on crab or lobster. The other part I'm not sure why it came to mind.	DF-A
3. Lungs and spinal cord, skeletal system, if these are lungs, kidneys down here.	3. This would be central vertebral—these lungs, these would be organs, kidneys, heart. I don't know. (?) A rib cage almost.	WFAt

IX. 10″

I have no idea. I don't see anything. Is there a heavy meaning in all this. Outlines don't take a familiar shape.

| 1. Only thing that stands out is there is something behind green and orange. 2 nostrils, little slits, like an animal nose as opposed to conventional nose. What kind of animal has a flat nose—a rhinoceros? | 1. The grey area (*Conventional nose?*) Not a human looking nose, but an animal's nose. | DF-Ad |

X. 11″

At least 6, 7 different colors.

| 1. My daughter's drawings at home. Early watercolor by Kathy. It's hard to believe people make money from these things. People actually see things in this? | 1. Like a child's attempt at experimenting with color. Is that significant? | WCF Art |
| 2. Long blue looks like spiders with all little legs but as far as anything else doesn't seem to represent anything. | 2. The shape again. | DFAP |

E X H I B I T 4

THEMATIC APPERCEPTION TEST

CARD 3BM   It's a girl crying, sitting against a sofa, a long bench seat. Looks like something on floor. I don't know what that is supposed to be if she is crying. No significance to it at all (?) Hopelessness, frustration. (?) Overfed in cafeteria. How can you expect me to make a story, when I have no idea . . . Seems to portray someone feeling hopelessly frustrated and gave up (?) I like happy endings. Whatever problem is, it will be solved. Hopefully life will get better.

CARD 4   (*Laughs*) Where did you get these people. This also looks like something out of 40s. She's holding him back from doing something. Cheesecake pictures in back? (?) I don't know, a war picture. Someone's going to go off to war. She's holding him back (?) Uncle Sam called and he has to go. (?) She? Don't go. (?) He'll come back as a decorated hero.

CARD 6BM   Definitely a dated picture. A mother and son picture. Mother looking out a window probably thinking of what happened and yet seems very concerned. Young fellow seems a little depressed. I don't know if he just offered some bad news. Just came in from outside and gave some bad news. (*Like what?*) Looks like something from Norman Rockwell. Maybe a son lost in the war. (Mother and son?) Maybe not related people. (?) Outcome doesn't look too big for her. (?) I don't know, again. Learn to deal with it.

CARD 7BM   It looks like a father and son having a very serious discussion. What was the discussion? The younger person has a concerned look and older person seems more relaxed, not as much tension in the face. Almost as if he has the wisdom of age, almost like he could empathize with this person (*Concern about?*) I guess, maybe some family situation or job. His wife is going to have the 14th kid and he lost his job. You're going to write that down, too? I'm only joking. (?) Outcome seems to be whatever the problems are, they will work out. Older person will provide guidance in solving the problems.

CARD 8BM   An operation of a sort, an incision made. Young boy being very reflective. I don't know if it's his father, brother, friend. He's contemplating whatever fate this person is going to have. I don't know if he was the cause of this operation. (?) Some kind of medical problem, if there's an incision. (?) A happy ending. I predict the patient will live and the operation is a success but it looks kind of primitive. Can you tell me a real story? Have

THEMATIC APPERCEPTION TEST

you made up a story? Looks like little Joseph Kerr, well groomed and proper, with tie, jacket, white shirt.

CARD 12M A young boy laying down. An older man reaching over to touch him. I don't know why he is, his hand is not touching, probably it's a priest offering a blessing or last rites. (?) Boy hit by car. (?) Appears to be unconscious, resting peacefully. (?) He's going to be all right. I don't know, I would never be a good script writer. If I were dead, I'd expect to be straight out.

CARD 13MF Definitely a close out. Where you get 12 for $1. Is there any titles to these? What do you do, make up your own title? This man is upset with this lady who's laying there partly clothed. I don't know if this is supposed to portray death. Because she's not moving. Arms extended and covers only partly up the chest. Man is hiding his eyes. I don't know what emotion that would be. I don't know if it's supposed to be sorrow. If she's dead, maybe denial. I don't know what led up to her being in this particular situation. (?) It don't look good. Have to call a doctor or an ambulance. It doesn't look like a happy ending. I get a sense of someone expired and this guy can't do anything for them.

CARD 14 Opening scene for Search for Tomorrow. This fellow is looking out the window, looking out into the world, with a sense of hope as opposed to someone who might want to jump out. Looking out and up as opposed to down.

CARD 15 Where do you get these pictures? This looks like one of those close outs. I don't know if this is a destructive person or an evil person. Seems to be distraught. He's in the middle of a cemetery with gravestones. (?) He's there to see someone or attempt to communicate with someone. (?) I don't know. He has stringy hair. From the garment, almost like a dress, I can't tell if it's a man or woman. (?) Someday he'll be in the cemetery. I don't know how I can make up another story. He'll have to deal with that in his or her life.

DISCUSSION

In this section, we contrast an adjustment disorder in a 38-year-old male to that of a 16-year-old high school female. In the former case, the major symptoms are depression and suicidal ideation, while in the latter case the disorder is accompanied by emotional disruption and conduct disturbance, symptoms often characteristic of young people.

For Mr. T, the rather common stressors of separation and impending divorce became an overwhelming set of circumstances. He was caught up in a cycle of hopelessness, depression, and alcohol abuse and imagined that the only "solution" was death. There are indications in the psychological testing as to why this man might be vulnerable to the stress of marital separation with its common psychological implications of rejection and worthlessness. While he is motivated toward adjustment to society and its norms, there are signs of impulsiveness and indications of mistrustfulness, as well as some difficulties in interpersonal relations. His periodic alcohol abuse is also an important element in this picture.

Despite a sense of underlying anxiety, Mr. T typically coped by denial and clung to the conventional and the routine. This coping style was seriously disrupted by his marital separation. His need for the comfortable customs of daily routine was exceeded only by his stronger needs for nurturance and support. While these very needs are challenged by the marital dissolution, throwing him into a depression, the same needs will most probably assist him in attaining a positive therapeutic alliance. His average intelligence, orientation to seeking and accepting support, and the clear precipitant of upset all suggest a positive therapeutic alliance and good prognosis in focused, supportive individual psychotherapy.

The case of Ms. K, like that of Mr. T, also involves family relationships. In this case, the recent divorce of her parents serves as the stressor. Exaggerated adolescent turmoil involving issues of psychosexual development, relationship to authority figures, and independence propelled Ms. K and her mother into an intensely intertwined battle over virtually everything. The spiral of escalation reached a climax in her threats to run away from home, the calling of the police, and temporary resolution by admission to the hospital. Her unusual physical appearance would perhaps make a psychiatric evaluator wonder if the extent of her rage and rebellion is beyond that of an adjustment disorder. However, when isolated from the overstimulating environment of home, she was quite perceptive about her depression following her parents' divorce, and admitted her own contribution to the constant battle with the mother. Notable in her psychological testing is a high level of intellectual functioning. However, this intellectual acumen is in sharp contrast to her sparse and unrevealing responses to the projective materials. One gets the sense of a highly intelligent young person who has a striking absence of inner creativity and imagination, and an impoverished development of the capacity to form meaningful attachments with others. All of the action is outside rather than inside for Ms. K.

This empty, vacant, inner experience of a person who is already 16 years of age bodes poorly for a productive therapeutic relationship, especially when combined with a suspicious attitude and oppositional stance towards authority figures. The testing was useful in highlighting potential difficulties in individual treatment and suggesting family intervention as an alternative. It is possible that the most efficacious therapeutic leverage might be found in interventions with the mother and daughter on a very behavioral level, so as to render home life less chaotic and frictional and more organized and structured. Only then would the possibility of developing Ms. K's relationship skills emerge. While the mother almost demanded that the daughter be involved in individual treatment, the testing was used to emphasize that the family rather than the daughter would be the most efficacious focus of treatment.

Given the time constraints noted in DSM-III-R, the diagnosis of an adjustment disorder is invariably a provisional one when the patient is in the midst of an adjustment crisis. If the adjustment disorder's symptoms do not resolve within six months, other diagnoses are made. For example, if her symptoms continued, Ms. K would probably be diagnosed as having a conduct disorder, and perhaps an antisocial or borderline personality disorder. For Mr. T, if the symptoms are not resolved, he might be given a diagnosis of major depression and complications such as renewed alcohol abuse and sexual difficulties could be anticipated.

SECTION

·II·

AXIS II DISORDERS

CHAPTER 7

Personality Disorders

A. PARANOID PERSONALITY DISORDERS

This Axis II condition is grouped in the so-called cluster A personality disorders which include not only paranoid but also schizoid and schizotypal personality disorder. All three disorders involve odd and/or eccentric behavior. The essential features of paranoid personality disorder are a long-standing and pervasive tendency to see others as threatening or demeaning. This often includes an expectation that others are exploitative and harmful. Thus, interpersonal behavior is characterized by mistrust and questioning of the loyalty and fidelity of others. While there are little data to this effect, there is a question by the authors of DSM-III-R as to the relationship between paranoid personality disorder and delusional symptoms and schizophrenia, paranoid type.

We present two cases of paranoid personality disorder, both involving young, single males. In both situations, the question arose as to the extent of the pathology beyond simply the aloof and suspicious presentation of self to others. Psychological testing was called for in both cases in order not only to explore the extent of healthy reality testing versus the dimension of thought disorder, but also to get some further information about the inner life of these individuals. It is not uncommon for patients to be referred for testing who, for either paranoid or other reasons, are unwilling or unable to form a trusting and open alliance with the therapist. In these situations, it is quite possible that the patient will be equally elusive and untrusting in the testing situation so that the testing is meager in its content and perhaps unhelpful. On the other hand, it sometimes happens that the testing situation, with its stimuli which are independent of a personal relationship (though in the presence of another), will elicit some clues as to the inner workings of the patient.

PARANOID PERSONALITY DISORDER

Mr. R is a 22-year-old, single, black male who entered outpatient treatment because "I've been feeling down. I don't make friends easily and I'd like to get rid of my shyness and be able to make eye contact with other people." He described himself as having difficulty making eye contact with other people since about the age of 11. At that time, his family had recently had a rather serious reversal in their financial situation and he was sent to live for several months with an aunt in a distant city. Since then, he had several periods of "extreme shyness," accompanied by a depressed mood for which he had not previously sought treatment.

Mr. R worked as a clerk, a job he had held for a few months after dropping out of college. He left college because he had been unable to attend his classes, becoming too preoccupied with seeing other people together while he remained alone. This had been his third attempt to pursue his college education. On previous occasions, he had always felt that there was something about the college which did not suit him and had left the area to live with other relatives and enroll in a new school.

He was presently living with a cousin but found this situation difficult as the cousin was "too traditional." He had also encountered difficulty at his job. He became angry with his coworkers for "invading his privacy" by listening in on his telephone conversations.

In interviewing Mr. R, the examiner found it extremely difficult to obtain any clear details of recent events. He seemed to be somewhat depressed and admitted to lacking energy and motivation for the last few months. He denied any difficulties with his sleep or appetite. Although he reported occasional thoughts of dying, he denied any suicidal plan. Although no clear diagnostic formulation emerged from this initial evaluation, his requests for help in overcoming his shyness and improving the quality of his social life were accepted as the basis for his treatment and he began attending individual psychotherapy sessions once a week.

Mr. R was seen in the outpatient department for the next four months with little change. An initial formulation of his difficulties as a mild depressive reaction to his inability to succeed in school and his career, combined with a growing conviction in the presence of an underlying psychosis partially masked by his paranoid and guarded style of thinking and relating, led to the recommendation of a course of neuroleptic treatment. Mr. R agreed to a trial of a low dose, high potency neuroleptic. He developed a severe dystonic reaction to the first medication and was shifted to a second medication which he tolerated better, but subsequently discontinued, claiming that it interfered with his concentration.

Towards the end of his fourth month of outpatient treatment, Mr. R raised the issue of discontinuing his treatment altogether during a periodic psychiatric consultation with the prescribing psychiatrist. On inquiry, he acknowledged that he had already made plans to return to his parents' home where he would be able to see his mother one more time before killing himself. He was transferred to the acute inpatient services of the clinic in order to forestall his plan and to reevaluate his future treatment plans.

DSM-III-R Diagnosis

Axis I: None
Axis II: Paranoid personality disorder
Axis III: None
Axis IV: Minimal—difficulties with coworkers
Axis V: Poor—Marked impairment in social relations (no friends or social contacts outside his immediate family

Treatment and Hospital Course

Mr. R was hospitalized for two months. During this time, his suicidal intentions vanished. He was shifted to a third neuroleptic treatment and complied with the treatment staff's recommendation that he give the medication trial a suitable period of time.

Upon discharge from the inpatient service, he was reevaluated in the outpatient clinic and was seen as little changed, apart from his suicidal intentions. He had stopped taking his medication, stating that "I don't need an antipsychotic drug, I'm not psychotic." In fact, as before, no clear evidence of psychotic symptomatology could be found. He was assigned to a new therapist in the outpatient department and no pharmacotherapy was prescribed for the time being.

However, over the course of the next few months, he made little progress in his treatment and his comments and remarks to his present therapist became more elliptical and cryptic. For example, he would often comment that his present therapist was "different from all the other doctors," but could not elaborate on why this was so, in his view. He continued to be extremely guarded in discussing how he spent his time or what he thought or felt. The therapist requested a psychological consultation in hopes of gaining some insight into how Mr. R's psychotherapy might be made to work more effectively.

Psychological Assessment

Mr. R met with the examining psychologist on two occasions and completed the WAIS-R, Rorschach, TAT, and DAP during the course of the evaluation. His testing was begun within a few days of his admission and there had been no change in his clinical status.

Mr. R achieved a full scale IQ of 120, with verbal and performance IQs of 130 and 100, respectively. His subscale scores ranged from very superior (*Vocabulary*) to low average (*Picture Arrangement*), with relative verbal inefficiency in his knowledge of common facts (*Information*), a finding perhaps explained by his initial anxiety as this was the first test administered and he volunteered the correct answer to questions he'd missed when he returned for his second appointment. His relatively poor *Arithmetic* score seemed largely accounted for by a deliberateness in his manner that resulted in his just failing to receive time credit for three of his responses. Among the performance subtests, he had the most difficulty with the *Picture Arrangement* subtest, a measure of anticipatory planning in social situations. He failed two of the first four items and received only partial credit for one other. His failures on this subtest stand out from the remainder of the timed performance subtests where his lowered scores did not result from mistakes but simply from inefficiency which lost him time bonuses.

On the Rorschach, Mr. R provided 17 responses on nine cards, rejecting *card VI*. His reality testing, as assessed from his overall ability to provide accurate and realistic percepts (F + % = 73) and frequently perceived figures (P% = 24%), were adequate. However, qualitatively, there was a hesitancy and tentativeness to his response style and an unusualness to several of his responses. He averaged over 20 seconds (24.6″) between being presented with the achromatic cards and his first response and on *cards I* and *IV*, waited as much as one minute before offering his first response. Moreover, his average reaction time nearly doubled when he was presented with the chromatic cards (48″), all of which may suggest that he is endeavoring to censor his reactions, especially when emotionally stimulated by the test material.

While nearly one-half of his responses are human or human-like, they were often peculiarly seen. For example, on *card II*, the popular human figures were perceived "in an argument" because of "cues hidden from view"; on *card VII*, he described the popular human figures as "alien dwarfs with large heads"; on *card VIII*, he found a "creature with a hideous grin" who was described as having horns and a protruding tongue. Qualitatively, these human responses suggested an idiosyncratic concern with malevolent and malicious qualities which appeared to persist in his percepts despite his extended response times.

None of Mr. R's test protocols contained any compelling evidence of blatant disruptions in or distortions of reality. His TAT stories stayed very close to the manifest content of the pictures. *Card 1* prompted a story of initial discouragement and final triumph; *card 2* concerned the usual conflict between past security and present ambition; *card 4* focused on the tension between the couple. On the TAT, as on the other tests, he guardedly hewed rather closely to the obvious and mundane. In the details of his stories, however, the same unusualness seen on the Rorschach appeared on the TAT. On *card 5*, he began by seeking reassurance that "I don't have to say what comes to mind, just make up a story?" He projected on *card 2* that the older woman in the background is "looking with some disdain at the girl on the left," left hanging a comment about the man's "eyes" on *card 4*, and after suggesting that the young boy on *card 8BM* used the rifle to shoot the older man, offered the personalized interpretation that the young boy had a look of "satisfaction" on his face.

It was only in his figure drawings that one was immediately struck with Mr. R's unusual view of reality. He initially requested to defer the test, which the examiner did. Later, when presented with the test again, in an evasive manner he asked if stick figures were acceptable and when asked to draw a person, he asked if a "sentient" would do. His first figure was of a "male sentient, capable of thought processes but not like a robot." The examiner questioned him about this distinction and was told that a sentient "could be man-made but not at the present time" and that "humans are sentient, too." This figure, with its exaggerated shoulders and proportionately tiny legs, was also drawn with a pointed chin, slanted, triangular eyes and squared-off head and gives the appearance of a robot or robot-like figure despite Mr. R's wish to distinguish it from a robot. His second figure, a female, was better proportioned and her facial features seem less sinister. Her lack of sexual characteristics was explained by his pointing out that, as sentients, "it doesn't make sense to differentiate them."

Mr. R's "sentients" appeared to represent a compromise view of human beings and their complex relationships. Preferring to relegate human relationships to the mechanical and logical as protection from the emotional and malevolent appeared to be the central issue for him. His suspicion of the motives and intentions of others was a dominant preoccupation and he struggled with the desire for emotional union and interaction which conflict with his prominent fears of infringement and annihilation.

Treatment Planning and Outcome

After his psychological evaluation while an inpatient, Mr. R was conferenced and a decision was made to transfer his psychotherapy to a female therapist in hopes that he would be able to develop a more trusting relationship with her. His refusal to continue taking a neuroleptic medication was respected and it was agreed that pharmacotherapy would no longer play a role in his treatment. He remained in the hospital for a few more days and then was readmitted to the outpatient clinic to begin working with the new therapist.

Throughout the remaining six months of his treatment, Mr. R reported himself as less depressed, although he still remained, for the most part, guarded and emotionally unavailable. He did, however, come to see his new therapist as "different from the other doctors" and related this to her warmth and interest in him. He could return her interest only by inquiring into her personal life. This effort was turned to advantage by his therapist as she indicated that Mr. R might wish to know others better if he felt comfortable with them and believed that they were interested in his welfare and respectful of his views. His therapist hoped that this formulation would encourage him to broaden his efforts in seeking out other friendships, but he proved unable to make this transition successfully.

At the beginning of the next summer, Mr. R began to make plans to return to live with his parents and reenroll in school. He revealed that he had begun to occasionally use Valium, which he purchased on the street near where he worked, in order to help him "relax." He was unwilling to consider other forms of medication, but did agree to consult with a physician after his move. He did not wish a referral to a psychotherapist, stating that he wanted his present therapist to be "my last therapist."

Mr. R carried out his plans to return to his parents' home and reenroll in school. Although his improvement was judged to be minimal, he did appear to find some relief in the reduction of his feelings of depression and his suicidal ideation and, at least with his therapist, was able to demonstrate some slight improvement in his interpersonal functioning.

EXHIBIT 1

Area of Assessment	Clinical Examination	Psychological Examination
I. Symptoms/Diagnosis		
Paranoid personality disorder		
Unwarranted suspiciousness and mistrust		
—guardedness/ secretiveness	Provides few details of his experiences	Adheres closely to minimal test requirements
—hypervigilance	None	Dilated response times; much attention to detail
—overconcern with hidden motives	None	Preoccupied with what may be "hidden from view"
Hypersensitivity		
—inability to relax	Complains of constant tension	Tension and vigilance interfere with fluidity of performance
—exaggeraton of difficulties	His failure as a student could bring his life to an end	Humiliated by aspects of his initial performance and corrects them at the first opportunity
Restricted affectivity		
—appears unemotional	Avoids feelings or any emotional turmoil	Intellect and rationality are of great importance
—lacks a sense of humor	None	Avoids spontaneity and is unsettled by surprise
II. Personality Factors	None	Extremely limited capacity to tolerate and/or express affect
III. Cognitive Abilities	Above average intelligence	Superior intelligence but limited ability to put his abilities to use

AREA OF ASSESSMENT	CLINICAL EXAMINATION	PSYCHOLOGICAL EXAMINATION
IV. Psychodynamics	None	Experiences others as potentially threatening
V. Therapeutic Enabling Factors	Recognizes his difficulty	Conflict over putting his mistrust of others aside to develop a working alliance with his therapist
VI. Environmental Demand and Social Adjustment	Functions best with minimal interaction with others	Has little understanding of his own or others' motivations
	Long history of poor social adjustment	Social relationship skills are very impaired

EXHIBIT 2

WAIS-R SUMMARY

Verbal Subtests	*Scaled Score*
Information	10
Digit Span	13
Vocabulary	16
Arithmetic	11
Comprehension	14
Similarities	15

Performance Subtests	
Picture Completion	10
Picture Arrangement	8
Block Design	12
Object Assembly	10
Digit Symbol	9
Verbal IQ	130
Performance IQ	100
Full Scale IQ	120

RORSCHACH SUMMARY

Number of Responses	17
Rejections	1 (Card VI)
Populars	4
Originals	0
Average R/T Chromatic	48"
Average R/T Achromatic	25"
F%	59
F+%	73
A%	29
H%	47
W:M	8:5
M:Sum C	5:2.5
m:c	2:0
VIII-X%	47
FK+F+Fc%	65
(H+A):(Hd+Ad)	12:1

RORSCHACH SUMMARY

Apperception	W	47%
	D	41%
	d	0%
	Dd + S	12%

EXHIBIT 3

RORSCHACH SUMMARY

Response	*Inquiry*	*Scoring*

I. 1′6″

This is meaningless to me. I don't see very much. (*Try to see something.*)

1. Shape reminds me somewhat of a bat.	1. Whole thing. Not really shape of bat, but reminds me of it. (*Anything else?*) Not really.	WFAP
2. There might be a person in the middle.	2. In the middle—hands, legs down here. (*Person?*) Shape. (*Anything else?*) Not really. (*Male or female?*) Female. (*Female?*) The shape.	DFHP

II. 33″

1. I guess it looks like two— well there's . . . (*Laughs*) . . . two, I guess beings—not exactly human—opposite each other with red heads—hands touching, right and left I guess, like in an argument.	1. Here—head, hands. They have some sort of cloak on—some sort of covering with red splotches that the black doesn't totally cover. (*Argument?*) I guess the red makes it look that way. Their hands, what looks like hands, are together. The cues hidden from view are they are going to swing. There's sweat coming off their faces, those little dots.	WM.FC(H)P

RORSCHACH SUMMARY

Response	*Inquiry*	*Scoring*
2. And then there's this wing shape taking off in the middle—the white part like a space . . . I don't know if I should use that part. (*It's entirely up to you*).	2. Some sort of space ship, could be alive, I don't know. (*Space ship or animal?*) Guess space ship and exhaust is coming out. (*Where?*) Red part. (*Exhaust?*) That's where exhaust comes out of back and the color I guess. It's what makes it look like the space ship is going.	S(D)Fm.CF Obj,Fire

III. 40″

1. Okay to see upside down? (*Yes*) Looks like some sort of giant insect with the card upside down.	1. Forearms, legs I guess— raised like they're arms. (*Head, arms?*) Like a human insect—those black spots there. Just top, waist up. (*Looks like human insect?*) Yes, waist up. (*What makes it look like?*) The sort of sharp points at the ends of the arms and what I saw as eyes. (*Waist here and arms here?*) Well body here and curve starts here—not elbow I guess. Do you give cards in same orientation? (*Yes*)	WF-A/H

IV. 60″

1. Upside down I see some monster thing. I guess aquatic probably.	1. Head, eyes, horns. Rest of it, an ill defined shape. That's why it has to be aquatic. Couldn't fly.	WF(A)

Rorschach Summary

Response	Inquiry	Scoring
2. Some sort of relative of Bigfoot.	2. Feet, big tail, small arms, back of head—can see a spine down there. (*Spine?*) Just looks like it. (*Anything about blot?*) I don't know, just reminded me of a spine.	WF(A)

V. 11″

1. That looks like a bat—as soon as you took it out—of course upside down.	1. Shape. (*Anything else?*) Well—not really. (*Why upside down?*) Just the shape looked better to me that way.	WFAP

VI. 2′

I don't know, doesn't look like anything.

VII. 38″

1. Upside down looks like some sort of . . . like an alien dwarf with a rather large head.	1. Legs, arms, head—this whole thing is the body. A whole piece is missing from the center. Nothing quite like that on earth right now. (*Dwarf?*) Well, the hands and the arms are stubby, I guess.	W(S)F(H)

RORSCHACH SUMMARY

Response	*Inquiry*	*Scoring*

VIII. 52″

1. Sideways—there's some sort of body—would be feline—and head looks like a rodent—of course, there's a piece missing, but . . .

1. If the head wasn't like a rodent's it could be of the cat family—a feline. (*Feline?*) Way it was—looks. (*Rodent's head?*) Just does. Must be a reflection of it over here. (*Reflection?*) Maybe it's reflecting in the water. Got to be some sort of reflection for two images to appear like that. (*Any-thing else?*) No. That's it. Well, maybe because I see this water over here makes me think of a reflection.

DFA

2. The blue is water.

2. Just that it's blue like water.

DCF Water

3. Looking at it I also see a creature with a hideous grin.

3. Eyes, monstrous tongue, horns. Just the face, or I guess it could be part of it-could be hands here. The white looks like teeth. (*Tongue?*) Just this oval shape in here. (*Hideous?*) Just looks triangular and looks like . . . the way the head is shaped and this could be the rest of the body.

W(S)M(H)

IX. 64″

1. I guess this thing here looks like a rather pudgy baby.

1. Head, eyes, arms, legs. The size of the head in relation to the body. It's sitting down. Looks like it's not old enough to talk. (*Eyes?*) That's where they should be.

DMH, Obj.

Rorschach Summary

Response	*Inquiry*	*Scoring*
2. This middle thing looks like a figure holding a . . . some sort of a . . . something—the only thing that comes to mind that would be held like that is a hedge trimmer.	2. Looks like a separate figure from the infant. The head here. (*Trimmers?*) It looks like it's holding something—some kind of tool. Hedge trimmers just came to mind. That's all.	DMH,Obj.
3. Third thing looks like a figure that is falling down holding something.	3. The round bottom made it look like those things kids punch that fall down and come up. They shape them in figures like clowns and things. This is some kind of figure like that. (*Holding something?*) An arm sticking out makes it seem like that.	DM.Fm,(H)
4. Of course, this could be water.	4. Just because symmetrical. It's sort of the form of a pool of water.	D(S)FWater
X. 50″		
1. Thing in the middle looks like a face.	1. White part—these are eyes—nose—here would be. (*Anything else?*) Not really.	dr(S)F-Hd

EXHIBIT 4

THEMATIC APPERCEPTION TEST

CARD 1   Okay a . . . I guess he was a, well he's feeling dismayed about practicing the violin. Later he gets over it and goes on to be a great violinist.

CARD 2   I guess this woman on the right is looking with some disdain at girl on the left who has some book. I guess she's going to school. She's thinking that she should be content to stay on the farm. Of course the girl feels differently and goes on to leave them all behind on the farm. (*Feel?*) Well she feels like she's doing the right thing.

CARD 4   Ah, I guess this guy's looking at some other female and she's tying to get him to look back at her. (*Who are they?*) A . . . husband and wife or boyfriend and girlfriend. (*Happens?*) I guess he finally turns around and they have some sort of fight, or quarrel, but she doesn't look like she would—as if she wants to quarrel—I don't know. They end up separating for a few weeks. (?) Well this guy looks like his eyes are really like, I don't know, looks like some, looks like he's like, I guess sort of stubborn. He doesn't like to be told what to do. He thinks his looking is insignificant and she's making a big deal out of it.

CARD 5   I guess this is a . . . I don't have to say what comes to mind? Just make up a story? (*Yes*) I guess I could say—that's a mother that's feeling sort of it's time to go to bed—looking in seeing the light on. (*Who?*) Children or child—whoever's playing the violin in the other picture. (*Happens?*) They go to bed.

CARD 8BM   I guess this guy in the foreground, he's thinking—that's his father—he's thinking that if the operation's not successful—of the responsibility he'll have to carry. That looks like a rifle or something there. Maybe he shot him. He wouldn't be there though. I don't know. (?) I guess the operation doesn't work and that's that. (*What operation?*) Can't tell. I just see a scalpel, that's all. He must have put the rifle there prominently for some reason. I mean the people who designed it. I guess they want me to think that or something. Guy looks like he has satisfaction on his face, now that I look at him.

CARD 12M   I guess this guy looks like he's dead or something . . . ah . . . ah . . . I don't think he's dead. His knee is lifted on the right side.

PARANOID PERSONALITY DISORDER

Mr. H, a 25-year-old, single male, had been living in his parents' house for the last year and a half. He was not employed during this time; in fact, he left the house on only two occasions for periods of an hour or two. Mr. H had returned home to live after working for two years as a proofreader, a job he took after dropping out of college during his sophomore year. He had done well during his freshman year getting straight As in an engineering program at an Ivy League university. However, he changed his major to philosophy and his grades had plummeted. He was finally forced to withdraw from school.

His family had little contact with him in the two years following his withdrawal from school and before his returning to live at home, but they were aware that he had developed an interest in "metaphysical sciences." This interest led Mr. H to "understand some things psychically which before I had only comprehended intellectually." Under the sway of this "understanding," he had called his parents, "sounding terrified," and they had told him he should come home.

During the first year of his returning home, he became progressively more isolated from his family. In the last few months before his admission, he was preoccupied with his need for "space." He communicated with his family exclusively by letter, noting that "my state of beingness at this time is such that I cannot harmoniously interact with anyone on a social level." His remonstrations to his family to recognize his need for complete physical isolation gradually took on more tyrannical overtones. He carefully observed the customary patterns of his family's movement and wrote out detailed schedules of their activities, which he expected them to follow, in order that there would be no chance of having to "physically interact" with them. He justified these schedules in long letters which he left for them about the house during the night. These letters spoke of his need to have "total and unrestrained access" to various areas in the house at specific times of day. His parents finally decided that he was in need of psychiatric attention and arranged for him to be admitted to the hospital.

Mr. H neither shared his parents' concern over his social isolation nor agreed with their suggestion that he be admitted for psychiatric evaluation and treatment. At the time of his admission, he presented his view of the situation as one in which his position was very much like that of "a political or ideological prisoner" in that he was forced to submit to the wishes of his parents who felt that they were acting on his behalf when the real issue was one of a fundamental disagreement over his personal freedom.

At the time of his admission, Mr. H was a tall, thin, pale young man with long hair and a long beard. His general appearance was disheveled, malodorous and unkempt. He described his mood as "fine" and his affect was noted to be flat and blunted. His speech was meticulous and precise and he clearly took some pleasure in using words, playing with their meanings and nuances, and seemed to be of superior intellectual ability. There were no abnormalities of attention, orientation, concentration, and memory noted during the mental status exam. He denied any present or past perceptual disturbances, including hallucinations, and gave no history of delusional thinking, suicidal or homicidal ideation. He evidenced significant impairment in his capacity for insight in that he was completely unaware that his behavior was in any way unusual. His judgment was grossly impaired in that he utterly failed to recognize the impact of his behavior on his family and had no idea of how they felt in response to his dictates regarding their use of their own home and restriction of their freedom.

DSM-III-R Diagnosis

Axis I: Rule out Schizophrenia, paranoid, unspecified
Axis II: Paranoid personality disorder
Axis III: Genital herpes, in remission
Axis IV: None—no obvious psychosocial stressor in the last year
Axis V: Grossly impaired—marked impairment in all areas of functioning—does not leave the house, is not employed, and avoids all social contact with his family.

Treatment and Hospital Course

Although Mr. H did not feel his admission was in any way warranted and he was admitted involuntarily, he made no attempt to petition for his release from the hospital. In fact, during his first month, he became much less reclusive than he had been at home and began to socialize with the other patients and even made some friends. His hygiene improved and he regularly attended his individual and group psychotherapy sessions which he seemed to enjoy.

During this period of evaluation, he was not begun on any medication. His psychiatrist wished to conduct the initial evaluation prior to beginning pharmacological treatment. At the time of his admission, his diagnosis was somewhat in doubt. His history revealed no clear evidence that he had any positive psychotic symptoms such as hallucinations or delusions. However, there had been a clear decline in his functioning since his late adolescence and possibly some transient disturbance in his sense of reality, related to hallucinogen abuse during his two years away from home and college.

Throughout his precollege years, he had been an extremely good student and graduated from a prep school where he was an active participant in an intramural athletics program and generally well liked by his peers. He portrayed this period of his life as significant in that until he had been sent to prep school by his father, he felt he had been merely an extension of his parents, conforming to their expectations rather than developing his own philosophy of life.

There was no history of psychiatric disorder in Mr. H's immediate family other than some occasional alcohol abuse on the part of the mother. Her father had died under somewhat questionable circumstances, a possible suicide, about one year after the death of his wife. Possibly he had suffered from a late-life depression in the context of his wife's death. Mr. H's paternal grandfather had also been a heavy drinker, an unusual behavior pattern for Jewish men of his generation. His family history, therefore, might give some reason to suspect a possible depressive illness.

Psychological Assessment

Considering the available information, Mr. H's treatment team was unable to arrive at a clear formulation of his diagnosis. His history of declining and, finally, grossly impaired functioning suggested a schizophrenic illness; however, there was no period of frankly psychotic symptomatology that had been observed or reported. His family history suggested the possibility of an affective disorder; however, no persistent disturbance in mood was seen and no associated features of a major affective disturbance were evident. Consequently, he was referred for psychological testing in the second week of his hospital stay, with a request for help in the differential diagnosis of a schizophrenic or affective disorder so that proper pharmacological treatment could begin. The psychologist administered the WAIS-R, Rorschach, TAT, SCT, and Bender Gestalt in order to address the diagnostic differential.

Consistent with the impression of his intellectual abilities reported during the mental status exam, Mr. H achieved a full scale IQ of 134, a score in the very superior range of intellectual functioning. His verbal and performance IQs were 143 and 118, respectively. This discrepancy of 25 points between his verbal and performance IQs reflects a great deal of intertest scatter. His verbal scores were all in either the superior or very superior range of intellectual functioning, while his performance subscale scores ranged from average to very superior levels.

Mr. H's relative strengths were to be found on the *Digit Span, Vocabulary,*

Comprehension, and *Block Design* subscales; his comparative weaknesses were on the *Picture Completion, Picture Arrangement,* and *Digit Symbol* subscales. This pattern of subscale scores suggests an absence of anxiety (*Digit Span* and *Block Design*) and social withdrawal or disinterest (*Picture Arrangement* and *Information*) characteristic of a schizoid style of relatedness. Although he was cooperative with the examination, in an intellectually detached fashion, he repeatedly attempted to engage the examiner in a debate concerning the validity of psychological testing. On the other hand, he frequently asked the examiner to confirm the correctness of his responses.

Mr. H's Rorschach performance demonstrated the same absence of anxiety in that there were no shading or black/white contrast responses. His test performance was quite good, with an adequate number of total responses (24) and with seven of these offered in response to the chromatic cards. His form level and number of popular responses, both general measures of reality testing ability, were quite satisfactory (F + % = 86; P% = 33) and consistent with his intellectualized style and intellectual ability, he produced several human movement responses (six), all of good form. Although he produced a form- and movement-dominated record, there were also responses where color was used, although these responses were principally of the less mature CF variety, as for example on *card IX* where the green areas are described as "bushes" in front of the deer.

The comparative lack of affective integration implied by this response where the foliage serves to hide the deer was seen more prominently in his TAT responses. To *card 15,* a card which typically provokes a story with a theme of depression or isolation, he produced a story of "an older person, maybe 40s or 50s, who doesn't look very happy standing in a cemetery." He reported that the man feels a "kinship" with the people in the cemetery because he feels "alienated" from the world. However, in a peculiar turn of phrase, he went on to say that "He feels alienated from the world and people he comes in regular contact with and feels more in contact with people he lives with who don't understand him or her."

This TAT story was one example in the test record where Mr. H gave evidence of peculiar thinking. Other examples included the WAIS Comprehension subscale item requesting reasons for why many foods need to be cooked ("people prefer to denature the food") and the WAIS *Similarities* subscale item requesting why air and water are alike ("elements in the mystical sense"). On the Rorschach, he referred to the central white area of *card II* as the "negative image" and referred to *card VI* as "a leaf with maybe a dragonfly coming out of the top, or the leaf is lying over the bottom part of the dragonfly."

There were places in the test protocol, particularly the SCT, where the problem of "contacting" others was also specifically raised. His usual response to contact with others is to set himself in opposition to others' wishes or to react with a passive, but begrudging, compliance. For example, on the SCT, he noted that he used to feel he was held back by "my parents' restrictive influence." He completed the sentence stem *while he was speaking to me* with the phrase "I wasn't listening," and wrote that: *if I had my own way, I would* "do as I pleased"; *when he was completely on his own, he* "enjoyed his freedom"; *his greatest wish was* "to have more freedom"; *more than anything else, he needed* "to be free." Demands made by others were reported as annoying (e.g. *I was most annoyed when* "they wouldn't let me do what I wanted to do") and, as he noted, *taking orders* "is not my cup of tea."

In fact, there was little sense of who Mr. H is or what he thinks or feels about most things on the SCT. He himself remarked on this fact when he wrote a note at the end of the test explaining that "these sentences don't necessarily represent my true feelings or my beliefs. Some things represent my personal situation or feelings, while others are just completions of the sentence for lack of anything better to write." Such sentence completions as being ashamed that "I hurt that person," feeling guilty about "having done that," and feeling he could murder a man who "could do something like that," were examples of his guardedness about himself even as he alluded to there being something to be revealed.

Treatment Planning and Outcome

The examining psychologist did not feel that there were significant indications of either schizophrenic or affective disorder in Mr. H's test record. The preservation of basic reality testing ability and, occasional ideational peculiarities aside, the absence of any serious examples of thought disturbance served to rule out a schizophrenic disorder. The predominant affective tone and intellectualized approach of the record were more in keeping with guardedness, secretiveness, and emotional avoidance rather than with depression. His hypertrophy of identity development and his defensive reaction of separating himself as a step towards perhaps building a more cohesive sense of himself were offered by the examining psychologist as the central issues to be addressed in his treatment plan.

Mr. H was discharged from the hospital after a three-month stay. Towards the end of his stay, he explained his reclusiveness and generally guarded style as solutions to his personal insecurity: "First, I must secure my personal integrity against outside forces, then I can be creative. It's like this: people who don't have enough to eat can't be philosophers. First they've got to solve the food problem. It's the same with me. I've got to secure my own borders before I can expand."

Mr. H was discharged and returned to live with his parents where he quickly reestablished his old manner of living. His parents once again had him hospitalized and on this occasion, he was treated with neuroleptics in an effort to address a possible underlying psychotic process. He responded no better to this course of treatment than he had to his last. As before, he was discharged as unimproved and arrangements were made for him to reside in a halfway house rather than return to live with his parents.

EXHIBIT 1

AREA OF ASSESSMENT	CLINICAL EXAMINATION	PSYCHOLOGICAL EXAMINATION
I. Symptoms/Diagnosis		
Paranoid personality disorder		
Unwarranted suspiciousness and mistrust		
—guardedness/ secretiveness	Revealed little about himself	Carefully guarded his thoughts and feelings
—avoidance of blame	Acknowledged no responsibility for his parents' anger	Accepts no responsibility for his present circumstances
—loss of appreciation of context	Could not see how his behavior conflicted with the social reality of family living	Argues about the validity of tests; wants only to provide "what you are looking for"
Hypersensitivity		
—inability to relax	Could not relax sufficiently to sleep with others in the house	Inordinately vigilant; marked absence of anxiety
—readiness to counterattack	Tenacious in defense of his own "rights"; met all criticism with an assertion of these "rights"	Guards against attack.
Restricted affectivity		
—takes pride in being rational and unemotional	Avoids any discussion of feelings	Largely restricts himself to the obvious and commonplace; adequate reality testing
—appears cold and unemotional	Appears cold and unemotional	Endeavors to control his affectivity
II. Personality Factors	Primary interest is in avoiding all anxiety	When emotionally aroused, he adopts an air of intellectual detachment

AREA OF ASSESSMENT	CLINICAL EXAMINATION	PSYCHOLOGICAL EXAMINATION
III. Cognitive Abilities	Above average intelligence	Superior intellectual abilities
IV. Psychodynamics	None	Severe identity disturbance, emphasizes boundaries with others, noncompliant with authority and avoids intimacy
V. Therapeutic Enabling Factors	Receptive to supportive efforts to allay anxiety	Reality appreciation is largely intact; occasional idiosyncratic thinking
	Passively cooperative with treatment if his "rights" are respected	None
VI. Environmental Demand and Social Adjustment	Emphasizes need for social withdrawal	Could perhaps function in a highly structured setting with minimal social contact
	Assumes no responsibility for self-care	None
	No externally directed ambitions	None

E X H I B I T   2

WAIS-R Summary

Verbal Subtests	Scaled Score
Information	13
Digit Span	193
Vocabulary	16
Arithmetic	14
Comprehension	16
Similarities	14

Performance Tests	
Picture Completion	11
Picture Arrangement	11
Block Design	19
Object Assembly	12
Digit Symbol	13
Performance Score	63

Verbal IQ	143
Performance IQ	118
Full Scale IQ	134

Rorschach Summary

Number of Responses	24
Rejections	0
Populars	8
Originals	0
Average R/T Chromatic	6″
Average R/T Achromatic	6″
F%	46
F + %	86
A%	33
H%	33
W:M	6.6
M:Sum C	6:2.5
m:c	4.1
VIII-X%	29
FK + F + Fc%	46
(H + A):(Hd + Ad)	15:1

RORSCHACH SUMMARY

Apperception	W	25%
	D	67%
	d	0%
	Dd + S	8%

E X H I B I T   3

RORSCHACH SUMMARY

Response	*Inquiry*	*Scoring*
I. 2″		
1. Looks like two people dancing.	1. Arms swinging out of each—like holding in the middle and sort of swinging around.	WMH
2. It looks like a person in the middle with arms raised up,	2. Arms up here reaching up like this.	DMHP
3. and two Christmas trees on the side.	3. You know how when you draw a Christmas tree, it looks like (*Demonstrates*), well that did too. (*Anything else?*) Just the angular up and out.	DF-Nat.
II. 3″		
1. Two people touching at the hand and at the knee and leg.	1. Head, arms, legs, and knees touching, touching from knee down.	WMHP
2. If you like—imagine it looks like a plane or jet	2. Some sort of flying object with pointed front wings and jet blast and	SFmObj
3. with rocket blast, pointed out at bottom.	3. redness coming out the back.	DCF.mF Fire
That's it. There are 10? Are the same cards used all over the world?		
III. 1″		
1. Two people holding something between them	1. Looks like two women here. There are their breasts.	DMHP
2. which might look like a large crab. Two females	2. (*Crab?*) Shaped like a crab and two things coming out like that could sort of be claws.	DFA

Rorschach Summary

Response	Inquiry	Scoring
3. with a big bowtie in the middle. (?) Have nothing to do with each other, but part of the same picture.	3. (*Bowtie?*) The shape.	DFClothP
4. This could also be a big butterfly.	4. Same part looks like a butterfly—the shape. Doesn't make sense. Doesn't fit in logically but if you take it in and of itself, piece by piece, it looks like that.	DFAP
5. And these could be two lamps here.	5. It's on a cord. The redness represents illumination relative to the blackness of the rest.	DFC-symObj

IV. 2″

1. A man with a jackhammer. Being taken from right down in front of feet and he's holding something in front of him that goes down to the ground. Shape of a jackhammer.	1. Like you are looking up, two feet, head, and feet much larger. Idea of perspective and this thing looks like a jackhammer	WMH,Obj
2. A man on a motorcycle. Taken from in front of the man, looking up.	2. Same man on a motorcycle. This is the front wheel and this is the handlebar.	WFH,Obj

V. 3″

1. Some sort of butterfly or moth.	1. The shape.	WFAP

VI. 22″

Doesn't look like anything much.

1. A leaf	1. The outline of a leaf, sort of a maple leaf.	DFPl

RORSCHACH SUMMARY

Response	*Inquiry*	*Scoring*
2. with maybe a dragonfly coming out of the top, or leaf is lying over the bottom part of the dragonfly	2. and this looks like a head. (*Coming out of top?*) Kind of merged into one, like no division between them. Then it looks like the back of the dragonfly is lying on top of a leaf. If you consider the dark part a continuation of the dragonfly. (*Kind of merged into one? I'm not sure what you mean?*) Visually, it looks like that—not realistic. Looks *as if*—it's an abstract picture. Looks like no separation between the two.	DFMA

VII. 3″

1. Two Indian squaws' grandmother's dancing.	1. This would be hand coming out. The dancing. The reason I say dancing people, a lot of these, it's the symmetry. It looks like a grandmother cause of the facial character from the sides and cause hair on the side seems like something I've seen on older ladies, maybe on TV. Reminds me of a grandmother type.	WMHP *Peculiar verbalization*

VIII. 15″

1. Two animals, I don't know what type, polar bears, or anything, four-legged, could be a bear,	1. The shape of them looks like they're stepping off a rock.	DFMAP

RORSCHACH SUMMARY

Response	*Inquiry*	*Scoring*
2. with one foot on a rock. The rest doesn't look like anything to me.	2. The jagged edges and solidness of it. (*Solidness?*) Aside from jaggedness it looks like a big thing. Craggy. (*Craggy?*) The indent on the side looks broken off, the way rocks look at times.	DCFN
IX. 8″		
1. Two deer or antelope	1. The rounded rump and horns.	DFA
2. with a bush in front of each one	2. Green, and relative to the antelope on the ground level. See, it's undefined, amorphous.	DCFPl
3. Not related, it looks like a nose with two nostrils.	3. Shape	D(S)F-Hd
X. 2″		
1. Insects, or close-up of insects or bugs, or microscopic creatures you might see in a sample of pond water.	1. These two things and these in here. Microscopic cause don't look like any insect I'm familiar with. I'd say microscopic cause I remember biology and looking at creatures you see in pond water.	drFA
2. Maybe a couple of spiders down below.	2. Shape of body and legs coming out.	DFA

E X H I B I T   4

THEMATIC APPERCEPTION TEST

CARD 1   There is a boy looking at a violin. He doesn't want to practice but his Mom wants him to. He's looking bummed out. (?) He will reluctantly pick up the violin, practice for a little bit, just as long as he can to satisfy his Mom, leave, and go off to do what he wants.

CARD 3BM   There is a person, perhaps a female, who seems quite sad about something and is sitting on the floor holding her head on her arm upon a couch and there is something on the ground by her. I can't tell what it is. It looks sort of like a gun. That's it. (?) After a while, she gets over her misery and she'll get up and go around in her normal way. Pain and sorrow won't go away immediately, that will take a longer time. The worst is over and she will be able to function in her normal way.

CARD 4   There's this guy, a handsome movie star like Clark Gable, without a moustache, in the 30s. There's this lady, an attractive movie-star-type lady, movie stars of the 50s perhaps. And he looks like he's going to go somewhere—determination in his eyes, his mind set. And she doesn't want him to go. She is holding onto him and looking at him. (?) He's saying he's going to go and he'll go.

CARD 15   There is a man, at least it looks like a man, I think. Then again, it could be a female. An older person, maybe 40s-50s. Doesn't look very happy. Standing in a cemetery. Perhaps he is depressed and gets solace from being in a cemetery in the sense that perhaps he feels a similarity or a kinship with the people. It's hard to phrase this, because it represents how he is feeling inside. He feels alienated from the world and the people he comes in regular contact with and he feels more in contact with the people he lives with who don't understand him or her.

EXHIBIT 5

SENTENCE COMPLETION TEST

1. *When he was completely on his own, he* "enjoyed his freedom."
6. *I used to feel I was being held back by* "my parents' restrictive influence."
9. *My father always* "hassles me."
19. *I was most annoyed when* "they wouldn't let me do what I wanted to do."
24. *When I think back, I am ashamed that* "I hurt that person."
29. *His greatest wish was* "to have more freedom."
36. *Taking orders* "is not my cup of tea."
37. *If I had my way, I would* "do as I pleased."
55. *He felt he could murder a man who* "could do something like that."
59. *While he was speaking to me I* "wasn't listening."
69. *I feel guilty about* "having done that."
83. *More than anything else, he needed* "to be free."

DISCUSSION

Mr. R was a young, single, black male who readily admitted to his shyness, an inability to make friends, and a fear of eye contact. His lack of a trusting therapeutic relationship with an outpatient therapist was climaxed by his responding only on inquiry, and in a rather bland way, that he was returning to his parents' home and saying goodbye to his mother before killing himself. This is precisely the type of clinical situation where one would be struck by both the guardedness and the untrustful relationship with the patient and the fear that there is much more serious pathology than meets the eye.

The first positive result of the testing is the relatively high IQ of this young man with a full scale IQ of 120. Secondly, and quite importantly, reality testing seemed adequate as reflected in accurate and popular perceptions on the Rorschach. His long reaction times are quite consistent with a pervasive sense of mistrust and screening of what he reveals about himself. This same pervasive need to not reveal was manifested in his TAT stories where he does little more than simply describe the details on the cards. It was only in a task that demanded his total creativity, the DAP, that we obtain some glimpse of his internal perceptions. He revealed a somewhat chilling one of robot-like human interactions characterized by thought and little or no feeling.

In comparison to Mr. R, Mr. H, a younger, 23-year-old male, seems more dependent upon his home base, more isolated, and more overtly involved in unusual ideas approaching schizotypal proportions. Upon admission to the hospital, he was in more overt conflict with others—in this case his parents—describing himself and his object representational world as akin to that of an ideological prisoner being forced to submit to hostile and intolerant others.

As with Mr. R, the treatment team raised questions as to whether or not Mr. H's presentation hid more pathological symptomatology, in this case a question of schizophrenic symptomatology, than appeared at the suspicious surface. Like Mr. R, Mr. H is an extremely bright young man with a full scale IQ of 134. Again, like Mr. R, his Rorschach protocol, which was more extensive than that of Mr. R, showed some idiosyncratic associations, but an absence of severe thought disorder and generally adequate reality testing. In his TAT stories, he articulated his sense of alienation from others. In fact, his TAT productions portrayed a core theme of meeting contact with others by setting himself in opposition with passive but begrudging compliance. His own verbalizations suggest that this way of relating to others is correlated with a profound sense of a need to shore up his own identity and integrity at the expense of pushing others away.

B. BORDERLINE PERSONALITY DISORDERS

The history of the borderline personality disorder concept is a long and torturous one. However, with the introduction of DSM-III, explicit and relatively behavioral criteria were consensually chosen, thus enabling clinicians to communicate reliably about patients who meet these criteria. The borderline patient as described in DSM-III-R is characterized by the relatively enduring traits of identity disturbance, labile moods, unstable and intense interpersonal relationships involving idealization and devaluation, impulsive and self-destructive acting out in the areas of sexuality, drug abuse, shoplifting, inappropriate and intense anger or lack of control of anger, and intolerance of being alone. These patients generally do not get hospitalized for stable and enduring "borderline" traits, but rather for acute events, such as suicide attempts and/or severe depressive episodes.

BORDERLINE PERSONALITY DISORDER

For the last two years, Ms. J, a serious student of music, has been unable to pursue her career plans because of several psychiatric hospitalizations. Her difficulties began almost three years ago, when she was 17, during her senior year in high school. She was intensively preparing for a series of orchestral auditions. She lost weight, in part intentionally, and spent all her spare time at a local recital hall where she had worked since she was 13. Her academic performance declined, she withdrew from her friends and family, and she began to cut her classes to have more time to practice. She began to abuse amphetamines in order to give her the energy she needed to practice several hours each day. Her auditions went well, but her family and her music teacher became concerned about her weight and encouraged her to seek psychiatric help.

She did consult a psychiatrist and her weight stabilized. She was able to spend the summer after graduation from high school touring with a chamber music group, but she could not eat regularly. When she was able to eat, she experienced frightening feelings of someone dying. She continued to lose weight and by the late winter her weight had dropped 23 pounds to 77 pounds. She was severely emaciated. She was hospitalized for three months and regained 18 pounds. One month later, she had lost nine pounds and, discouraged with her progress, she made a serious suicide attempt, resulting in coma and a second hospitalization.

After being discharged, she reported that she was very depressed and constantly preoccupied with thoughts about food and her weight. She also experienced several intense and protracted episodes of depersonalization and again attempted to take her life. She was found comatose the next morning by her roommate and rehospitalized. Despite a course of ECT and treatment with several antidepressants, she continued to feel depressed and began to cut herself. She was now plagued with obsessions about food and developed several compulsive rituals to ward off her feelings of depression and depersonalization. While in the hospital, she made a serious suicide attempt by severing the arteries in both arms. After this attempt, her family demanded a transfer to another hospital. They were thoroughly discouraged with her lack of progress and angry at her hospital psychotherapist whom Ms. J claimed had taken to referring to her as "Miss Frankenstein" because of the prominent sutures on both her forearms required to close the deep wounds left from her suicide attempt.

At the time of her admission, she was described as an attractive, petite young woman with partially healed, but nevertheless noticeable, scars on both forearms. Although she was cooperative with the interview, she was disdainful in her attitude, especially on learning that she would not be treated by the hospital's senior psychiatrists. She spoke in a droning monotone and claimed to have no active suicide plans at present although she expressed a strong wish to die. She described her mood as "okay" now. The examining psychiatrist noted no disturbances in attention, concentration, memory, or other intellectual functions. She could give no reason for requesting admission other than to state that because of her failure to improve at the previous hospital, she was requesting admission "because I have to." She was accompanied on admission by her mother, who corroborated her history.

DSM-III-R Diagnosis

Axis I:	Major depression, recurrent, with psychosis
	Obsessive compulsive disorder
Axis II:	Borderline personality disorder (Primary diagnosis)
Axis III:	None
Axis IV:	Severe—graduation from high school; repeated psychiatric hospitalizations
Axis V:	Very poor—marked impairment in both social relations and occupational functioning

Treatment and Hospital Course

Although Ms. J's obvious disturbances in appetite, weight, and mood regulation had resulted in previous diagnoses of anorexia and major depressive disorder, the progression of her illness and her failure to respond to previous treatments had led to the impression of severe character disorder as the primary psychiatric difficulty.

She was admitted to the hospital and immediately gave notice of wanting to leave. She was informed that the hospital staff felt very strongly that she was a danger to herself and, if necessary, would take her to court and request that she be retained in the hospital against her wishes. She retracted her notice, but remained sullen and unwilling to engage actively in her treatment. Thus, the first weeks were taken up with gathering a history from her and her family and obtaining the records from her previous hospitalizations and outpatient therapists.

Ms. J and her family, including her two older sisters, had little to contribute to helping the hospital staff to understand her difficulties. For her family, the onset of her difficulties was a great surprise. She was described by them as a happy child who made friends easily, was active socially, did reasonably well academically, and excelled at music, which she loved. She had taken up music at age four and her mother had been a constant source of encouragement and support since then. As her interest in music had grown, her attachment to her teacher had grown as well; in between hospitalizations, she had been living alternately with her teacher and her family.

Although the family could find no reasons for Ms. J's difficulties, her family history was interesting on two accounts. First, there was a great deal of psychiatric illness on both the paternal and maternal sides of the family. A paternal cousin and a maternal great-uncle had both committed suicide; a paternal aunt and the patient's mother had made suicide attempts, with her mother's attempt occurring when Ms. J was 8 years old and after her father had learned of Mrs. J's extramarital affair from Mrs. J's "close friend." A maternal great-aunt and a maternal great-uncle were psychiatrically hospitalized for bipolar disorder and "homicidal tendencies," respectively.

Secondly, Ms. J and her mother bore a close physical resemblance to one another and it became quite clear that Ms. J's success in music was of immense gratification to Mrs. J, who had wanted to become a musician herself but instead married Mr. J when she found herself pregnant. At that time they had moved in with her husband's parents where they remained until their daughter's graduation from high school. Mrs. J found this living arrangement convenient as Mr. J's mother was "sickly" and she devoted a great deal of time to caring for her. She found taking care of her mother-in-law draining but gratifying as she and her husband fought a good deal and did not seem to have a particularly close or gratifying marital relationship.

Ms. J provided little information about herself except to make it clear that she felt no one "really cared" about her and she was convinced that she would be better off dead. The records of her previous treatment made it clear that it would be difficult to engage her in psychotherapy. She previously had stated quite clearly that her illness gave her a special status that mobilized the concern of others and she was adamant in her wish to retain her special status at whatever risk to herself.

Psychological Assessment

Ms. J had been extensively assessed by the psychology staff during her previous psychiatric hospitalizations. Overall, she was found to be of average intelligence, but with cognitive inefficiencies evident in her inability to execute planful activity and a diminished ability to benefit from task-derived feedback. The possibility of frontal lobe dysfunction was raised but finally ruled out because of the absence of confirmatory neurological findings and the presence of profound depression. The presence of psychomotor retardation, a listless, apathetic and indifferent attitude towards the examination, difficulties in concentration, and profound hopelessness about the future were felt to be the primary factors compromising her performance and best understood in the context of her depressive disorder. The final summary suggested a diagnosis of major depression in the context of a borderline personality disorder.

Her present psychological examination was carried out three weeks after her admission and two months after her previous examination. She was given the WAIS-R, MMPI, SCT, and Benton Visual Retention tests to help in establishing her diagnosis and in determining her capacity to profit from an intensive exploratory psychotherapy. The examiner also administered the Rorschach, which Ms. J initially refused to take, but subsequently completed.

Her present intellectual functioning was in the average range, with full-scale, verbal and performance IQs of 90, 85 and 100, respectively. Her sub-scale scores indicated a significant amount of intertest scatter, ranging from borderline to high average levels of intelligence. Her relative strengths were on those subtests where her performance could be enhanced by careful attention to details of the test materials. Her relative weaknesses were on those subtests which required her to make use of previously learned information, particularly as it applied to conducting conventional social relationships. Her performance on the WAIS-R was marred by her inability to expend any effort in those instances where she could not immediately find the correct answer. As a consequence, there was a significant amount of intratest scatter in the majority of her subtests.

Her WAIS-R performance was consistent with a profound depressive disturbance and her symptomatic presentation on the MMPI also revealed significant affective disturbance. Two of the clinical scales were extremely elevated (*scales 2* and *8* > 90) and three additional clinical scales were sufficiently elevated to warrant clinical attention (*scales 3, 4* and *1* > 70). Her main symptomatic difficulties included depression, alterations in her sense of reality, emotional disorganization and lability, and difficulties in impulse control. The severity of her disturbance is clearly evident on examination of her SCT. Ms. J reports that *most of all I want* "to be dead," that *I felt most dissatisfied when* "I didn't die," and that *I feel happiest when* "I think I'm going to die." That her entrenched desire to be dead is related to her affective state is clearly attested to when she notes that *I was most depressed when* "I tried to kill myself" and *I am afraid of* "feeling."

While her self-directed aggression seems clearly related to her affective state, it seems rooted in her relationship with her mother. In her previous psychological examination, she was given the TAT and told a story of a desperate young woman who commits suicide. Yet from the organization of the story it was clear that the focus of the story was not on the suicide itself, but rather on the impact of the young woman's death on the mother. The SCT from the current examination included her observation that *when with her mother, she felt* "as if she had to put on an act about how she was feeling." Her mother is described as someone who always "tries to make everyone happy," but she does not see her mother as a happy person (e.g. *I wish that my mother* "was happy.").

It would appear that Ms. J feels herself caught between living her life in a way that would satisfy and please her mother or, instead, leading a more independent and perhaps less gratifying life. Her wish to please her mother shows up in her acknowledgment that as a child her greatest fear was "not being able to play as well as my cousin" and expresses her pride that "she could play well," although not as well as her cousin (i.e. *she felt inferior when* "she accompanied her cousin"). Her ambivalence about her music is made evident when she asserts that *she often wished she could* "be a dancer."

Choosing an alternative career is one avenue of independence from her mother and her family. A second avenue that might help to shore up her identity would be a man. Ms. J feels that *most women* "behave according to what their man says" and she feels that *she couldn't succeed unless* "she had him standing by her side." What sort of man to choose, however, seems to be a problem. Someone like her father would appear to be a poor choice since she feels "uncomfortable" around him and "disappointed" in him generally. Additional difficulties seem likely to crop up as well. Although *more than anything else, she needed* "to know she was loved," she feels that *most marriages* "end in divorce" and that *most people are* "very self-centered." Perhaps this explains why she finds it very difficult to actually carry through with the compliant and obedient posture that would earn her the love she so desperately seeks (e.g. *taking orders* "makes me angry" and *I dislike to* "be told what to do").

Based on the examination of these results, the diagnostic picture which emerged seemed most consistent with a major affective disorder in the context of severe borderline personality disorder. Additionally, there were strong narcissistic and antisocial elements present in the test findings.

Treatment Plan and Outcome

Ms. J's treatment plan was developed with three treatment goals in mind. First, given her initial level of cognitive disorganization and lack of enthusiasm for the hospitalization, her individual psychotherapy and milieu management would focus on establishing a supportive relationship within the context of appropriate limits on self-destructive behavior. Subsequently, she and her parents would be involved in family therapy, with both her individual psychotherapist and a family therapist sharing responsibility for the treatment. This stage of her treatment was planned to help her and her family to effect a productive separation and to develop mutually satisfying means of supporting one another while working towards this goal. Finally, Ms. J's individual psychotherapy would then be developed along more exploratory lines as it became evident that she was better able to monitor her own affective state and could tolerate a more intensive examination of her own motivations and goals.

The first stage of this plan occupied the first five months of Ms. J's two-year hospitalization. During these months, she continually complained that the hospital staff were unresponsive to her needs and emotionally unavailable to her. She frequently became enraged and attempted to harm herself, which required the staff to intervene in order to protect her. She evaded her staff escort while away from the hospital for an optometrist's appointment and purchased a number of over-the-counter medications which she used in an attempt to kill herself. Medical attention was mobilized by a passerby. Following the attempt, she revealed that she had planned it weeks in advance and felt no remorse. She had wanted to express how angry she felt with the hospital staff for "being too professional with me."

Following this attempt, Ms. J reported a marked reduction in her feeling of anxiety and tension and also diminished suicidal ideation. Her obsessive ruminations regarding food and eating and their relationships with death, nightmares with violent themes and a recurrence of episodes of depersonalization all offered opportunities for interventions which she experienced as helpful. She was given a regular program of activities off the unit and expressed some feelings of pleasure in participating in them.

Her family work began shortly after this with an initial focus on her role in the family. It quickly became clear that Ms. J had always been an emotional support for her mother who treated her more as a close friend and confidant than as a child. Her mother frequently turned to her for comfort and friendship to compensate for Mr. J's perceived unavailability. Mr. J was portrayed by Ms. J and her mother as "tyrannical," but on closer examination, neither she nor her mother could provide any convincing examples of his tyranny. The myth of Mr. J's unavailability was apparently largely propagated by the mother and believed by Ms. J; the two women had for years operated their own closed emotional system, leaving Mr. J to fend for himself.

As this became clearer to Ms. J and her family, Mr. J began to look forward to the family sessions as they provided his only avenue for an emotional engagement with his wife and daughter. Mrs. J began to develop a closer relationship to her husband, but was fearful of acknowledging this to her daughter for fear that it would "hurt" her. In a complementary fashion, Ms. J came to the conclusion, after taking a pass for the weekend to her parents' home, that returning to live at home would not be good for her. After informing her parents of her decision, she worried that she had "deeply hurt" her mother.

Neither mother nor daughter were able to address in the family sessions their fears of hurting one another. Instead, they both successfully managed to engage the hospital staff in rushing ahead with plans for Ms. J's discharge. The staff was anxious to capitalize on Ms. J's apparent improvement and to avoid the anticipated disruption which would ensue in a few weeks as her individual therapist, to whom she had become quite attached, would be leaving the hospital and would be unable to continue working with her.

In this context, two months after beginning the family therapy, Ms. J made another suicide attempt. Allowed to attend off-unit activities without a staff escort, she had signed out to a scheduled activity and gone instead into town, bought several cleaning products, and ingested them. She later reported that after ingesting the cleaning products, she realized that she had not wanted to die but only to relieve her anxiety and dysphoria, and so had called the hospital. Discharge plans were suspended. She was transferred to a new therapist and her family work continued.

For the next year, Ms. J's hospital course was characterized by her struggle to achieve an effective separation. Although progress was made by both her and her mother in expressing their guilt and anxiety about such a separation, Ms. J did not seem ready to actually proceed with her discharge plans. She was transferred to another inpatient unit where she could continue to work with her current hospital psychotherapist. Although initially agreeable to the transfer, she quickly began to idealize the treatment staff of her former unit despite her earlier and continued devaluation of them prior to her transfer, and to devalue the treatment staff of her new unit. Her family became alarmed at her renewed anger and dysphoria and encouraged her to leave the hospital against the advice of the hospital staff. Ultimately, the family was persuaded of the need for continued hospitalization but, as they had previously done with her transfer to the present hospital, insisted that her treatment be continued at a different hospital.

EXHIBIT 1

AREA OF ASSESSMENT	CLINICAL EXAMINATION	PSYCHOLOGICAL EXAMINATION
I. Symptoms/Diagnosis		
Borderline personality disorder		
Two unpredictable or impulsive and potentially self-damaging behaviors		Prefers action-oriented problem solving; poor impulse control
—substance use	Amphetamine abuse	
—self-injury	Mutilated forearms	
Unstable and intense interpersonal relationships	Rapid shifts in relationships with treatment providers	Easily feels exploited and used by others
Lack of control of anger	Easily angered and then inflicts self-injury	None
Identity disturbance	Uncertain career choice and uncertain family loyalty	Relies on others for self-definition and direction
Affective instability	Marked emotional lability	Prone to emotional over-reaction
Intolerance of being alone	Feels desperate and empty when alone	Depends on others' praise for emotional gratification
Self-mutilation and suicide gestures	4 suicide attempts—twice by overdose, twice by cutting	None
II. Personality Factors	Able to persevere to achieve long-term goals	None
III. Cognitive Abilities	None	Difficulty integrating feedback and sustaining goal orientation
IV. Psychodynamics	Symbiotic relationship with mother, with anger and resentment at fulfilling her mother's narcissistic needs	Ambivalent relationship with mother with death of self seen as only means of separation and individuation

AREA OF ASSESSMENT	CLINICAL EXAMINATION	PSYCHOLOGICAL EXAMINATION
V. Therapeutic Enabling Factors	None	None
VI. Environmental Demand and Social Adjustment	Highly reactive to environment	Relies on external appearances to fit in
	Dislikes rules and orders	Rebellious and obstinate
	Aware of secondary gain from her disruptive behavior	Risks her life to get others to care for her

EXHIBIT 2

WAIS-R Summary

Verbal Subtests	Scaled Score
Information	6
Digit Span	12
Vocabulary	6
Arithmetic	7
Comprehension	5
Similarities	9

Performance Tests

Picture Completion	12
Picture Arrangement	12
Block Design	10
Object Assembly	10
Digit Symbol	8
Verbal IQ	85
Performance IQ	100
Full Scale IQ	90

MMPI Summary

F'LK: 28*34"1'7069-5

Rorschach Summary

Number of Responses	20
Rejections	0
Populars	9
Originals	1
Average R/T Chromatic	18
Average R/T Achromatic	21
F%	70
F+%	89
A%	55
H%	20
W:M	3:1
M:sum C	1:1.5
m:c	3:1
VIII-X%	30

Rorschach Summary

FK + F + Fc%		70
(H + A):(Hd + Ad)		12:3
Apperception	W	15%
	D	70%
	d	5%
	Dd + S	10%

EXHIBIT 3

RORSCHACH SUMMARY

Response	*Inquiry*	*Scoring*
I. 7″		
1. The whole thing reminds me of a butterfly.	1. The whole thing. (*Butterfly?*) I don't know, it just did. Shaped like a butterfly, like it had wings and a body in the middle.	WFAP
2. I see like a body from the back.	2. Right in the middle, with hands and feet. (*Body?*) I don't know, it looked like it had feet. Like a body from the back, like looking at it from the back, with like two hands.	DFHP
That's it.		
II. 10″		
1. I see another butterfly	1. Right here, the red. (*Butterfly?*) Same thing as the other, like it had wings and like a body in the middle. (*Anything else?*) The color.	DFCAP
2. and a spaceship	2. The white. (*Spaceship?*) It was just sort of shaped like some sort of satellite, and like the red on the bottom made it look like it was taking off.	SFmObj
3. with fire coming out the bottom	3. (*Fire?*) Just because it is red. (*Anything else?*) No, that's all. Looks like flames burning.	DCF.mF Fire
4. and two animals. I don't know what kind of animals, but two animals.	4. This, the red, like an animal standing up on its back legs. (*Look like two animals?*) They had two legs, and standing on its back legs, like when a dog begs. Just reminds me of some animal, but I'm not sure what one.	DFMA

Rorschach Summary

Response	*Inquiry*	*Scoring*

III. 18"

1. I see two people facing each other. They look like they're almost like standing over a fire, like trying to warm their hands.

1. Right here. When they make these up, do they make them so you see a certain thing or just put ink on the page? (*Questions later.*) OK. (*People?*) A head and arms, and legs, and shoes. (*Fire?*) Right here. It doesn't really look like fire. It looks like smoke, but it looks like they're trying to warm their hands. (*Smoke?*) It looked like smoke to me, I don't know. (*Smoke?*) I don't know.

WM.KFH, SmokeP

That's all.

IV. 41"

1. I see two feet, two boots I guess.

1. Right here. (*Boots?*) It looked like it had feet and a heel. (*Anything else?*) No. (*Feet and a heel?*) Yes, like a foot and a heel, just like a boot.

DFClothP

2. Two ears, like of an animal. That's it.

2. Here. (*Ears?*) It looked like how animal ears flop down.

dF-Ad

V. 15"

1. Looks like a butterfly.

1. The whole thing. (*Butterfly?*) The same as the others; it looked like it had wings and a body in the middle. (*Anything else?*) Uh-uh.

WFAP

That's it.

RORSCHACH SUMMARY

Response	*Inquiry*	*Scoring*

VI. 26″

1. I see a cross with a body on it.

1. Right here. The body is that dark part in the middle, and it looked like it's got a cloth like hanging. (*Body?*) The dark area looked like an abstract body, like a head and a body but not, like not outlined, just an abstract. (*Cloth?*) Sometimes they hang a cloth on a cross, like a poncho type. (*Cloth?*) It was like light, and it was like white.

DFC′.H,Cloth

That's it.

VII. 19″

1. I see two heads, no four heads

1. One here, one here, one here, and one here. (*Four heads?*) Each of them looked like they had a nose and a mouth, and two of them had eyes. (*Only two had eyes?*) Yeah, and two to me looked like women

DFHd

2. and two looked like they were pigs to me. (*Look like pigs?*) Had a nose like a pig.

DF-Ad

3. and a butterfly.

3. Down at the bottom, right here. (*Butterfly?*) It had a body and wings.

DFA

VIII. 10″

1. I see two bears

1. Right here and right there. (*Bears?*) Just the shape of the body, like the head looked like the head of a bear, and it had like four legs.

DFAP

RORSCHACH SUMMARY

Response	*Inquiry*	*Scoring*
2. and like a backbone of a body, and like ribs	2. Here, and there's ribs here. Like it just looked like the inside of a body to me. (*Backbone and ribs?*) I don't know how to explain; it just looked like a backbone to me. (*Blot reminded you?*) Just that dark area looked like a backbone, looked like a backbone, that's all I can say.	di(s)FAt
That's it.		
IX. 35″		
1. The only thing I see is, I think they call it your pelvic bone. I'm not sure.	1. Blue, this whole thing right here. (*Pelvic bone?*) To me, like what I remember from books and stuff, like it seemed like it was sort of shaped the same way.	DFAt
X. 18″		
1. I see a lot of bugs, insects.	1. Blue, this looked sort of like a crab or a lobster. (*Crab or lobster?*) It just looked like it had a lot of legs and claws. (*Anything else?*) Uh-uh.	DFAP
	2. The black hue	DFA
	3. and the black up here is like some kind of bug, maybe like a roach or . . . I don't know, but they looked like bugs. (*Bugs?*) They looked like they had legs too, and antennas. (*Anything else?*) (*No.*)	DFA
	(*I noticed you sort of cringed when you described the crabs and bugs, what was your feeling?*) I see so many cockroaches on the unit. They make me cringe . . . I don't like them.	
That's it.		

E X H I B I T 4

SENTENCE COMPLETION TEST

2. *She often wished she could* "be a dancer."
7. *She felt proud that* "she could play well."
8. *As a child my greatest fear was* "not being able to play as well as my cousin."
12. *I was most depressed when* "I tried to kill myself."
36. *Taking orders* "makes me angry."
37. *I dislike to* "be told what to do."
39. *Most women* "behave according to what their man says."
44. *She felt she couldn't succeed unless* "she had him standing by her side."
52. *Most of all I want* "to be dead."
58. *Most marriages* "end in divorce."
60. *My mother always* "tries to make everyone happy."
70. *When my father came home, I* "was disappointed."
74. *I felt happiest when* "I think I'm going to die."
83. *More than anything else, she needed* "to know she was loved."
84. *Most people are* "very self-centered."
87. *I am afraid of* "feeling."
88. *When with her father she felt* "uncomfortable."
94. *When with her mother, she felt* "as if she had to put on an act about how she was feeling."
99. *I wish that my mother* was happy."

BORDERLINE PERSONALITY DISORDER

In the six months prior to her admission, Ms. W had been seen in psychiatric consultation on three previous occasions. Each of these consultations followed her report that she had been attacked by a black man. On the first occasion, she reported an attempted rape which she was able to thwart by assaulting her attacker. The second occasion involved her being held at gunpoint by her original attacker, who burned her with cigarettes and punched her after finding her alone at home. Finally, she subsequently reported a brief abduction by this same man, who proceeded to set fire to several of her stuffed animals and who threatened to do the same to her if she revealed the incident. At each consultation she acknowledged being emotionally upset by the incident, but her parents, strangely, found her unusually calm otherwise. After the first two incidents, she refused the psychiatrist's recommendation of additional consultations, stating that she was fine and could manage on her own. Following the third incident, the psychiatrist and her family convinced her to enter a local hospital to undergo further evaluation.

These events unfolded against a background of a seemingly well-adjusted, well-liked, and physically gifted 17-year-old girl who, prior to these events, had given no evidence of psychological difficulty. Although she was an indifferent student with average grades, she was active in school athletics and would have been elected captain of her high school district's women's athletic league had not hospitalization prevented her from returning to her senior year. She belonged to many different social groups and always had friends, although she admitted feeling close to no one. Two features of interest were noted in her personal and family history. One involved a suicide attempt by one of her older brothers two years prior to the onset of her difficulties and the other was a history of drug abuse in a younger sister. In her personal history, both sleepwalking and sleeptalking, which during childhood had been associated with "bad dreams," had persisted well into adolescence.

Ms. W came from an upper middle class background and had developed a pattern of drug abuse typical for her peer group. She used drugs occasionally, preferring stimulants such as cocaine and amphetamine to hallucinogens, and periodically used marijuana. Although she denied any history of drug use at the time of admission, routine urinalysis for drugs was carried out because of sudden behavior changes in the week prior to her admission. During the week, she had become increasingly hyperactive and irritable, with periods of restlessness and distraction alternating with periods of social withdrawal and despondency. She had begun to talk about taking her own life. No detectable level of drugs was found in her urine. During her hospitalization, her parents pressed for a clear diagnosis and rapid recovery. Becoming dissatisfied with their daughter's progress and unable to tolerate the ambiguity reflected in the hospital staff's formulation of their daughter's difficulties, they had her transferred to a large teaching hospital where they hoped she would receive a more thorough evaluation.

DSM-III-R Diagnosis

Axis I: Rule out Amphetamine delusional disorder
            Rule out Bipolar disorder, manic
Axis II: Borderline personality disorder
Axis III: None
Axis IV: Extreme—repeated physical and sexual abuse
Axis V: Good—slight impairment in social functioning, i.e. no close
            friends

Treatment and Hospital Course

At the time of her transfer to the teaching hospital, Ms. W presented as a thin, very well groomed girl who appeared to be the epitome of good health and clean-cut good looks. Her manner was somewhat cool and disdainful, leaving the interviewer with the impression of a maturity beyond her years. She stated that she had agreed to come to the hospital because "my doctor recommended it," but she had no complaint herself. She expected to be released after a brief period of evaluation since she did not see herself as being in need of any further treatment. Most remarkable was the bland manner in which she carefully recounted the details of her sexual and physical abuse.

As part of her evaluation, she was given a battery of psychological tests during the third week of her hospitalization. The results of her psychological examination were felt to support the treatment staff's clinical impression of Ms. W as attempting to present a tightly knit facade of mature functioning which masked significant emotional turmoil. Long-term inpatient treatment was recommended in order to confront her posture of denial and establish a treatment situation in which she could begin to address her underlying emotional distress. Upon being presented with this recommendation, Ms. W rather blandly accepted the offer of long-term hospitalization. In the months following, her facade began to crumble. As she revealed more of herself, she began to speak of a "dark side" to her personality which she had always kept concealed from others. Significant difficulties in managing sexual, aggressive, and depressive experiences became apparent and often led to periods of depersonalization and derealization during which she made frantic attempts to inflict injury on herself.

Psychological Assessment

Ms. W was given the WRAT, Bender Gestalt, Rorschach, TAT, and Object Sort Test shortly after admission. Because she had been given the WAIS only two months previously, this procedure was not repeated. However, the results were available and were incorporated into her evaluation. The examiner was asked to provide a diagnostic assessment, including an evaluation of possible residual effects of amphetamine abuse, and treatment recommendations.

Although Ms. W was generally cooperative with the examination, she expressed the fear that "testing will be used against me this time as well because if the tests don't come out good and the evaluation doesn't come out good, then I'm stuck here." Her efforts to control her anxiety over the outcome of the evaluation were expressed in an aloof, but superficially charming and flippant attitude towards the examination.

Her previous examination with the WAIS revealed a full-scale IQ of 116 with verbal and performance IQs of 114 and 116, respectively. Her scaled subtest scores ranged from average to very superior levels, indicating a moderate degree of intertest scatter and reflecting some intellectual inefficiency. Her performance on the WAIS was consistent with her lackadaisical attitude towards school, with her *Vocabulary* and *Information* subscale scores among the lowest. The results of the WRAT provided further support for this view as her achievement scores in reading, spelling, and arithmetic were all noticeably below the 12th grade level. Her knowledge of social conventions (WAIS *Comprehension* subscale) represented a relative strength consistent with her ability to make a good impression.

Her approach to the unstructured tests in the battery, the Rorschach and TAT, was characterized by rigid and virtually unrelieved attempts at avoidance, emotional withdrawal, and blatant denial. For example, seven of the 16 TAT cards administered resulted in stories in which the main character is tired, asleep or unaware. Her Rorschach protocol, consisting of only 14 percepts, is replete with efforts to avoid having to give any response, reflecting her fear that it will again be "used against" her to keep her in the hospital. When confronted about her attitude, she continued to avoid engaging with the test by reporting what she saw during her previous testing and remarking that "it doesn't look like that now."

Her rather transparent attempts to maintain an image of herself as a "nice girl" by denying the possibility of any negative feelings about herself or others raised questions about her potential for transient psychotic regressions under emotional stress. Her compulsive efforts to bring order and control to her experience were evident in such an emotionally undemanding task as the Bender. In copying the nine designs, she numbered each and drew a line down the lower middle of the page to separate the last two designs from the remainder. In the more emotionally demanding and less structured testing situation of the Rorschach, she attempts to control the experience and minimize its impact on herself by limiting the number of her percepts. However, despite her inhibiting efforts, she is unable to make a convincing presentation. Her percepts are often somewhat at odds with the consensual reality appraisal made by healthier individuals and suggest a rather fragile hold on reality.

The energy involved in warding off negative aspects of herself and of her experience served as a source of interference in her intellectual performance. She was at her best when she was able to keep an emotional distance from the test stimuli and from the examiner, especially when she felt she had engaged the examiner in viewing her as she would like to be seen. Thus, concern over her ability to tolerate a closer look at herself formed the basis for the recommendation for continuing her treatment in a structured inpatient setting. Her test results were seen as most consistent with a diagnosis of borderline personality disorder with narcissistic and paranoid features.

Ms. W was tested a second time, three years after the testing reported above. She was preparing for discharge and the examination was requested to assess the degree of change in her psychological functioning and to comment on those issues which remained to be addressed in her outpatient treatment. The examination consisted of a WAIS-R, Rorschach, TAT, and MMPI.

At the time of the second testing, she was functioning in the average range of intellectual ability with a full scale IQ of 109 and verbal and performance IQs of 96 and 127, respectively. Compared to her previous results, her full-scale IQ was five points lower, her verbal IQ 10 points lower and her performance IQ 11 points higher. These disparities represent sizable, but not uncommon, shifts in intellectual performance under the impact of an extended treatment intervention aimed at a major reorganization of personality dynamics. As before, the subscale scores ranged from Average to Very Superior. Among the verbal subtests, the most noticeable shifts (lower on second testing) are on the *Arithmetic* and *Comprehension* subtests. These shifts were interpreted as indicating that at that time emotional factors were having an impact on her ability to concentrate and, in other respects, problem-solve. Previously, her ability to ward off emotional factors had contributed to her higher scores. During the second testing, once she began making errors, she became distracted and preoccupied and had difficulty shifting her attention to new items. Additionally, she indicated that she had been considering correct responses but had withheld them because of her uncertainty.

On the projective tests, the weakening of her formerly rigid and compulsive defenses allowed the occasional eruption of fantasy material which she was struggling to master. The potential for depersonalization and derealization experiences when confronted with her own aggressive wishes was also mirrored in her performance. Such experiences would most likely occur in the context of loss where her guilt over such wishes was easily mobilized. Her efforts to master these feelings and incorporate them into a view of herself which she could accept remained tentative. She demonstrated abrupt shifts in affect, relied on disavowal and repudiation of such wishes when consciously recognized, and otherwise retreated into her former disdainful and devaluing stance. The latter posture, however, was less in evidence than formerly.

The overall impression of this examination, when contrasted with her previous examination, was of a young woman still having significant difficulty in establishing a well articulated self-definition. The availability of previously denied aspects of herself and the sporadic direction of her efforts to incorporate these aspects were seen as positive trends. These trends can be noted in two examples.

In the first test protocol, her response to *card II* of the Rorschach featured a response of "some kind of bottle" (central white space) from which some liquid (the upper and lower red areas) was seen as squirting or spilling. Her second testing produced a response to the same area, but was now reported as "a scary horror movie mask" with bloody eyes and a hole for the actor wearing the mask to breath through. Her former emphasis on emptiness and depletion has been replaced with a recognition of an inner life which is as yet poorly integrated, but nevertheless able to make contact with the surrounding world.

The second example is taken from the TAT, *card 3GF.* When first tested, she saw the young woman in the picture as having been injured when the wind blew a door against her face. Her second testing produced a story in which the young woman was seen as holding her head after awakening with a hangover. This shift from a disclaimed injury arising from adventitious circumstances to one which conveys a greater sense of personal involvement in the face of poor impulse control indicated the general trend towards acknowledgment of responsibility for her own behavior.

Treatment Planning and Outcome

The results of Ms. W's first examination focused the treatment staff's attention on her concealment of significant emotional turmoil and led to the recommendations of long-term hospitalization and intensive individual psychotherapy. As she was repeatedly confronted with the discrepancies between her self-reports and her behavior, she was forced to acknowledge aspects of herself which she had previously concealed from herself and others. This eventually provoked a severe behavioral regression associated with multiple episodes of attempted self-injury. When necessary, the hospital staff intervened to insure her physical safety but continued to insist that she explore the impact of her behavior on herself and others and assume responsibility for it.

Ms. W remained in the hospital for 3½ years, during which she repeatedly alternated between periods when she was able to assume her former posture of aloof maturity and other periods when she was engulfed by the "dark side" of her personality. Her efforts to reconcile these various aspects of herself were at the center of her psychotherapy and progress had been made at the time of discharge. She was better able to manage her destructive impulses and had given up her former drug abuse and self-mutilation. Her trust in others gradually increased and she finally admitted she had made up the attacks which had first brought her to psychiatric attention. She was able to complete high school and accumulated some college credit during her hospitalization.

The determination of the hospital staff to deal directly with her "dark side" without collaborating with her in its suppression and denial was instrumental in helping her learn to increase her trust in others and, ultimately, in herself. As a consequence, she made progress in being able to acknowledge and accommodate aspects of herself that had been disavowed completely. At the time of her discharge, significant difficulties in adaptively integrating these aspects remained, but the balance of forces had indeed shifted in favor of realistic efforts to address these difficulties in the context of a relationship on which she had come to rely and in which she had placed a great deal of trust. She was discharged to a structured living situation and continued outpatient treatment with her hospital psychotherapist.

EXHIBIT 1

AREA OF ASSESSMENT	CLINICAL EXAMINATION	PSYCHOLOGICAL EXAMINATION
I. Symptoms/Diagnosis		
Borderline personality disorder		
Two unpredictable or impulsive and potentially self-damaging behaviors		
—substance use	Stimulant and marijuana use	None
—self-injury	Multiple contusions	None
Identity disturbance	Struggles with values, loyalties and self-image	Attempts to ward off, repudiate, and deny unwanted thoughts and feelings
Affective instability	Marked mood shifts	Integrative efforts disrupted when emotionally stimulated
Self-damaging acts	Cuts on neck, torso, arms and legs	None
II. Personality Factors	No intimate relationships	Avoids emotional involvement
III. Cognitive Abilities	Average intelligence	Average intelligence
IV. Psychodynamics	Difficulty integrating positive and negative aspects of self-image	Struggles with integration and management of aspects of self
V. Therapeutic Enabling Factors	Difficulty trusting others	Difficulty trusting others but has some insight into her difficulty
VI. Environmental Demand and Social Adjustment	Academic work below ability	Academic work below grade level and ability
	Family prizes emotional restraint	Prefers to remain uninvolved and detached
	Active participation in athletics	None

EXHIBIT 2

WAIS-R Summary

Verbal Subtests	Scaled Score
Information	10
Digit Span	10
Vocabulary	8
Arithmetic	7
Comprehension	11
Similarities	10

Performance Subtests	
Picture Completion	11
Picture Arrangement	11
Block Design	15
Object Assembly	18
Digit Symbol	13

Verbal IQ	96
Performance IQ	127
Full Scale IQ	109

Rorschach Summary

Number of Responses	14
Rejections	0
Populars	3
Originals	0
Average R/T Chromatic	39"
Average R/T Achromatic	1'47"
F%	43
F+%	90
A%	29
H%	21
W:M	6:1
M: sum C	1:4.5
m:c	4:2
VIII-X%	36
FK+F=Fc%	43
(H+A):(Hd+Ad)	5:2

RORSCHACH SUMMARY

Apperception   W   43%
D   43%
d   0%
Dd + S   14%

EXHIBIT 3

RORSCHACH SUMMARY

Response	*Inquiry*	*Scoring*

(Patient recognizes Rorschach. E. tells her instructions and adds that it doesn't matter whether she sees now the same thing as before, but to tell everything that it looks like to her now.)

I. 38″

1. I guess it looks like a bat or a butterfly. More like a bat.

    1. Doesn't include these. *(A bat?)* The way the wings or whatever are out. And it was black. — WFC′AP

I'm done. I don't see anything else in it.

(If you take your time, there may be other things that it might look like.)

It looks like an inkblot to me. I really don't see anything on that one.

II. 1′5″

(Smiling slightly.) Now that's the one I saw that was a seal before (turning ring on hand).

1. All right. Here's a new one for you. This one here, the white space looks like some kind of bottle and it looks like it was silkscreened so that the white is the shape. The color isn't the shape but the white part.

    1. *(Silkscreened?)* Because it was not a dark picture on a white background but a white picture with a dark outline. — SFC′Obj

Rorschach Summary

Response	*Inquiry*	*Scoring*
2. All right. Here's a good one. And it's squirting stuff up here (*pointing to upper red*) and some of it has spilled underneath it.	2. (*Squirting?*) The different color, I guess . . . (*Anything else?*) No. Just that It was a different color.	DCF.mFObj. *Fluid*
3. The seals. (*What about the seals?*) Oh, I don't know (*rubbing eyes*).	3. Here's the head, the neck, the flippers. (*Seals?*) The shape. (*Anything else?*) No. (*Patient sits back in chair, rolls eyes back, and looks disgusted.*)	DFA

I don't see anything else.

III. 59″

| 1. I guess that looks like two people on either side of a washing basin throwing up clothes, the red thing right there (*pointing*), and work-ing or preparing food or something. | 1. Two people here—head, body, legs. It looks like they are doing something like washing clothes, making food or something like that. | WMHP |

That's it.

IV. 2′10″

(*Patient sitting still and star-ing at card with chin resting in hand.*)

I don't see anything (*pushes card away*).
(*Are you afraid to say what you see or are you afraid to see anything?*)

RORSCHACH SUMMARY

Response	*Inquiry*	*Scoring*

I remember what I saw the last time and I don't know why I saw it. I really don't see much of anything. There's no good shape. I don't know. I remember what I saw last time on this one but it doesn't look like it.

(*And you don't see anything else now?*)

No.

(*What did you see the last time?*)

It looked like something from a . . . that looked like a cartoon character or a monster or something. I remember seeing one of them from before that looked like a cartoon character monster. I don't even know if it was this one.

1. This one has three legs.

    1. Whole thing. The cartoon monster character had two legs but this one doesn't even have a head, and that's another leg. (*What would this one be?*) I don't know. It didn't look like the cartoon figure. It had three legs. I don't know.   WF(A)

What if I turned it upside down? Can I do that? But it still doesn't look like anything.

RORSCHACH SUMMARY

Response	Inquiry	Scoring
I don't understand. Do you have to give a response? Can't I say nothing? I don't see anything on it and I don't want to make up anything if I don't see anything.		
(*Examiner interrupts testing and asks patient to discuss her feelings about the test. Patient relates how the test could be counted against her, as it was during her last hospital stay, where "they thought I saw too many things that weren't what I was supposed to see." E. briefly discusses purpose of testing encourages patient to relax.*)		

V. 27"

1. That one looks almost like the first one, like a bat or a butterfly, except for the two outside things.	1. (*Bat or butterfly?*) The little antennaes on the top and the wings. (*The antennaes made it look more like a bat or butterfly?*) More like a butterfly.	WFAP
I don't see anything else.		

VI. 3'46"

1. I don't see much. I just see a little thing but it doesn't look right. (*Do you want to tell me what it is?*) That looks like half of the sun and these are the beams coming out of it, but I don't know what's over it or around it. I can't make anything out of it.	1. That's the sun cut in half. I don't know what's over it (*running finger up and down area covering it*) and these are the rays coming out. (*Half a sun?*) Just that it was half a circle. (*And the rays?*) Just because they were coming out of the half circle. (*Looks very irritated at E.*) (*Anything else?*) No.	DFNat.

RORSCHACH SUMMARY

Response	Inquiry	Scoring

VII. 1'55"

1. I guess just two faces. This is the nose and the mouth here. One face here and one here.

(Pushes card away.)

When I see it, I remember what the old images looked like, and I just don't see anymore why I saw them. The other psychologist just said okay and flipped it over and that was that.

1. *(Runs finger around.)* I guess this could be a hat, but I didn't think of that before *(smiles). (Are you including it now?)* No. Just this here. Here are the eyes, the nose, the mouth.

DFH

VIII. 1"

1. That and that and the two greens look like a tree. That's the top of the tree, a Christmas tree or something.

1. Here's the top and here's the stem. *(A tree?)* I guess the shape and the color.

DFCPl

2. And that looks like it's some kind of rocky mountain, the rocks underneath it, the yellow and red there.

2. Probably just the color, the yellow or brownish color. *(The color of rocks?)* The yellow was kind of brownish and that reminded me of rocks. I don't know. *(Anything else?) (Nods no.)*

DCFGeo.

That's it.

IX. 12"

That still looks the same as the last time.

RORSCHACH SUMMARY

Response	*Inquiry*	*Scoring*
1. It's a UFO or some kind of flying saucer. It's like in "Close Encounters of the Third Kind." Did you ever see it? It's a movie. And that's a dome on top, and it's like taking off, and all the rest is like the flames, like after a spaceship takes off to the moon, there are always big clouds and dust and stuff.	1. (*UFO?*) Just the dome on the top, and the shape like round. (*Show me where dust and flames.*) All of it. All of it is dust and flames. (*Dust and taking off?*) Because of the line in the middle, it looked like it was going off. And it was on the top of the card. ("*It*" *is the dome?*) Yes, and there are clouds of dust and flames around it. (*Fingering mouth, yawns.*)	WFm.CF.KF Obj, Fire, Cloud

That's it. (*Yawns.*)

X. 59″

| 1. That looks like a moustache with two eyes there and there. | 1. (*Where are the eyes?*) Just the orange here. (*Moustache?*) Just the way it was shaped. (*And the eyes?*) Cause the moustache and the nose were there, the eyes were there. | drF-Hd |
| 2. And the whole thing looks like fireworks. All different colors. | 2. Just because there were so many different colors. (*Fireworks?*) Because Explosion fireworks are usually splattered like that with all sorts of bright colors and different shapes. (*Splattered?*) Just because there was space in between all the different colors. | WCF.mF Explosion |

EXHIBIT 4

CARD 1   5"All right. This is a little boy who . . . (*Someone enters room*) . . . is practicing his violin and he couldn't seem to get some of the notes so he put it down and rested for a while . . . uhmmm . . . picked it up, got the notes, played his song, and . . . was happy again. (*Thoughts?*) Well, he was upset because he couldn't get the notes that he had gotten before so he was just concentrating on getting the notes and he did it, so he was happy.

CARD 2   11" All right this is a city girl who came to the country for the summer to work on her Aunt and Uncle's farm and she's feeling scared because it doesn't look like much fun and she doesn't think that she can do it. But after a few days of working on the farm she likes it so she stays there all summer. (*Why does she decide she likes it?*) Because she's used to the city and not really working outside and she's not used to doing any physical labor so she thinks it's fun.

CARD 3GF   6" Okay. This lady . . . just came into a room from a dark hall-way and when she was opening the door the wind from the windows was blowing it back. (?) Like the wind from the windows blew the door back at her. And the door hit her in the side of her face and she's holding it because it hurts so she goes to the bathroom and puts some ice on it and (*grimaces upturned nose and mouth—like "so that's all"*). All she ends up with is a little lump on her face. That's it. (*Any particular thoughts?*) It hurts. (*What led up to it, her coming into the room?*) I guess it was the kitchen and she was hungry and she wanted to get something to eat. (*Yawns*)

CARD 5   4" All right. This lady just came home from work and when she opened the door she was surprised to see the flowers on the table that her husband sent her. What? Do I need an end? (*Pushes blouse sleeve up arm*). She put the flowers in the vase and went to cook dinner. (*Thoughts?*) She was surprised and happy.

CARD 8BM   14" (*Holding thumb in hand bent backwards*) Okay. This little boy just got out of the hospital. (*Talking in a little girl voice*) He had his appendix removed. And he's thinking about what happened in the hospital or what could have happened to him in the hospital. He couldn't remember their cutting him or anything. He was under anaesthesia. And he feels happy because he's out of the hospital and he's got his clothes back and he's on his way back to school. (*He's happy because he got his clothes back?*) Usually

THEMATIC APPERCEPTION TEST

in the hospital you have to wear pajamas and he's all dressed up so he looks like he likes to wear nice clothes.

CARD 9GF   24″ This lady is standing on the ledge of the first floor of a building on the porch looking out at the water where someone just caught a really big fish and all the people are running to see the fish and she's excited because she heard something happening and heard a lot of people running and so she went out of her room to see what was going on. (*Any particular outcome?*) I guess the guy on the beach caught a really big fish and she saw it and all the people went back to their houses and hotels, went back to what they were doing. (*Excited because she heard something?*) She heard people running and talking or whatever. (*Why do you think that made her excited?*) Because she wanted to see what was going on. (*Any thoughts?*) No, she just wanted to see what was happening and then she went back to whatever she was doing. (*What was she doing?*) She had a book in her hand. Maybe she was reading or writing a letter or something.

CARD 10   26″ (*playing with bracelet on left hand*) All right. This is a kid who just got back from uh . . . a basketball game (*said quickly*) and is really tired and on his way to bed so he gave his, I guess his father a kiss and a hug good night and went to bed. And he's feeling tired because he just played basketball and hencely (*unclear*) upset because he lost. (*Did you say hencely?*) No, just upset.

CARD 12F   10″ uhmmmm. . . . This girl is with her grandmother and they're in a store shopping for a wedding dress because she's going to get married and the grandmother is really happy and so is the girl and they buy one they both really like and go home to try it on. That's it.

CARD 12M   7″ This guy just got back to his room where his roommate is sleeping and he's asking him if he's awake and he's just about to touch him on the shoulder and shake him to wake him up cause he wants him to get up to help him do his homework. (*Playing and mouthing gold chain with cross on it*) . . . (*Shrugs shoulders*) . . . And he's feeling bad because he has to wake up his friend who had a hard day at school just because he needs him to help him with his homework. (*Yawns and is playing with ring*). And his friend gets up and helps him with his homework and they both go back to bed and (*shrugs and grimaces*) that's it. (*Laughs, starts playing with hair, yawns.*) (*Why does he need him to help him with his homework?*) I guess because he promised him he would help him after he got back . . . It's like a college dorm or something. (*And what kind of a hard day did the other one have?*) He had a lot of classes and when he got back to the dorm he had a lot of homework to do so he was tired and went to sleep. (*And didn't do his homework?*) Which one? (*The one who slept*) The one who is sleeping did his and the one who isn't didn't do his and is asking the guy who is sleeping to wake up. (*Looking at E fixedly*) (*In what field is the homework in do you think?*) Spelling (*laughs, rubs hands over eyes and stretches*). (*They have to go back to bed?*) After they finish that guy's homework.

CARD 13MF   5″ Okay. This is a picture of a guy who just got up and got dressed to go to work and he's still tired so he's rubbing his eyes and trying to be quiet so his wife can sleep. And he's feeling like he wants to go back to bed because he's tired. That's it. (*What's the story?*) (*Looks back at examiner hard*) (*You've given more of a description of a scene than a story*) He went out to a party the night before, got home late, and had to get up early and go to work; (*Shrugs shoulders*) and he's tired. (*The outcome?*) The wife gets to sleep till 10 and he has to be at work at 9. (*And his thoughts?*) That he shouldn't have stayed out late because he had to get up for work.

CARD 14   15″ Uhmm . . . This is a guy who's in a dark bedroom and he woke up and went to the window because it was so light outside but when he got to the window it turned out, it was just a spotlight . . . that was turned on outside of his window so he felt tired, closed the window and went back to bed . . . (*stops*) (*Is that it?*) (*Nods*) (*Thoughts and feelings?*) He wondered what the light was and when he found out he just went back to bed. (*No particular thoughts?*) No. He just found out what the light was because he was wondering because he was in a dark room.

CARD 15   9″ Uhmmm. All right. This guy is in uh . . . a veteran's cemetary where his best friend was shot and killed in the war so he's praying at his grave. And he feels sad . . . that's it. (*Outcome?*) Oh . . . uh . . . he put flowers in front of the grave and went home to go to bed. (*Any thoughts?*) Already said he was sad.

CARD 16   7″ (*laughs*) Uhmmm. (*Laughs and stretches back in chair with arms spread out*) This is a story of one piece of a cloud. It doesn't have a silver lining. It's not a dark rain cloud. It's just the everyday, average white cloud who blocks the sun so you can't get a good tan. And the cloud doesn't have any feelings and . . . just floats on by. Bet you never heard that one (*smiling at E.*). (*Picks up card, turns it over and puts it back on the pile herself*). (*One piece of a cloud?*) It doesn't have the rims. (*Motioning with hands*) It's like you cut

THEMATIC APPERCEPTION TEST

it out (*Chopping motion with sides of hands*) and because it's just one white piece of paper. The only reason I said it was a cloud was because it was white.

CARD 18GF 28″ (*arms folded against chest*) Uhmm (*scratches head*). This is a lady's mother . . . who just fell down and is having a little trouble standing up so the daughter is helping the mother stand up and she's worried that the mother's so old that she might have broken a bone but she stands up and walks around a little bit and she's fine. (*scratches elbow*) (*Why did she fall down?*) I guess she just slipped because she was having trouble walking. (*Scratches hand*) (*Any particular thoughts the daughter is having?*) She was worried that mother was so old that she might have broken a bone but she realizes when she walks around again that nothing really happened. (*Said in monotone voice, though not irritated, just repeats what she said before.*)

DISCUSSION

Ms. W, a 17-year-old, single female living with her parents, and Ms. J, a 20-year-old, single female meet criteria for borderline personality disorder. As is typical of many borderline patients, both are young, single females. Although similar, it is their differences that are important for treatment planning.

Ms. W had no clear-cut Axis I disorder and had a relatively good prior adjustment as noted on Axis V. While borderline, she met only five of the eight criteria for the diagnosis. She was not actively suicidal, nor did she have a past history of suicide attempts as many BPD patients do. However, her physically self-destructive behavior was extreme. Ms. W's treatment was intensive, with much investment of therapeutic time and expense. She was treated on a long-term, inpatient unit followed by individual, long-term, dynamic psychotherapy with relatively ambitious goals. This was due, apparently, in large part to a relatively good prognostic picture. Her projective tests were marked by avoidance, emotional withdrawal, and denial, and a rigid and desperate attempt to keep a "nice girl" image. This became the focus of treatment, which resulted in a more relaxed and integrated sense of self with some acceptance of the other aspects of herself.

Ms. J was more seriously disturbed than Ms. W. in diverse ways. She met all eight of the criteria for borderline personality disorder on clinical examination, including a history of anorexia and serious suicide attempts. In addition, she had a clear diagnosis of major depressive disorder with psychosis on Axis I. Her Axis V rating was very poor, indicating marked impairment in social and occupational functioning prior to the present episode.

The treatment of Ms. J was long and difficult, marked by improvement and then declines when she would reengage in self-destructive behavior. The testing material suggested overinvolvement and fusion with the mother, and this became a major focus in the family treatment. A central family therapy goal was some growing differentiation from other family members. In addition, she received individual psychotherapy during her inpatient treatment. Her relationship with this therapist created intense feelings and it would appear that she began to see the therapist much as she saw her father—a negative person in her environment. Inasmuch as her treatment could not be completed successfully at the admitting facility, future therapeutic efforts would need to take into account her capacity for the development of intense transference feelings and plan her treatment accordingly. This might include a treatment plan which combined individual with group psychotherapy.

C. NARCISSISTIC PERSONALITY DISORDERS

Narcissistic personality disorder is characterized by a longstanding pattern of grandiose fantasy and behavior, a lack of empathy toward others, and a hypersensitivity to the evaluation of self by others. The specific diagnostic criteria involve reacting to criticism with rage and shame, taking advantage of others, an exaggerated sense of one's own self-importance and competence, preoccupation with fantasies of unlimited success, a sense of entitlement, eliciting constant attention and admiration from others, an inability to recognize the needs and experience of others, and preoccupation with feelings of envy. Individuals with these characteristics seem destined to encounter difficulties in interpersonal relations.

NARCISSISTIC PERSONALITY DISORDER WITH ORGANIC DELUSIONAL SYNDROME

Mr. C was 28 years old at the time of his first psychiatric admission to a large, urban psychiatric hospital where he was first seen in the emergency room by the psychiatric resident on call. He was driven to the hospital by his father who had received an incoherent phone call from Mr. C in the early hours of the morning. The father went to his son's apartment and after repeated reassurances to his son that he was alone, he was admitted into the apartment. Mr. C told his father a rambling and largely incoherent story about being "spied on" by people on the street. He would not leave the apartment, but his father eventually persuaded him to accompany him to the hospital. He rode in the back of his father's car, keeping well out of view until they arrived at the emergency room.

The father was quite surprised to find his son in such a disorganized and "paranoid" state. Mr. C worked in his father's business and so had daily contact with him. They had been arguing a great deal lately and Mr. C seemed unusually irritable. His irritability and a rather dramatic weight gain of some 10-20 pounds in the last few weeks were, however, the only significant changes noted by his father. He attributed both these changes to his son's distress over the death of his mother, in unexpected and traumatic circumstances, a few months earlier. Although Mr. C lived alone in his own apartment, he had spoken with his mother daily and had frequently visited his parents in their nearby apartment before her death.

When seen in the emergency room, Mr. C could give little pertinent information about his recent life. He spoke at length about his conviction that someone was "spying" on him and, on further questioning, connected this

fear with his concern that "certain people" from whom he had been pur-
chasing large amounts of cocaine might be "out to get him." He was admitted to the inpatient psychiatric ward for further observation and evaluation
with a provisional diagnosis of organic delusional syndrome resulting from
his extensive (in excess of one gram per day) cocaine abuse.

Within 72 hours of his admission, his mental status had cleared sufficiently for him to provide a more coherent account of his recent activities
and for his paranoid delusions to have completely evaporated. He admitted
to a history of escalating cocaine abuse since the death of his mother in
an effort to ward off the despair he felt over losing her. She had died of
kidney failure which she developed after falling from a stepladder. She had
spent four months in a coma before her death. Mr. C, against the advice
of his father, had his mother transferred from hospital to hospital as he
found each new team of doctors "a bunch of incompetent assholes."

During the period of his mother's coma, Mr. C frequented prostitutes
where he was introduced to cocaine. He found that cocaine heightened and
prolonged his sexual pleasure and, as the weeks wore on, his cocaine abuse
escalated since little else gave him any pleasure. In the final weeks before
his admission, his life consisted of desultory periods in which he attempted
to work, punctuated with episodes of binge eating and vomiting and sado-
masochistic sex and drug orgies with many different prostitutes. As he
became increasingly irritable and paranoid, he spent less and less time out
of his apartment. In the final few days before his admission, he left his
apartment only to purchase food and cocaine. Finally, he took to his bed
where his daily life consisted of 5-10 episodes of binge eating and vomiting
interspersed with cocaine ingestion. Television was his constant companion;
he was too "wired" to sleep. Developing, first, ideas of reference and, finally,
frank paranoid delusions, he called his father when he became certain that
someone was trying to break into his apartment to steal his cocaine.

DSM-III-R Diagnosis

Axis I: Organic delusional syndrome
Axis II: Narcissistic personality disorder
           Rule out Dependent personality disorder
Axis III: None
Axis IV: Extreme (death of mother)
Axis V: Good

Treatment and Hospital Course

Mr. C quickly recovered from the acute effects of his cocaine abuse and his delusions rapidly abated. As they did so, however, he became increasingly depressed. Because of this, his psychiatrist recommended transfer to another hospital where he could receive a more extended period of inpatient evaluation and treatment for his depression. Mr. C accepted the recommendation of his psychiatrist and five days after his emergency room admission was transferred to another psychiatric facility. At the time of his admission there, he presented as a somewhat overweight young man with an outwardly jovial manner. He recounted the events leading to his admission and transfer with a somewhat ironic air and a bemused expression as if to help the psychiatrist understand that such behavior was hardly characteristic of him.

When asked about his mother's death, he was able to elaborate on his feelings of anger towards the medical staffs who had been unable to help her. He acknowledged the sadness he felt at her death. Initially, he was reluctant to explore his feelings about his mother in any detail, always returning to his angry feelings. He was angry at the doctors who had cared for his mother and he was angry at his father who, within a few months of his mother's death, had begun a relationship with a widowed friend of his mother's.

Mr. C required much encouragement before he reluctantly agreed to discuss his mother. As he did so, his jovial manner dissipated and was replaced with an air of sadness and great longing. His mother had been his "best friend." As far back as he could remember, she had known his innermost thoughts and feelings, almost before he himself had known them. She had been a constant source of encouragement and support and it was her love for him and her faith in him that had carried him through the rough times in his life. Since losing her, he had felt empty and ashamed that he had made so little of himself, considering her hopes for and faith in him.

On this and other occasions when Mr. C could be persuaded to speak about his mother, a genuine sense of melancholy seemed evident. However, at all other times, he seemed to have no difficulties. He went about his daily routine in the hospital with a lighthearted air. He ate and slept well and offered no complaints. He enjoyed spending time with the staff or other patients. Puzzled by the striking difference between his public appearance and his inner grief, the psychiatrist referred him for psychological testing to help her better understand the discrepancy.

Psychological Assessment

Mr. C was given an MMPI, WAIS-R, Rorschach, TAT and DAP. The examination began three weeks after his emergency room admission. The referral form requested help with his Axis II diagnosis. The psychiatrist felt Mr. C had both narcissistic and dependent personality features, but was unsure as to whether he indeed had a personality disorder. The psychiatrist also requested an evaluation of Mr. C's "mood disorder."

Mr. C cooperated with the examination which began with the MMPI. His MMPI profile was primarily remarkable for the relative absence of any indications of severe psychopathology. All the validity and the clinical scales had T-scores below 70, except for Mf scale. His profile peaks were obtained on *scales 6 (Paranoia)* and *9 (Mania)* (T-scores of 67 and 68, respectively), consistent with some mistrust and irritability noted in his clinical presentation and perhaps related to the residual effects of his cocaine-induced psychosis.

On the WAIS-R, Mr. C achieved a full-scale IQ of 98, with verbal and performance IQs of 107 and 87, respectively. This 20-point discrepancy between Mr. C's verbal and performance IQs is rather large and can be traced primarily to his very poor performance on the *Block Design and Object Assembly* subtests (scaled scores of six). Apart from these two subtests, his scaled scores all fell between nine and 12. When one inspects the details of his performance on the *Block Design* and *Object Assembly* subtests, it appears that Mr. C's difficulties are traceable to time pressure difficulties. On the easier items of both subtests he was able to quickly grasp the final product required and completed each design well within the time allotted for the item. However, on the last three items of the *Block Design*, he required an additional 1-10" beyond the allotted time limit for the item, thus losing credit for his correct performance.

Similarly, on the *Object Assembly* subtest, he rapidly completes the first three items but, although he knows the last item is an elephant, cannot manage to correctly assemble more than the head and the trunk in the time allotted for the item. Finally, in both subtests, there were minor difficulties (e.g. inverting the ear on item two of the *Object Assembly* subtest) which further reduced his score. In the examiner's notes for these two subtests, Mr. C appeared to be reduced to a rather inefficient trial and error strategy when his initial attempts met with failure, and he persisted in this strategy on later items.

On the projective tests, Mr. C showed the same persistence noted in his WAIS-R performance. He produced 51 Rorschach responses. The record is notable for its multiple indications of overproductivity. These include a low number of responses using the whole blot, few popular responses, a sizable proportion of unusual detail responses, and yet an overemphasis on easily perceived animal responses. The underutilization of determinants other than form also testify to the inherent impoverished quality of the record, despite his outer productivity. These quantitative indices suggest an individual whose ambitions overreach his abilities and indicate a predisposition to emphasize quantity over quality in his performance. His emphasis on quantity is, in fact, purchased at the expense of quality. His deemphasis of the commonplace and usual (e.g. low P% and W%) and his attention to the unusual represent the countervailing trends in this regard.

Qualitatively, his ambitions are represented in both the content and sequence of his responses. For example, he begins his Rorschach with the response "Butterfly. No, actually like a bee combination. The middle looks like a bee and the outside looks like a butterfly." These themes of the dangerous (the bee) and the harmless (and at other times, comically so) are constantly reworked in his nine responses to *card II*. His initial response to *card II* relies on the large, black details to become "two men slapping hands together, or something strange in the mirror. In fact, someone looking at his own reflection." This response is followed by "witches" in the upper red details, a "pig or rabbit" in the large, black details, "a face . . . with a big nose" as an edge detail and the same face (inverted) as "a clown" on the opposing side.

Returning to an unusual area in the large, black details, Mr. C next reports "a little boy. Very interesting, I see a man inside." It is the red in the black that reminds him of the boy because of "the expression on his face." Turning his attention to the lower red detail, he next reports "a sad face, maybe a crab." The former because of "sad eyes and looks like tears. It looks like he is crying." Finally, "two black bears" because of "the black and the shape."

This sequence of responses illustrates Mr. C's fluidly shifting euphoric-dysphoric mood state with elements of grandiosity and exhibitionism intertwined with denigration and a powerless passive-dependency. Fundamentally, Mr. C sees the world as having a kaleidoscopic, unstable flavor, with the relatively innocuous readily transformed into the threatening. The initial butterfly on *card I* becomes a bee and, later, his rats on *card VIII* change into much more formidable mountain lions.

These protean, conflictual aspects, while more subtle on the Rorschach, come into prominence in his TAT stories. In his first story to *card 1*, Mr. C moves immediately from mastery concerns related to the young boy's "worry about what his parents think about him" to "standing ovations" and an ultimate outcome as "a world-famous musician." He concludes the story by noting that "happy endings are great." In fact, in 12 stories, eight end happily. His preferred theme is that of an epic triumph in the face of overwhelming adversity: a young man from a small town moves to the big city and becomes "president of the United States of America" (*card 14*); the son of a used car salesman is accepted to medical school (*card 7BM*); a young serviceman survives the war and returns home with his foreign lover whom he "sweeps off her feet and takes her back to the U.S. to get married"; a young boy miraculously recovers after a three-day coma through the intercession of his father's prayers and the father is "enraptured . . . as he thanks God for the return of his son." Although cast as sweeping drama, these stories are nevertheless trite and cliché-ridden. All human interaction described in the stories is forced to come about by the press of external forces and the characters in these stories are described as merely reacting, albeit most often heroically, to these forces.

The stereotypy of these stories also appears in Mr. C's presentation of male and female responses to these natural tragedies. Men, as noted in the examples of heroism cited above, triumph. Women, on the other hand, are characterized by their frightened forbearance. For example, the mother on *card 10* is "proud" and "happy" that "her little boy has grown up to be a man" but now that he is marrying and moving out on his own, her only real solace lies in her son's "retaining many of the values that his mother taught him." And poor solace it must be, for in the conclusion of the story she "dies of natural causes."

Mr. C's characteristic denial of the ominous is to be found in his story to *card 5* in which a woman home alone at night bravely opens a door into a room where she suspects a burglar is present, only to discover that she had "left the window open and to find a tree banging on the open window." Finally, when war again provides the backdrop for a story of a heroic son enlisting "after hearing news that his country is under attack by foreign enemies," the mother is presented as "worried and very scared of the unknown forces of the war that may take her son's life and shatter her ideals and age her terribly . . . the only thing that is left in her life will disappear."

In these stories, Mr. C's preoccupations with boundless success, entitled achievement in the face of overwhelming odds, an egocentric assumption of being at the focus of all forces, natural and unnatural, and an exhibitionistic display of his astonishing talents are all interwoven into his presentations. In the face of such relentless self-aggrandizement, there is little room for an empathic appreciation of others. His empathic disability can easily be gleaned from his human figure drawings. Both figures are mere primitive sketches rushed off in a haphazard manner. The male figure shows no identifiable gender-specific characteristics. Its nonfunctional hands, nonexistent feet, and total absence of bodily articulation suggest an ineffective child much in need of nurturance and support. The female figure, with her bald head and tiny lower appendages, is shown in profile, perhaps to emphasize her only noticeable sexual characteristics, her full bosom and skirt.

Treatment Plan and Outcome

The report of Mr. C's psychological examination results ruled out the presence of a significant mood disturbance and emphasized the narcissistic and dependent elements to his personality. His rapid recovery from his cocaine-induced delusions and the absence of a prominent Axis I mood disorder led his treatment team to formulate a treatment recommendation for an outpatient psychotherapy rather than to extend his inpatient stay.

Upon being presented with this treatment plan, Mr. C could identify no reason for continuing under psychiatric care. His father was of the same opinion. His psychiatrist attempted to point out that to the extent that he was unable to resolve his grief over his mother's death, he remained at risk for further decompensations such as the one which had led to his hospitalization. Mr. C acknowledged the relationship between his mother's death and his decompensation but felt that he now knew how to avoid further episodes of decompensation, by refraining from further cocaine abuse.

Unable to persuade Mr. C to accept the recommendation for outpatient treatment, the psychiatrist suggested that the examining psychologist go over the results of his evaluation with Mr. C. The psychiatrist hoped that by doing so, Mr. C could be helped to see more clearly the ineffectiveness of his coping strategy. The psychologist reviewed his results with him and pointed out his tendencies to blame his problems on things outside himself, his indifference to anyone's problems but his own, and his inordinate needs for admiration and attention. In doing so, the psychologist was careful to also support Mr. C's real needs for attention and impart to him a sense of encouragement.

Mr. C appreciated the efforts of the psychologist and the psychiatrist and did feel as if he had been understood. He agreed to accept the recommendation for outpatient treatment and was discharged from the hospital. On followup contact two weeks later, Mr. C had not contacted the psychiatrist to whom he had been referred. When called by his former hospital social worker, he reluctantly admitted he had begun abusing cocaine again. Within a few weeks, he had decompensated again and was admitted to another hospital for detoxification and referral to a substance abuse program.

EXHIBIT 1

Area of Assessment	Clinical Examination	Psychological Examination
I. Symptoms/Diagnosis		
Narcissistic personality disorder		
A. Grandiosity	Focuses on the unique nature of his relationship with his mother	Constant themes of unmitigated victory in the face of adversity
B. Preoccupation with fantasies	None	Preoccupied with unlimited success
C. Exhibitionism	Admits to "clowning around" to get attention	Self-esteem overly dependent on the approval of others
D. Cool indifference or marked reaction to indifference, criticism or defeat	None	Denigrates the goal when defeat is imminent
E. Relationships disturbed by:		
—entitlement	None	Expects to be the constant focus of others' attention
—lack of empathy	Fails to understand father's wish to remarry	Unable to appreciate others' needs except as they relate to his own
II. Personality Factors	None	Poor use of ego resources; relies on making a good impression
III. Cognitive Abilities	Average intelligence	Average intelligence
IV. Psychodynamics	Idealized bond with his mother	Expects support and admiration regardless of accomplishments
	Poor impulse control	Relies on external affective controls; very prone to shifting mood states

AREA OF ASSESSMENT	CLINICAL EXAMINATION	PSYCHOLOGICAL EXAMINATION
V. Therapeutic Enabling Factors	Acute, relatively brief period of major symptomatic disturbance	Quick recovery with acknowledgment of difficulties
VI. Environmental Demand and Social Adjustment	Prefers to get by with the minimum amount of effort	Exploits the environment to serve his own needs
	No close personal relationships outside his immediate family	Marginal adjustment to external demands to avoid confrontation

EXHIBIT 2

WAIS-R SUMMARY

Verbal Subtests	*Scaled Score*
Information	12
Digit Span	12
Vocabulary	10
Arithmetic	12
Comprehension	11
Similarities	12

Performance Subtests

Picture Completion	10
Picture Arrangement	11
Block Design	6
Object Assembly	6
Digit Symbol	9

Verbal IQ	107
Performance IQ	87
Full Scale Score	98

MMPI Summary

LK/F: 5′96-4231/87:0#

Rorschach Summary

Number of Responses	51
Rejections	0
Populars	8
Originals	1
Average R/T Chromatic	4″
Average R/T Achromatic	3″
F%	62
F + %	84
A%	45
H%	27
W:M	9:6
M:Sum C	6:3

Rorschach Summary

VIII-X%		33
FK + F + Fc%		65
(H + A):(Hd + Ad)		25:12
Apperception	W	18%
	D	45%
	d	10%
	Dd + S 27%	(Pure S)

EXHIBIT 3

RORSCHACH SUMMARY

Response	*Inquiry*	*Scoring*

I. 1″

1. Butterfly. No actually like a bee. Combination of the middle looks like a bee and outside looks like a butterfly.

1. The shape, the wings.

WFAP

2. Middle looks like bee outside like butterfly. Maybe it's a housefly. No wings of housefly go backwards. No it is not a housefly.

2. Only the middle, the shape, the head, the eye and the stinger.

DF-A

II. 5″

1. Two men slapping hands together or something, looking in the mirror. In fact, someone looking at his own reflection is about it.

1. The connection between the hands, the arm meeting on the center. (*Anything else?*) The shape of the shoulder, other shape of their bodies, could have been their body. (*Reflection?*) The way it looked like a drawing cut in half but when I studied them closely they are two distinct drawings.

WMHP

Do I have to say more about it (*As you wish*). How did they make these cards? Well they must have made it with ink. If I put the picture together it looks like someone in reflection but if I look at it separately the red looks

2. like an old witch, two of them and the black looks like

2. The shape of nose and chin. (*Old?*) Well all witches are old.

DF(Hd)

RORSCHACH SUMMARY

Response	*Inquiry*	*Scoring*
3. a rabbit or like a grown pig or rabbit	3. The ears, shape.	DFA
4. but if I turn the card I see a face over here with big nose.	4. The nose, the chin.	drFH
5. And the bottom on the other side could be a clown.	5. Looks like he is smiling. (*Smiling?*) Shape of mouth.	drMHd
6. I see a little boy. Very interesting I see a man inside.	6. It looks like a boy, the expression of his face. I saw the head and the nose. (*Man inside?*) I thought that. I mean the boy looks like a boy and a man.	drMHd
7. I see a sad face	7. Sad eyes, tears, looks like it's crying.	DM-Hd
8. or maybe a crab.	8. The shape.	DFA
9. The two blacks can be two bears.	9. The black and the shape.	DFC'AP
III. 2″		
1. I see two monkeys hanging upside down.	1. The tail, the drawing, looks like they are hanging from a branch.	DFMA
2. A butterfly.	2. Wings.	DFAP
3. A skull, no a mask.	3. Looks like a religious mask. I do not know whether it has a sad or happy face. The shape has openings and someone could look into it.	D(S)FMask
4. Also a crab.	4. The shape. Claws.	WFA
5. Two people talking.	5. Head, legs, body.	WMHP
IV. 6″		
1. This one is interesting. I see two hands.	1. The shape. A finger here and here.	dFHd

RORSCHACH SUMMARY

Response	*Inquiry*	*Scoring*
3. Face like Jimmy Durante.	3. The nose.	drFHd
4. I see a dog.	4. Head, nose, front paws.	DF-A
V. 1″		
1. A bat, a butterfly.	1. (*Bat or butterfly?*) The shape makes it look like either.	WFA
2. A horse's leg.	2. Actual shape of it.	dFAd
3. A half man and half horse.	3. Leg like horse but the head looks like a man, mythological character.	drFH/A
4. A bull.	4. The outline looked strong.	DF-A
5. Clouds.	5. The white and the dark, the white against the black.	WC′FCloud
VI. 5″		
1. Again like a crab, no not like a crab. An animal with a claw, not a snake.	1. Eyes, the shape, the claws.	drFA
2. I see a lamppost.	2. The black color, the separation and the light and the darkness, the separation of light and dark.	DFCObj.
3. I also see a penis.	3. The shape of it. It is erect also, the head is.	drFmSex
4. And if I see that, here I see a vagina symbol.	4. The opening looks like an ass and vagina.	drFSex
VII. 1″		
1. A river through a valley.	1. Looked like setting of sun on landscape. An opening, the gray area looked like water or reflection of the sun.	dFm.FKNat.
2. A vagina again.	2. The opening.	dFSex
3. An angry dog's face.	3. The nose, he has a thick nose. (*Angry?*) Looks like it's growling.	DFMAd
4. A wolf.	4. The mouth, the eyes.	DFAd

RORSCHACH SUMMARY

Response	Inquiry	Scoring
3. An angry dog's face.	3. The nose, he has a thick nose. (*Angry?*) Looks like it's growling.	DFMAd
4. A wolf.	4. The mouth, the eyes.	DFAd
5. Two people.	5. Not people only two faces, the shapes.	DFHdP

VIII. 6″

Hmm, much more detail here.

Response	Inquiry	Scoring
1. Two rats or mountain lions.	1. Just the shape.	DFAP
2. Human heart and veins from heart.	2. Shaped like human heart. The red is the veins of the heart.	diFCAt
3. A man's face or body.	3. I saw the whole body, the legs, arm and the face.	diFH
4. I see a baby, a fetus.	4. The outline is the shape of the baby. The full formation had not occurred, he is waiting to bust out.	drFm(H)
5. Animal head.	5. The shape, a prehistoric animal.	DFAd

IX. 6″

Response	Inquiry	Scoring
1. I see a human skeleton, like a pelvis.	1. The way it's shaped.	DFAt
2. A reindeer on top.	2. Well I did not see the deer only it's antler. (*Antler?*) It has the shape of a deer's antlers.	dFAd
3. Looks like a forest landing deep in something. I also see the core of the earth. I see different coloration.	3. I was imagining a cross section of the earth. Color looked like drawings from a textbook showing an oil drill going down pushing things. (*Forest landing?*) I don't know what made me say that, maybe the colors remind me of the forest.	WKF.CFGeo.

RORSCHACH SUMMARY

Response	*Inquiry*	*Scoring*
4. Ocean with land around it.	4. Shape, looks between Europe and North America, the land is around the ocean. (*Anything else?*) Color blue.	DFC-Geo.
5. A lady upside down.	5. (*A lady upside down?*) Shape, arms, legs and body.	drF-H

X. 3"

(*This is the last card*)

Oh I'll see all kinds of things.

1. I see parrots.	1. The shape, their tails.	DF-A
2. I see tulips.	2. Shape of the buds on the top.	ddFPl
3. Overall a butterfly.	3. Put it together, the overall shape would be butterfly, all the colors.	WFC-A
4. Helicopter and tank.	4. The shape and the color, Army helicopter.	DFCObj
5. Rabbits.	5. The shape of the ears.	DFA
6. Crab.	6. The overall shape.	DFAP
7. Monkey in a tree.	7. The tail. It looked that it was on a tree inside the tree eating something off the tree. (*Tree?*) Branches sticking out.	drFMA,PlO

E X H I B I T 4

CARD 1   2″ The young protégé studying his new piece of music that he wants to play in rehearsal next Saturday night. He is very concerned whether he can master this but he learns to master it and will get a standing ovation on the concert. They live happily forever after. (*Who is they?*) Him and his parents. (*Feelings?*) He feels worry about whether he can accomplish this on Saturday and what his parents think about him but he just motivates himself and he goes on to become a world famous musician. Happy endings are great.

CARD 3BM   5″ Looks like, this is a sad, cruel sort of woman who is about to take her own life. Her husband and children were killed in a car accident leaving her all alone, broken hearted, alone and scared. Feeling that she has nothing to live for, she is about to pull the trigger and broke down crying and she discovered that she does not have the courage to pull the trigger to take her own life. She realizes that life must go on and she is strong enough to endure these hardships, but she endures the pain. I would say she is happy but she realizes the challenges and is ready to meet the challenge.

CARD 4   3″ This is a love story in Italy during WWII when a young serviceman falls in love with the hospitality of young Italian woman. Their love and passion were strong in times of war. News came in that war was over, that he is coming back to America and she does not want to let him go, she pleads her case for the love she has for him and that their love is very strong. He is torn between his love for her or whether his feelings are true or just flaring up during the war. Passions are hot during the war. He then picks her up, I mean he sweeps her off her feet and takes her back to the US to get married. They both are very happy now.

CARD 5   3″ She was home alone last night. She thought there was a burglar in the other room. She opened the door quickly to surprise the would-be intruder. She is very scared and nervous that her life may be in danger. When she opened the door she was startled that she left the window open and to find a tree banging on an open window—she was relieved that there was no burglar in the house.

CARD 6BM   11″ O.K. What do I do with this one? I have not decided whether this is going to be good news or bad news. Let's see. . . . young George comes home after hearing news that his country is under attack by foreign enemies. He went by the recruiting station on the way from home and enlisted to do his part as his father and his father's father before him did to protect the great land. His mother on the other hand is very worried and very scared of the unknown forces of the war that may take her son's life and shatter her ideals and age her terribly. Now the guy is confronted with the true tragedy of the war and about the death of his father that he never knew. She is scared, lonely, that the only thing that left in her life will disappear.

CARD 7BM 5″ Son you are old enough I want you to come into the used car business. I am proud and eager that my own flesh and blood will be standing next to me selling cars the way I have for the past 35 years. Now some one will carry on the family name for generations to come. The son had bad news for the father. He said I do not know how to break the news but I am not going to sell cars. I was just accepted in MD school which fulfills my dream as a doctor. He is very happy and excited to fulfill his dreams and goals but concerned and sad that he let his father down. But his dream is final. He will go to medical school. The father, he was excited but became disappointed but then he turned out to be happy because his son's fulfilling his dream.

CARD 10 10″ This is the story of Joe and his mother. Joe is very happy and very sad at the same time. You see. . . . (*pause*). This is the day that he is supposed to get married. His mother is so proud of him she is so happy that her little boy has grown up to be a man and he is boy enough to seek advice and assurance from his mother. It is a very happy day. He gets married and lives happily ever after. He will retain many of the values that his mother thought of him. She dies of natural causes. (*Patient appears very anxious moving in his chair*)

CARD 12M 5″ This one is terrible, this is the worst possible thing to happen in life. A parent thinking about burying a child, that his child will die before him and the task of burying the child is inconceivable for him as he worked and struggled all his life so children will live a better or longer life than he did. The son has not been awake for three days but his father has not left his bedside praying that he will save the life of his child. The son opens his eyes finally and says to his father that he is hungry. Tears of joy erupted from the father's eyes as he thanked God for return of his son.

CARD 13MF 7″ This is a terrible sad story marking the death of one's loved ones. They have been married 50 years when a sudden heart attack

THEMATIC APPERCEPTION TEST

took the life of their beloved one's. (*What do you mean?*) Well she had a heart attack. She died at home in his arms happy and content. He is trying to decide what to do, who to call, wrestling with his family. On the one hand he is miserable and in agony that his wife is gone. On the other hand he is happy and greatful that they shared 50 years.

CARD 14 3″ This is the story of a young man named Jim who just graduated from college. He is very excited to start his new life. He decided to leave the small town where he was raised and leave to go to a big city to try his chance in fame and fortune. He was happy and excited about the chance of starting his adventure but at the same time he was scared and nervous about the obstacles and unknown that may lie ahead, a fight for which he was not prepared to win but he must win them. He is a champion and a winner. He must overcome the odds to prove his destiny. He will become the president of the United States of America.

CARD 15 10″ This was devil's nightmare on Halloween night. This guy is very happy and excited that he finally gets his chance to wake up the dead. There he stood chanting the poem. (*Patient is smiling and laughing*) That gives him a charge, excitement which sends chills through his body. Period and paragraph. It did not work, he felt terrible. You see he was nuts to begin with. He froze to death, a very ironic story (*smiling*).

NARCISSISTIC PERSONALITY DISORDER

Mr. A was a 21-year-old student who had just returned to college for his junior year. Despite a chronic history of academic underachievement and a sophomore year at college that had resulted in academic probation, he anticipated no problems during his junior year. Although he resolved to bring up his grades under pressure from his father, he quickly fell into his usual pattern of applying himself only in those classes which he enjoyed. Shortly after the beginning of the semester, he was accused of having broken into several dormitory rooms and stolen stereo equipment and was put on probation again pending the outcome of the police investigation. He adamantly denied any involvement in the thefts. His family was unpersuaded by his denials and unmoved by his consternation. They had suffered through several such thefts and denials during his high school years when he had needed to support his compulsive gambling habits.

Feeling rejected by his family and recognizing the inadequacy of his academic performance, Mr. A began to feel increasingly hopeless. He began to have difficulty socializing as word of his alleged involvement in the thefts began to circulate around campus. He lost all interest in women and sex, a matter of some concern to him since he had always prided himself on his sexual abilities and was given to boasting of his sexual exploits. In fact, during his senior high school year, his sex life had been a fairly reliable means of bolstering his self-esteem. For a period of several months, he had been fascinated with prostitutes and had often used his father's credit cards to rent hotel rooms where he could act out his rape fantasies with them. He became bored with these adventures and turned to aggressive and anonymous homosexual encounters from which he derived "an animal-like relief." He discontinued these escapades only because he feared that exposure of his activities might jeopardize his chances of using the college's ROTC program to gain admission to officer's candidate school after graduation. Although he did join the ROTC, a congenital heart defect, which he had neglected to report, resulted in his rejection from the program after his first week.

Things continued to go poorly for Mr. A. After he learned of formal charges being brought against an accomplice in the stereo thefts, he became more hopeless about improving his own situation. At about this time, he wrote to his parents describing his feelings and telling them that his present problems were all their fault. Finding it difficult to sleep, he consulted the school physician and was given 20 tablets of a sleeping pill. However, he left the office with the impression that he had been given tranquilizers and within a period of two hours had consumed them all. He was found comatose in his dormitory room and was taken to a local hospital where he made a quick recovery after emergency medical treatment. His school counselor recommended he leave school and hospitalize himself for psychiatric treatment. He returned home and received the same advice from a former therapist whom he had consulted previously regarding his compulsive gambling. He agreed to the hospitalization and his former therapist arranged his admission.

On admission, Mr. A stated that he was seeking hospitalization because "I'm depressed and not functioning and I overdosed on sleeping pills." Although he described his mood as depressed, his affect was of full range and normal intensity. There were no disturbances noted in his thinking; no perceptual disturbances were revealed on examination. His speech was normal in rate and flow, but was remarkable in its content in that he continually remarked on how other's acts related to him without any seeming awareness of his own role in bringing about his difficulties. His attitude at such times indicated that he expected others to feel sympathetic with his plight and acknowledge the special nature of his problems. For example, the impact of his accomplice's arrest on his "hopelessness" and on his poor academic performance were presented as obvious and he felt the overdose was actually the physician's fault for not adequately informing him of the dangerous potential of overusing the drug. He reported that at the time he had overdosed, he had not felt suicidal and he reported no present suicidal feelings.

DSM-III-R Diagnosis

Axis I:	Dysthymic disorder
Axis II:	Narcissistic personality disorder (Primary diagnosis)
	Rule out Antisocial personality disorder
Axis IV:	Mild—new school year
Axis V:	Fair—some impairment in both social and occupational functioning

Treatment and Hospital Course

Mr. A quickly adjusted to the routine of the unit and seemed to fit in easily with the other patients. He demonstrated no difficulties in sleeping and always appeared to be in good spirits. He continued to complain of feeling depressed despite any objective evidence of abnormal mood or changes in neurovegetative functioning. The lack of objective evidence to support Mr. A's complaints of depression led his psychiatrist to consider a diagnosis of a personality disorder as Mr. A's primary diagnosis. Mr. A had no family history of affective disorders. His father abused alcohol and his brother abused drugs, but neither of them had ever been treated for these substance abuse problems. He admitted to using marijuana and alcohol on many occasions, but was convinced his substance use had never presented a problem for him. His parents were concerned about his difficulties, but were also angry at him and found it difficult to understand how the hospitalization could be helpful.

Psychological Assessment

In order to help in establishing Mr. A's personality disorder diagnosis, he was referred for psychological testing. The psychiatrist requested information regarding his intellectual abilities and the nature and degree of his depression. In light of his history of academic underachievement, the psychiatrist also requested that he be evaluated for any learning disabilities or other neuropsychological difficulties. He received a neuropsychological screening exam, an MMPI, a WAIS-R, Rorschach, TAT, Sentence Completion Test, and Bender Gestalt.

A review of the results from his screening exam revealed no significant neuropsychological findings. His academic difficulties seemed more likely to be related to motivational and other psychological difficulties than to neuropsychological ones. He achieved a full-scale IQ of 108, which reflected the average of markedly discrepant verbal and performance IQs of 124 and 86, respectively. His subscale scores ranged from the Borderline and Low Average levels (*Picture Completion, Block Design* and *Picture Arrangement*) to the Very Superior levels (*Similarities* and *Comprehension*). Among the verbal subtests, his relatively poor performance on the *Digit Span* and *Arithmetic* subscales was partially a reflection of anxiety and diminished concentration.

His performance subtests were lowered by his tendency to work quickly and to settle on the first approximate solution to be achieved without giving proper attention to a final check of the details. For example, he completed the eighth item of the *Block Design* in 100 seconds, but inverted the red triangle in the lower left-hand corner of the design. This deficit was particularly noticeable on the *Picture Completion* subtest, which assesses discriminative judgment, where he gave his weakest performance. His relative strengths were apparent on those subtests requiring the exercise of abstract reasoning, knowledge of social conventions, and the application of some modicum of social judgment. Mr. A did well on these subtests despite some mild intrusions of his own idiosyncratic concerns.

Bearing in mind that the WAIS-R is a highly structured evaluation during which the examinee is required to produce responses with a high degree of factual or consensual validity, Mr. A's mild intrusions take on diagnostic importance. For example, on the *Comprehension* subscale, which elicited his second best performance on the WAIS-R, elements of grandiosity and entitlement were woven into his generally quite adequate answers. In explaining how one should act if one is the first person to see smoke and fire in a movie theater, he thought it best to inform the usher and call the fire department and then "get the people out calmly." Interestingly, despite his clear recognition that those in a position to take responsibility for clearing the theater and controlling the fire should be notified, he felt that he must be directly involved himself in order to insure an adequate outcome. Likewise, when asked to explain the meaning of the proverb "Strike while the iron is hot," he focused on the preparedness of the agent ("Strike when you're ready, not later or before") rather than, as is more usually the case, the availability of the opportunity. His responses to those *Comprehension* items involving relationships between individuals and agencies also reveal the same egocentric focus. Borrowing money from banks rather than from friends was seen as advantageous because "friends aren't always there, banks are"; people should pay taxes in order "to get services from the state."

While Mr. A clearly recognizes his own needs, he feels that some degree of guile and duplicity is necessary in order to meet them. His first percept on the Rorschach is of "a fox," an animal associated in mythic lore with craft and wiliness in the pursuit of his own needs. But also like the fox of Aesop's fable who contemptuously disparages the grapes he cannot reach, Mr. A must find some way to protect himself from the humiliation of failure. Constant praise is required to maintain his self-esteem (e.g. *when someone looks at me, I* "feel good"; *after he made love to her he* "felt good"). In seeking it in the arena of social relationships, however, the threat of not receiving it and the humiliation engendered by openly desiring it are the risks. On the *Sentence Completion Test*, Mr. A acknowledges that *he felt proud that he* "was smart," but also notes that he can be made to "feel stupid" if he is criticized or if he fails an examination.

His preferred attitude to such situations is to hold himself back from any gratifying emotional engagement with others. In his very constricted Rorschach, he manages only 13 responses, a level of productivity that is inconsistent with his intellectual abilities. Of note, both of his human responses are "two females staring at each other" (*cards III* and *VII*). He generally limits himself to the obvious and mundane. Almost one-half of his responses are popular responses (P% = 46), an equal proportion are based solely on perception of form (F% = 46), and with few exceptions they are limited to easily perceived animals (A% = 85). His Bender also reflects detachment in his minimally invested, perfunctory copies of geo-metric designs.

On the TAT, he tells trite stories that, like his Rorschach responses, avoid the emotional nuances of the interaction. For example, his story to *card 10* deals with the 15th anniversary of "a man and a woman" who "hope to live a good life the next 15 years. It's just a nice family, the American dream." When actually caught up in the emotional content of the card, he offers endings involving suppression and denial of strong affects (*cards 13MF, 3BM* and *7BM*) or a retreat into reluctant compliance and formalistic "duty" (*cards 1* and *6BM*, respectively).

Shame is to be particularly avoided, as Mr. A notes in his story to *card 13MF*. The card depicts a woman with bare breasts lying on a low, narrow bed with her face partially turned towards the wall. In the foreground is a man dressed in shoes, pants, shirt and tie who is holding his right arm across his face and is standing beside a small table containing books and a lamp. He opened his story, after a long pause, with the comment that "this is bringing back lots of bad memories." He went on to state that "this guy had picked up a hooker in a cheap hotel room. She's a stone cold junkie, flat on her back. He'll leave feeling lower than before. He'll wander the streets and try to forget." Amnesia seems to be the only possible solution to "bad memories." The possibility that emotional difficulties could be worked through with the help of someone is treated with contempt. His story to *card 12M* involves a hypnotic treatment for cessation of smoking by a client who "doesn't think it's going to work, but $25.00 isn't too much to pay." The hypnotist is, as predicted, unsuccessful in immediately helping the client to deal more satisfactorily with his oral needs and the experience simply becomes "something to talk about with the guys at the office."

Although Mr. A's dysphoria and low self-esteem were quite real features of his current psychological state, he seemed more prone to address these difficulties through an action orientation designed to provide immediate relief. His MMPI profile showed its peak elevations on *scales 2* and *4* (both > 80) with *scales 3, 7* and *8* also showing clinically significant elevations (> 70). However, despite his awareness of these difficulties, he showed little concern over them (e.g. *F scale* < 60).

The examining psychologist summarized these test findings as most con-sistent with a narcissistic personality disorder, specifically highlighting his detached view of others, his insensitivity to their feelings, his own sense of entitlement and specialness, with some evidence of sociopathic charac-teristics given his willingness to exploit others for his own needs. These latter feelings about himself were felt to be features of his personality disturbance that would make it especially difficult to engage him in a psychotherapeutic treatment where he could acknowledge his more painful feelings of depreciated self-worth and address the defensive purposes of his entitlement and contempt for others.

Treatment Planning and Outcome

Mr. A was informed of the results and formulation of the psychological testing and responded by being quite pleased that his difficulties could be given a name. Despite his acceptance of the diagnosis and his agreement with the formulation of his difficulties, he continued to speak of his problems in terms of the fault resting with others. In his individual psychotherapy, this attitude was gently confronted and he was encouraged to accept some responsibility for his problems and his treatment. He paid lip service to the need for him to do so if he were to alter his situation in life, but invested no real effort in the task. The only change recorded during his subsequent treatment was that he ceased complaining of his "depression."

As Mr. A began to feel less "depressed," he began to push for a discharge from the hospital. The hospital staff, feeling that there was no longer any need for Mr. A to continue his treatment in the hospital, began to allow him passes from the hospital to arrange for his discharge. He used these passes to reacquaint himself with several recently discharged, female patients with whom he developed social, and in some cases intimate, relationships. When the hospital staff became aware of these liaisons, they confronted him with their impropriety. He was unable to recognize or accept that these activities were yet another example of how he continually got himself into trouble by acting out his difficulties rather than seeking alternative, and more constructive, solutions.

He was discharged from the hospital with a referral for individual psychotherapy and with recommendations that he enroll in a local college and live independently of his family. In order to help his family continue to work on their own difficulties in allowing the separation, they also were referred to a family therapist.

EXHIBIT 1

AREA OF ASSESSMENT	CLINICAL EXAMINATION	PSYCHOLOGICAL EXAMINATION
I. Symptoms/Diagnosis		
Narcissistic personality disorder		
Grandiosity	Emphasizes the special nature of his problems	Projects a view of himself as unique
Preoccupation with fantasies	None	Preoccupied with proving his intellectual brilliance while having basically low self-esteem
Exhibitionism	Requires the admiration of others to maintain adequate self-esteem	Intensely focussed on his own needs and desires
Response to criticism is rage, humiliation, or feelings of inferiority	Poor academic performance leaves him hopeless; humiliated and enraged by alleged theft	Avoids becoming affectively involved with the examination
Entitlement	Surprised no one believes his innocence	Believes his own needs are always paramount
Exploitativeness	Readily exploits other patients for his sexual needs with complete disregard for rules	Some sociopathic tendencies
Lack of empathy	Cannot understand how his parents, hospital staff or other patients feel	Indifferent or unable to recognize how others feel. Detached from others.
II. Personality Factors	Personality features consistent with a narcissistic personality disorder	Personality style consists of alternating impulse ridden periods and anhedonic despair
III. Cognitive Abilities	Possible learning disability or neuropsychological difficulties	No learning disabilities or neuropsychological difficulties; average or above average intellectual ability but functions very inefficiently

AREA OF ASSESSMENT	CLINICAL EXAMINATION	PSYCHOLOGICAL EXAMINATION
IV. Psychodynamics	Poor frustration tolerance	Performance highly susceptible to disruption by anxiety
	Feelings of shame and humiliation prevent acknowledgement of any responsibility for his problems	Use of avoidance, denial and externalization to maintain self-esteem
V. Therapeutic Enabling Factors	Provisional acceptance of recommendation for treatment	Accepts recommendation but is not motivated to change and expects failure
	Above average verbal skills	Above average verbal skills
VI. Environmental Demand and Social Adjustment	Chronic history of poor academic performance with recent academic probation	Consistently achieves below abilities unless assured of ultimate success
	Active social life with no close friends	Sees others largely in terms of their ability to fulfill his own needs

EXHIBIT 2

WAIS-R SUMMARY

Verbal Subtests	*Scaled Score*
Information	12
Digit Span	9
Vocabulary	13
Arithmetic	9
Comprehension	14
Similarities	16
Verbal Score	73

Performance Subtests	
Picture Completion	6
Picture Arrangement	8
Block Design	7
Object Assembly	10
Digit Symbol	9
Performance Score	40

Verbal IQ	124
Performance IQ	86
Full Scale	108

MMPI Summary

FKL/ 24"7853'6-901/

Rorschach Summary

Number of Responses	13
Rejections	1 (Card IX)
Populars	6
Originals	0
Average R/T Chromatic	12"
Average R/T Achromatic	8"
F%	46
F + %	77
A%	85
H%	15

RORSCHACH SUMMARY

W:M		9:2
M:Sum C		2:1
m:c		4:0
VIII-X%		31
FK + F + Fc		46
(H + A):(Hd + Ad)		12:1
Apperception	W	69%
	D	31%
	d	0%
	Dd + S	0%

E X H I B I T   3

RORSCHACH SUMMARY

Response	*Inquiry*	*Scoring*
I. 10″		
1. A fox.	1. The whole thing; you know, spaces were eyes, ears were at the top. Just the shape.	W(s)FAd
(More?)		
2. A butterfly.	2. The whole thing. Looks like wings on the side, butterfly body in the middle.	WFAP
II. 21″		
1. I see groundhogs in the black part . . . that's all I see.	1. It was the black parts on the sides. Just short, stumpy little animals laying on their sides. (?) You know, laying down, like facing each other.	DFMA
III. 9″		
1. The black part is two females staring at each other, putting their hands on a table.	1. The black parts on the side. Looks like females because of shape, breasts, female form.	WMHP
2. The red part is a butterfly.	2. That was red part in the middle. Just looked like a butterfly.	DFAP
IV. 11″		
1. This looks like a butterfly this way.	1. The whole thing. The sides look like wings, top part was the head. Just the shape.	WF-A
V. 5″		
1. This looks like a butterfly, too.	1. The whole thing. Just the shape, wings, antennae, head.	WFAP

RORSCHACH SUMMARY

Response	Inquiry	Scoring

VI. 4″

1. This looks like a mashed pussy cat (*laughs*).

1. The whole thing. Looks like somebody ran over it and mashed it. Top part is head with whiskers, rest is shaped like a mashed cat.

WFA

VII. 8″

1. This looks like two females staring at each other.

1. The whole thing. Top parts was the heads, and rest looks like bodies. (*Staring?*) Yeah, they were facing each other.

WMHP

VIII. 7″

1. This is two bears climbing a tree.

1. The bears are two figures over the sides; the green part is shaped like a tree and the rest is part of the tree or rocks. (?) It was the shape.

WFMA,Nat.P

IX. 17″

I don't see anything in this one. It just looks like an inkblot.

Rejection

X. 8″

1. This looks like Sea World.

1. The whole thing. It was the colors . . . and the shapes (*points to different figures.*) It looks like different things swimming around.

WFM.FCA

2. The blue is angel fish.

2. It just looked like a colorful fish to me, like an angel fish swimming.

DFM-A

3. The red in the middle is shrimp, just the colors. They're swimming around.

3. It looked like a shrimp swimming around in the water, not the cooked kind.

DFM-A

E X H I B I T 4

THEMATIC APPERCEPTION TEST

CARD 1 Well. His parents wanted him to take violin lessons, but he doesn't like it. He doesn't want to be put through that torture. (*What will happen?*) He'll get used to it, learn to like it or he'll give up.

CARD 3BM She's just despairing. I don't know about what. Life's gotten to be too much for her. (*What's she despairing about?*) I don't know. (What will happen?) She won't kill herself. Hopefully she'll get over whatever it is.

CARD 4 A scene out of a movie . . . He's going off to some great adventure, something very, very dangerous. She could give him happiness but he has to do something to prove his machismo. (*What will happen?*) He'll probably end up getting killed or something.

CARD 5 Mother heard a noise . . . she opens the door and sees nothing's wrong. (*What's she thinking?*) She's worried about a child. She heard something fall on a table but she found out it was just a cat fooling around.

CARD 6BM Just a mother and son at a funeral. Someone somewhat close to them has died but not all that close. They're waiting around to pay their respects. Then they'll go home. Just a family duty one has to perform.

CARD 7BM Just two businessmen talking at a bar about everything. They're drinking a little too much and they're a little bored. They're doing something more pleasurable than going home to their wives. They'll get in their cars, go home, and hopefully not kill anybody on the way.

CARD 10 Just a man and a woman on their 15th anniversary. They hope to live a good life the next 15 years. It's just a nice family . . . the American dream.

CARD 12M This man is being hypnotized to quit smoking. He doesn't think it's going to work, but $25 isn't too much to pay. He won't succeed but it'll be something to talk about with the guys at the office.

CARD 13MF (*long pause*) This is bringing back lots of bad memories. This guy has picked up a hooker in a cheap hotel room; she's a stone cold junkie flat on her back. He'll leave feeling lower than before; he'll wander the streets and try to forget.

CARD 14 Just a man looking out a window . . . overlooking a sidewalk on a hot summer day; people are going by. He's planning to go out tonight. He's doing a healthy form of contemplation.

THEMATIC APPERCEPTION TEST

CARD 15 (*Laughs*) I never saw this one . . . Hmmm . . . (*Long pause*) This looks like something out of a horror movie . . . (*frowns*) . . . The person is at a grave, someone has died, there's emptiness in this picture. Can't even tell if it's a male or a female. Almost something like visiting a graveyard after WWI . . . like those images of people going to see their dead sons who are never coming back. Somebody who was 18 years old, went off to war and was blasted to bits and this person outlived their own children and they'll die a lonelier death. This picture could almost be used for propaganda. (*How so?*) You know, war, death, its waste. (*Sighs*) I've read so much about it. (*And?*) Well, you know, some wars are useful but nothing was gained after WWI. So many people had sons that never came back. Of course, she's lucky in a way, lucky enough he came back to her to be buried.

EXHIBIT 5

SENTENCE COMPLETION TEST

3. *It looked impossible, so he* "stopped."

7. *He felt proud that he* "was smart."

8. *As a child my greatest fear was* "being alone."

18. *Usually he felt that sex* "was needed."

29. *I used to daydream about* "being successful."

32. *Love is* "needed."

38. *When someone looks at me, I* "feel good."

40. *After he made love to her, he* "felt good."

42. *When I am criticized, I* "feel stupid."

48. *When he found he had failed the examination, he* "felt stupid."

63. *Whenever he does below average work, he* "feels stupid."

DISCUSSION

The two patients we have chosen to illustrate this personality disorder are both young men. Both of these young men were hospitalized not for interpersonal behavior characterized by narcissism, but for situational depression and behaviors that were illegal (stealing, using cocaine) and could be conceptualized as inappropriate attempts to handle anxiety and other difficulties. Both Mr. A and Mr. C manifest difficulties in relating to others, not exclusively related to or captured by the narcissistic label. Mr. A seems quite shallow and manipulative in his relationships, and his behavior has antisocial characteristics. Mr. C seems to have a more salient and meaningful connection with his mother, at least, but remains superficial in many of his contacts. And, most crucial for treatment planning, both of these young men manifest personal attitudes and interpersonal behavior that are threats to the formation of a viable treatment alliance. Both are inclined to blame their troubles on external factors and want little assistance beyond immediate symptom relief. Psychological testing is called for in both cases to pinpoint these threats to the treatment alliance, and to use the data in order to confront the patients with their particular deficits.

Mr. A was a 19-year-old college sophomore who came to the attention of the mental health community because of a series of behaviors that led to a drug overdose (possibly suicidal in nature). A resolve made to his father to achieve in school was followed by his studying only what pleased him. This was followed by possible theft and trouble with the authorities, which led to depression and further dysfunction. Thus, after a series of behaviors involving acting out and, most probably, lack of honesty about his own behavior, he was hospitalized with depression that seemed situational, with the overriding issue of his personality traits that chronically got him into trouble.

The projective materials were noteworthy for their content that was obvious, mundane and trite. The general picture emerged of a young man who solved difficulties by action designed to give immediate relief, built on a basic attitude of insensitivity to others and a sense of his own specialness and entitlement. The testing results portrayed in clear detail the serious problems in beginning a therapeutic approach with such an individual. The difficulty of establishing a therapeutic alliance in which the patient recognizes, at least to some degree, his own difficulties, his contribution to these difficulties, and his need for assistance to change is greatly amplified by this man's basic character traits involving acting out, disregard for others, and a false sense of his own specialness. At best, the testing assisted the therapist in articulating and confronting the patient with these difficulties quite early in treatment.

Mr. C, a 28-year-old, unmarried male, came to the attention of the mental health field, as did Mr. A, not because of his personality disorder *per se* but in an organic state due to cocaine abuse in the context of depression and grief following the death of his mother. Following his hospitalization, the organic delusional syndrome cleared quickly and the treatment team was faced with assessing his personality strengths and weaknesses. In fact, the treatment team was struck by his public appearance of normality, which was in sharp contrast with his profound sense of loss and grief over his mother's death as revealed in psychotherapy sessions. His testing results in some ways mirrored this dichotomy. For example, his MMPI was in the normal range on all scaled scores. While it does happen that psychiatric inpatients yield a normal MMPI, this is a relatively rare event. While Mr. A's Rorschach was significant for its banality, that produced by Mr. C was extensive, with very few populars and an emphasis on unusual details. Themes of dangerousness, countered by undoing and with a focus on percepts that were harmless, were noted in the Rorschach. It was in the TAT, however, that Mr. C revealed his preoccupation with fantasies of success and epic triumph.

References

Adams, K.M., & Heaton, R. (1985). Automated interpretation of neuropsychological test data. *Journal of Consulting and Clinical Psychology, 53*, 790–802.

American Psychiatric Association (1952). *Diagnostic and Statistical Manual of Mental Disorders* (1st ed.). Washington, D.C.: Author.

American Psychiatric Association (1968). *Diagnostic and Statistical Manual of Mental Disorders* (2nd ed.). Washington, D.C.: Author.

American Psychiatric Association (1980). *Diagnostic and Statistical Manual of Mental Disorders* (3rd ed.). Washington, D.C.: Author.

American Psychiatric Association (1987). *Diagnostic and Statistical Manual of Mental Disorders* (3rd ed. rev.) Washington, D.C.: Author.

Anastasi, A. (1988). *Psychological Testing* (6th ed.). New York: Macmillan.

Aronow, E., & Reznikoff, M. (1976). *Rorschach Content Interpretation.* New York: Grune & Stratton.

Bellak, L. (1975). *The TAT, CAT, and SAT in Clinical Use* (3rd ed.). New York, Grune & Stratton.

Bellak, L., & Bellak, S.S. (1973). *Manual: Senior Apperception Technique.* Larchmont, N.Y.: C.P.S.

Bender, L.A. (1938). A visual motor gestalt test and its clinical use. *American Orthopsychiatric Association, Research Monographs,* No. 3.

Beutler, L.E., & Clarkin, W.F. (1990). *Systematic Treatment Selection: Toward Targeted Therapeutic* Intervention. New York: Brunner/Mazel.

Butcher, J.N., Keller, L.S., & Bacon, S.F. (1985). Current developments and future directions in computerized personality assessment. *Journal of Consulting and Clinical Psychology, 53*, 803–815.

Cameron, N. (1938a). Reasoning, regression and communication in schizophrenia. *Psychological Monographs, 50*, 1–34.

Cameron, N. (1938b). A study of thinking in senile deterioration and schizophrenic disorganization. *American Journal of Psychology, 51*, 650–664.

Clarkin, J.F., & Hurt, S.W. (1988). Psychological assessment: Tests and rating scales. In *Textbook of Psychiatry,* Talbott, J.A., Hales, R.E., & Yudofsky, S.C. (eds.). Washington: The American Psychiatric Press.

Cronbach, L.J. (1949). *Essentials of Psychological Testing.* New York: Harper & Brothers.

Dahlstrom, W.G., Welsh, G.S., & Dahlstrom, L.E. (1972). *An MMPI handbook. Vol. I. Clinical interpretation.* Minneapolis: University of Minnesota Press.

Dollin, A., & Phillips, W. (1976). Diagnostic referral questions in psychological testing: Changing practices in the fifties, sixties and seventies. *Psychological Reports, 39,* 850.

Dollin, A., & Reznikoff, M. (1966). Diagnostic referral questions in psychological testing: Changing concepts. *Psychological Reports, 19,* 610.

Elwood, D.J. (1969). Automation of psychological testing. *American Psychologist, 24,* 287–289.

Eron, L.D. (1950). A normative study of the Thematic Apperception Test. *Psychological Monographs, 64* (9, Whole No. 315).

Eron, L.D. (1953). Responses of women to the Thematic Apperception Test. *Journal of Consulting Psychology, 17,* 269– 282.

Exner, J.E., Jr. (1974). *The Rorschach: A Comprehensive System,* Vol. 1. New York: Wiley.

Fairbank, J.A., Keane, T.M., & Malloy, P.F. (1983). Some preliminary data on the psychological characteristics of Vietnam veterans with post-traumatic stress disorder. *Journal of Consulting and Clinical Psychology, 51,* 912–919.

Fowler, R.D. (1985). Landmarks in computer-assisted psychological assessment. *Journal of Consulting and Clinical Psychology, 53,* 748–759.

Garfield, S.L. (1983). *The Study of Personality and Behavior* (2nd ed.). New York: Aldine.

Garfield, S.L., & Kurtz, R. (1976). Clinical psychology in the 1970s. *American Psychologist, 31,* 1–9.

Golden, C.J. (1979). *Clinical Interpretation of Objective Psychological Tests.* New York: Grune & Stratton.

Goldstein, G., & Hersen, M. (Eds.) (1984). *Handbook of Psychological Assessment.* New York: Pergamon Press.

Goldstein, K. (1939). *The Organism: A Holistic Approach to Biology Derived from Pathological Data in Man.* New York: American Book Co.

Goldstein, K., & Scheerer, M. (1941). Abstract and concrete behavior: An experimental study with special tests. *Psychological Monographs 53* (2, Whole No. 230).

Goodenough, F.L. (1926). *Measurement of Intelligence by Drawings.* Yonkers, N.Y.: World Book Co.

Hammer, E.F. (Ed.) (1958). *The Clinical Application of Projective Drawings.* Springfield, Ill.: Charles C. Thomas.

Harris, D.B. (1963). *Children's Drawings as Measures of Intellectual Maturity: A Revision and Extension of the Goodenough Draw-A-Man Test.* New York: Harcourt Brace Jovanovich.

Hathaway, S.R., & McKinley, J.C. (1942). A multiphasic personality schedule: The measurement of symptomatic depression. *Journal of Psychology, 14,* 73–84.

Hathaway, S.R., & Meehl, P.E. (1951). *An Atlas for the Clinical Use of the MMPI.* Minneapolis: University of Minnesota Press.

Hevern, V.W. (1980). Recent validity studies of the Halstead-Reitan approach to clinical neuropsychological assessment: A critical review. *Clinical Neuropsychology*, 2, 49–61.

Holt, R.R. (1967). Diagnostic testing: Present status and future prospects. *Journal of Nervous and Mental Disease, 144*, 444– 465.

Holtzman, W.H. (1968). Holtzman Inkblot Technique. In A.I. Rabin (Ed.), *Projective Techniques in Personality Assessment* (pp. 136– 170). New York: Springer.

Hulse, W.C. (1952). Childhood conflict expressed through family drawings. *Journal of Projective Techniques, 16*, 66–79.

Hyer, L., O'Leary, W.C., Saucer, R.T., Blount, J., Harrison, W.R., & Boudewyns, P.A. (1986). Inpatient diagnosis of post-traumatic stress disorder. *Journal of Consulting and Clinical Psychology, 54*, 698–702

Jung, C.G. (1910). The association method. *American Journal of Psychology, 21*, 219–269.

Klopfer, B., & Kelly, D.M. (1942). *The Rorschach Technique.* Yonkers, N.Y.: World Book Co.

Koppitz, E.M. (1964). *The Bender-Gestalt Test for Young Children.* New York: Grune & Stratton.

Koppitz, E.M. (1975). *The Bender-Gestalt Test for Young Children: Research and Application, 1963–1973.* New York: Grune & Stratton.

Korchin, S.J. (1976). *Modern Clinical Psychology.* New York: Basic Books.

Lachar, D., & Alexander, R.S. (1978). Veridicality of self-report: Replicated correlates of the Wiggins MMPI content scales. *Journal of Consulting and Clinical Psychology, 46*, 1349–1356.

Lubin, B., Larsen, R.M., & Matarazzo, J.D. (1984). Patterns of psychological test usage in the United States: 1935–1982. *American Psychologist, 39*, 451–453.

Lubin, B., Larsen, R.M., Matarazzo, J.D., & Seever, M. (1985). Psychological test usage patterns in five professional settings. *American Psychologist, 40*, 857–861.

Luria, A.R. (1973). *The Working Brain.* New York: Basic Books.

MacAndrews, C. (1965). The differentiation of male alcoholic outpatients from non-alcoholic psychiatric patients by means of the MMPI. *Quarterly Journal of Studies in Alcohol, 26*, 238– 246.

Machover, K. (1949). *Personality Projection in the Drawing of the Human Figure: A Method of Personality Investigation.* Springfield, Ill.: Charles C. Thomas.

Marks, P.A., Seeman, W., & Haller, D.L. (1974). *The Actuarial Use of the MMPI with Adolescents and Adults.* Baltimore: Williams & Wilkins.

Matarazzo, J.D. (1972). *Wechsler's Measurement and Appraisal of Adult Intelligence* (5th ed.). Baltimore: Williams & Wilkin.

Meehl, P.E. (1954). *Clinical versus Statistical Prediction: A Theoretical Analysis and a Review of the Evidence.* Minneapolis: University of Minnesota Press.

Morgan, C.D., & Murray, H.A. (1935). A method for investigating fantasies: The Thematic Apperception Test. *Archives of Neurology and Psychiatry, 34*, 289–300.

Murray, H.A., et al. (1938). *Explorations in Personality.* New York: Oxford University Press.

National Computer Systems (1984). *1984 catalog* [Professional Assessment Services Division]. Minneapolis: Author.

Pascal, G.R., & Suttell, B.J. (1951). *The Bender-Gestalt Test: Quantification and Validity for Adults.* New York: Grune & Stratton.

Pfohl, B., & Andreasen, N.C. (1986). Schizophrenia: Diagnosis and classification. In A.J. Frances & R.E. Hales (Eds.), *American Psychiatric Association, Annual Review, Volume 5* (pp. 7–24). Washington DC: American Psychiatric Press.

Pitrowski, Z.A. (1964). A digital computer administration of inkblot test data. *Psychiatric Quarterly, 38,* 1–26.

Rapaport, D., Gill, M., & Schafer, R. (1945–1946). *Diagnostic Psychological Testing* (Vols. 1–2). Chicago: Year Book Publishers.

Rapaport, D., Gill, M., & Schafer, R. (1968). *Diagnostic Psychological Testing* (rev. ed. edited by R.R. Holt). New York: International Universities Press.

Reitan, R.M., & Davison, L.A. (Eds.) (1974). *Clinical Neuropsychology: Current Status and Applications.* New York: Halsted.

Rohde, A.R. (1946). Explorations in personality by the sentence completion method. *Journal of Applied Psychology, 30,* 169– 181.

Rorschach, H. (1942). *Psychodiagnostics: A Diagnostic Test Based on Perception* (P. Limkau & B. Kronenburg, Trans.). Berne: Huber. (Original work published, 1921: U.S. distributor, Grune & Stratton).

Rotter, J.B., & Rafferty, J.E. (1950). *Manual for the Rotter Incomplete Sentences Blank, College Form.* New York: The Psychological Corporation.

Schacht, R., & Nathan, P.E. (1977). But is it good for psychologists? Appraisal and status of DSM-III. *American Psychologist, 32,* 1017–1025.

Schafer, R. (1948). *The Clinical Application of Psychological Tests.* New York: International Universities Press.

Schafer, R. (1954). *Psychoanalytic Interpretation in Rorschach testing.* New York: Grune & Stratton.

Schmidt, H.O., & Fonda, C.P. (1956). The reliability of psychiatric diagnosis: A new look. *Journal of Abnormal and Social Psychology, 52,* 262–267.

Spitzer, R.L. (1980). An in-depth look at DSM-III (interviewed by J. Talbot). *Hospital & Community Psychiatry, 31,* 25–32.

Spitzer, R.L., & Fleiss, J.L. (1974). A reanalysis of the reliability of psychiatric diagnoses. *British Journal of Psychiatry, 125,* 341–347.

Spitzer, R.L., Forman, J.B., & Nee, J. (1979). DSM-III field trials: Initial diagnostic reliability. *American Journal of Psychiatry, 136,* 815–817.

Spitzer, R.L., Williams, J.B., & Skodol, A.E. (1980). DSM-III: The major achievements and an overview. *American Journal of Psychiatry, 137,* 151–164.

Tendler, A.D. (1930). A preliminary report on a test for emotional insight. *Journal of Applied Psychology, 14,* 123–136.

Wechsler, D. (1939). *The Measurement of Adult Intelligence.* Baltimore: Williams & Wilkins.

Wiggins, J.S. (1973). *Personality and Prediction Principles of Personality Assessment.* Reading, Ma.: Addison-Wesley Publishing Co.

Wolk, R.L., & Wolk, R.B. (1971). *Manual Gerontological Apperception Test*. New York: Human Sciences Press.

Zubin, J. (1967). Classification of behavior disorders. *Annual Review of Psychology, 18*, 373–406.

❖

Name Index

Subject Index